2ND EDITION

# So *that's* what they're for!

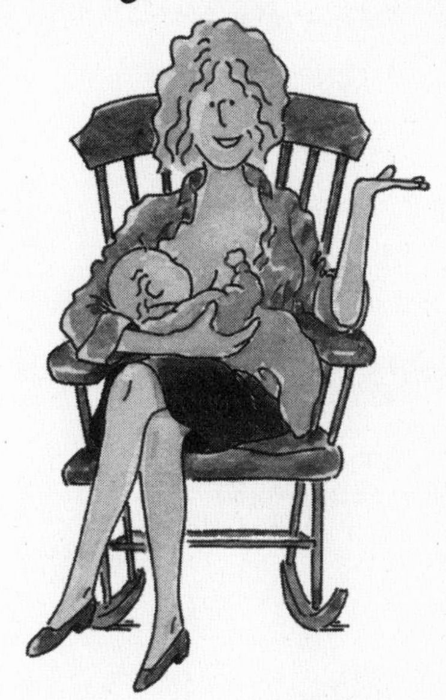

## BREASTFEEDING BASICS

Janet Tamaro

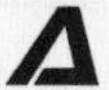

ADAMS MEDIA CORPORATION
Avon, Massachusetts

Published by Adams Media Corporation
57 Littlefield Street, Avon, MA 02322. U.S.A.

ISBN: 1-58062-041-8

Printed in Canada.

J I H G F

**Library of Congress Cataloging-in-Publication Data**
Tamaro, Janet.
So that's what they're for! : breastfeeding basics / by Janet Tamaro
p. cm.
Includes index.
ISBN 1-58062-041-8 (pb)
1. Breast feeding—Popular works. II. Title.
RJ216.T33 1996
649'.33—dc20 96-13657
CIP

This publication is designed to provide accurate and authoritative information with regard to the subject matter covered. It is sold with the understanding that the publisher is not engaged in rendering professional advice. If advice or other expert assistance is required, the services of a competent professional person should be sought.



*This book is available at quantity discounts for bulk purchases.*
*For information, call 1-800-872-5627.*

Visit our home page at *www.adamsmedia.com*

*For Olivia and Julia, who'll always be my babies.*
*And for my husband, Steve Natt,*
*for all the times he could've*
*been a baby but wasn't.*

# Contents

## Part III Everything Else You Wanted to Know But Were Too Tired to Ask

# Preface

Almost five years ago, I had one little baby named Olivia, and I had no idea the first time she cried for food that breastfeeding would be so darn complicated. And the bookstore didn't solve my problems. I was put off by the tone of a lot of the books on breastfeeding. It was either the onslaught of too many hormones in my mother cocktail or early Alzheimer's, but I started feeling like I had too many homework assignments, too much to think about, and was already falling dangerously behind in Mommy 101. I wanted to know, "Is this going to be on the midterm?" I didn't want a thick manual. I didn't want to be preached to. I wanted someone to make me laugh—and pass along what I needed to know. Somebody, somewhere must have already written a humorous book on breastfeeding, I'd thought.

It turns out that somebody had to be me. Since I'm a journalist, I was already an information junkie. All I needed was to spend two years reading the literature on breastfeeding while also getting certified as a lactation educator. So now I have a B.A., a M.S. (Master of Sciences) degree and, most importantly for my readers, an L.E. (Lactation Educator) certification. (All of those degrees pale in comparison to my years of on-the-job training as the family restaurant, thanks to my two little girls.)

But most of all, I needed to interview hundreds of mothers and fathers, and include real life experiences. That, in effect, became *So That's What They're For!* I can't take full credit for writing a funny book on breastfeeding, (Though I might add I did win "best sense of humor" in the sixth grade . . .) I credit the people who told me their stories. The reason the book is funny is because reality is almost always stranger and funnier than fiction. As you will soon see, though parenting is exhausting, it is also the most amusing chapter of life.

After the first edition of *STWTF!* came out, and I had a second baby, Julia. I decided to put all of my training and know-how to work. This time around, I would be the master of my breasts. I would not struggle through the early weeks of breastfeeding the way I had the first time. But, as it turns out, Julia took no notice at all of my L.E. certification, couldn't care less that I'd written a book on breastfeeding and gave me fits (and amazingly painful nipples) when I tried to feed her. I had to swallow my pride and take myself to the nearest and best lactation consultant I knew: Lois at the Lactation Institute in Encino, California. In her office, I let her examine both me and Julia, who we'd dubbed "the washboard" thanks to her exuberant work on my nipples. Lois gave me lanolin (which worked on my sore nipples), and examined Julia's suck. To my relief, Lois asured me I wasn't doing it "wrong." Julia had an unusual palate and had an inefficient (and painful) way of "naturally" breastfeeding. We had to re-train her to suck!

Lois put my husband to work. He re-read the chapter in my book, "Problems: from Small Ones to Big Ones," the one neither of us had ever expected to actually need to know. Then with the help of Lois, my husband learned how to "finger feed" pumped breastmilk to Julia (you'll learn about that technique in this book).

I became in effect, the dad, because I was no longer Julia's source of food. Oh sure, I pumped, but Steve was the one with the magic finger. Julia would open her mouth and crane her little neck toward the sound of *his* voice, not mine. I found out firsthand what it felt like to have a breastfeeding problem. It tested even my level of commitment, and renewed my feelings of empathy for new mothers who have trouble (and for fathers who feel left out in the early weeks). But we conquered Julia's suck problem, and she eventually made her way happily back to me.

That said, I've received hundreds of letters from women who said they had *no* trouble breastfeeding at all, thanks to the tips, stories, diagrams and do's and don'ts contained in this book. The book was intended to prevent problems, help you understand how to avoid pitfalls, and understand what's a big problem and what's a small one.

I've been overwhelmed by the kind and effusive reactions I've received from people who've been helped by this book. First time mothers found the book, read the unintimidating directions, and went about inserting Breast A into Mouth B. Sisters and friends who'd successfully breastfed picked it up to give as a shower gift to women they knew were reluctant to breastfeed. Husbands even tell me they've stumbled on it when there was nothing else to read in the bathroom and actually enjoyed it and were spurred into becoming breastfeeding proponents themselves.

Since the book came out in 1996, there has been even more research and information on the irreplaceable value of human milk for a baby's health, development, avoidance and reduction of illness, his social skills, even his IQ! I've added everything that's new and revised a few things, making this the most current book on breastfeeding out there. Here then, is the updated, newly revised, and hopefully funniest breastfeeding guide you'll find.

# Acknowledgments

Always, there are too many people to acknowledge, but I'd like to thank those who were so generous with their time and knowledge. My thanks go to: Laura Haynes Collector, my lifelong friend and dedicated La Leche League Leader for her help and support. I'd like to thank all of those committed to breastfeeding, who took the time to pass on so much of what they know, particularly Chele Marmet, Ellen Shell, Sandra Jansen, Corky Harvey, Ruth Gruen, Dr. Jay Gordon, and Dr. Jane Heinig. I'd like to also thank Dr. Robert Hamilton, who was so gracious with his time and expertise. And then I need to thank Selma Lewis for thinking this was a good idea, Sasha Goodman for getting this off of my computer, Pam Liflander for all of her help, and Nancy Bacal for sharing her gift. To Vicky, for loving and taking such good care of my daughter when I had to write. To all of the mothers who shared their stories. And to my own mother Therese for all her years of mothering.

# A Word to the Wise

Even though I have two daughters, just for simplicity's sake I've chosen to use the pronoun *he* when I talk about babies. That's my only reason. I like girls and women, I happen to be female, and I hope you don't take my use of this pronoun as gender preference. It was just awkward to keep writing *he/she*. Plus, *he* has fewer letters to type than *she*.

Also, except for the experts quoted here, I've used only the first names of the women, men (and babies) that I interviewed. When it was requested, I also changed the name; so if you know someone with the same name, don't assume you're reading his (okay, or her) story.

## Introduction

# Getting Going

Congratulations. You're about to discover what I did. After years of being tormented by the size of my breasts (36B on a good, or bloated, day), I can't tell you how happy I was find to out that this part of my body was actually good for something other than torturing me. (Why is it that your breasts are never the style featured in *Cosmopolitan*?)

Well, finally you're about to meet one person in your life who'll love your breasts no matter how flat, round, small, large, firm, flabby, fashionable, or lopsided they may be: your new baby.

You are completely normal if you never thought about breastfeeding before you got pregnant. You're also normal if you know next to nothing about it. After all, you don't need to know how to fly a plane if you're a passenger, unless everyone but you keels over. You don't need to know how to breastfeed until you have a baby to feed.

You are not a bad person if you are ambivalent, think it may be embarrassing, strange, even icky. Even if you've been dying to have a baby, you may not be dying to breastfeed. That's normal, too.

The good news for your expected baby is that you've picked up this book. Hopefully, by the time you've read through the material here, everything you will have learned will convince you that there really is no good alternative to mother's milk.

### Myth Busting

The biggest myth about breastfeeding is that it's easy from the start. It isn't. However, having said that, you should also know that it isn't nearly as difficult as your friends will tell you it is. Breastfeeding requires both practice and some know-how. Eventually, it is easy and natural. But it takes some getting used to and, yes, it takes a little work. (By the way, I hope I'm not the first to tell you that babies are a little work in general.)

If you needed to turn on a light in a darkened room, but you didn't know where the light switch was, you'd do a lot of fumbling around. You might trip over furniture, bang into a wall, even scrape your knuckles on an exposed nail. But if you knew where the light switch was, you would just go to it and turn it on. With breastfeeding, you need to know a little something about it before you fumble around trying to find the switch, which makes sense if you think about it. Just because something is natural doesn't mean it doesn't require some time, effort, and practice. Walking is natural, but it still requires lots of practice before you can do it well. Check with your mother if you don't believe me, and then maybe she'll be able to explain how you got those permanent dents on your forehead.

## It Used to Be Easy Because Everyone Knew What It Looked Like

Until you are a nursing mother, you may never have seen a baby doing it up close and personal. In countries where breastfeeding is still considered the cultural norm, you will see this phenomenon on a daily basis. You'll sit next to nursing mothers on a bus, stand behind them in lines, and eat lunch near them. That means you will see many, many times how breastfeeding is accomplished even if you haven't done it yourself.

In this country, breastfeeding is a mysterious process to us. So is cooking your ancestors' dishes, if your mother has never shown you how. I remember watching my grandmother make *gnocchi* (Italian dumplings). My grandmother learned how because her mother taught her. And her mother taught her. And so on. You may be a few generations removed from a mother who breastfed. If so, it's doubtful that your great-grandmother will be around to help. But you'll often find that you might get help from the most unlikely sources. Caitlin, a new mother, was trying to breastfeed in public for the first time in a dentist's waiting room when her daughter Emily was three weeks old. "I wasn't that good at breastfeeding yet, and there was an elderly woman waiting, too." The seventyish woman sat there primly, clutching her handbag and looking at everything in the room but Caitlin. "I was so embarrassed for myself and for her that I took a blanket and put it over Emily, but she screamed because she didn't want it. Then I tried to go under the blanket myself, but Emily was still screaming because the blanket was in the way of my breast." Finally, Caitlin came out from under the blanket for air, dripping with perspiration. The woman looked at Caitlin and said, "Would you like some help? I breastfed fourteen children."

You can often get help from friends and relatives, but they are not always the best source of information. The most logical person to go to for help might seem to be your doctor. But in this book, you will frequently be referred to a lactation consultant. A lactation consultant is likely to be a nurse, a physical therapist, a dietitian, or someone initially trained in a medical field. Two women in the forefront of this field are Chele Marmet and Ellen Shell, who started the first accredited program in the country for a degree in lactation at the Lactation Institute in Encino, California. They tell the story of a young woman who came to them for breastfeeding help. When they solved her baby's sucking problem, they felt like geniuses who'd just discovered a new tool in science. But the young woman called them later and said, "My grandmother told me that's what she used to do."

I prefer the advice of a lactation consultant over that of a traditional doctor, not because all consultants are perfect and can solve every problem. (They aren't, and they can't.) And not because all doctors don't know how to ease breastfeeding worries. (Many do.) But in general, lactation consultants are much better prepared to handle breastfeeding problems than your doctor is. Research has shown that about one-half of the doctors who take care of mothers or babies admit that they don't know enough about breastfeeding. Plus, consultants are used to setting aside an hour or two of their time in order to fix what's wrong. Most doctors simply don't have that kind of time. The AAP encourages doctors to get more knowledgeable about breastfeeding and insurance companies to get with it and start paying for the services needed to support women, like lactation consultants.

The good lactation consultants have had very specific training and are usually certified. A reputable consultant who has a lot of experience getting babies on their mothers' breasts is often the last stop for women who don't know where else to turn. Doctors, nurses, or hospitals can all refer you to a good consultant. So can your childbirth educator and the organizations listed in the Appendix of this book. BEWARE if your doctor isn't referring you to anything but a can of formula. The recent changes in the American Academy of Pediatrics guidelines admits that some doctors are, in fact, "obstacles" to breastfeeding because of "physician apathy and misinformation." Be proactive and make sure you find the help you need.

## So *That's* What This Book Is For!

When you get right down to it, breastfeeding requires a fair amount of complex choreography. This book will get you off to a good start. *So*

That's *What They're For!* will give you those dance steps you'll need for your tiny new partner. You'll want to know how to breastfeed correctly from the beginning so that you can avoid being one of the horror stories you've likely heard from your friends. You'll need ammunition to persuade a reluctant husband, mother, or mother-in-law. Or maybe you yourself aren't yet convinced about what is so darned special about breastfeeding. Keep reading. You will be.

## Remember

If you can remember one-tenth of what is in this book when it is your turn to get started, you'll be in great shape. The one thing you must remember above all else is this: you can breastfeed. You *can* do it. Your body made a *baby*. Trust that nature has given you the perfect equipment to feed your new baby.

Even after you get the hang of breastfeeding, you may still have other questions such as: When will I stop feeling like a *National Geographic* special? Can I ever leave the house? Is it normal to have this little suction cup attached to me every waking moment? And the questions don't stop even after you get fully comfortable, typically by the end of the first month.

You'll have questions that only someone who's been in the same boat can answer, such as: How do I get my baby to learn to go to sleep by himself after I've become the human pacifier by nursing him to sleep? How do I stop my milk from ejecting and staining my silk suits every time I glance at a photograph of my sweet baby? What do I do if I forget my breast pump on a trip and either have to find a substitute or risk turning into a 50DDD? And what if when my baby gets teeth, he decides to practice his new chompers on my nipples?

## You Can Do It

I hope this book gives you courage and help and reminds you to keep your sense of humor about this stage in your life. You will likely look back on these days fondly. Each time you breastfeed, your child will thank you with an expression of euphoric bliss you will never before have seen on a human face. No one but my daughter, before or since, has ever been so happy to see my breasts—and sometimes even me along with them.

I know you'll discover what I discovered as a parent: children are the most valuable things we have in our lives. Breastfeeding is an expression of that value, so *any* breastfeeding that you do is valuable. Good luck.

# Part I
# The Learning Curve

# Chapter 1
# How Did Breastfeeding Get So Complicated?

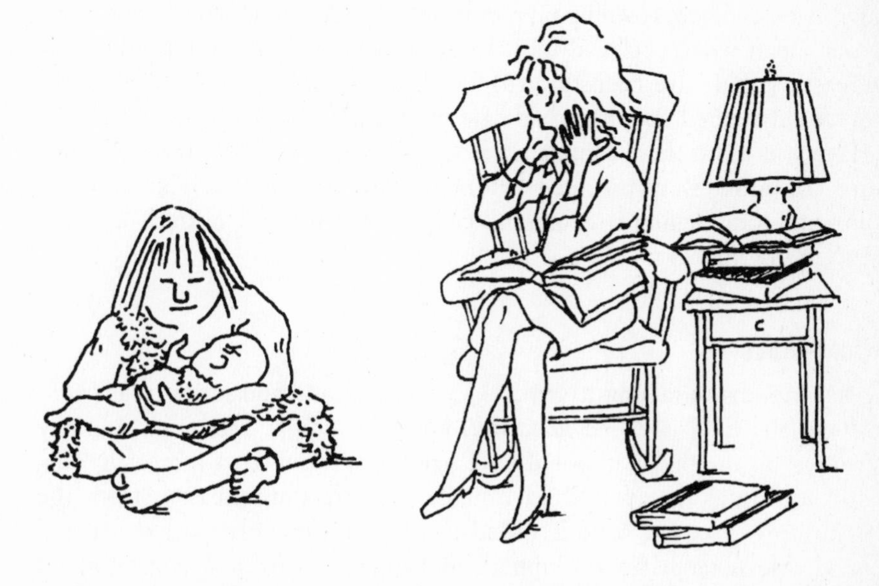

When my first daughter, Olivia, was a few weeks old, I had a minute to realize I was overwhelmed by the abrupt addition to my life. Nine months is enough time to prepare a room, but as my neighbor who'd had three children kept yelling at me from her porch, "Nothing prepares you for a baby!" Nothing in my life as a television correspondent, investigative reporter, writer, slacker, aerobiciser, coffee drinker, lazy housekeeper, worrier, prepared me for Olivia. I hasten to add, "as wonderful as she is."

And the one thing that I'd counted on being easy was actually the most difficult part of caring for my newborn. That thing was breastfeeding. After three weeks of struggling with my breasts; her mouth; my bra; her head, arms, and legs; my nipple; and her jaw, we finally got the hang of it, and I was able to feel confident that my body could feed my baby. But I went through a lot to get to that place, and even when I thought I was doing it right, I still ran into problems. It took me two years of research to discover that the stuff that happened was largely unnecessary and, in most cases, preventable.

## "My Friends Say It Hurts"

I had turned to my peers for help, but during those first weeks and even after, I not only *heard* all the horror stories, I *became* the horror story. I had sore, cracked, bleeding nipples (sorry, I forgot to tell you to put down your lunch while you read this). I was so engorged, if you tapped on my breasts, you'd have been rewarded with the sound a drum makes. And I eventually ended up with a bad case of *mastitis* (that's a breast infection). Have you heard these complaints from other people? All of these ailments are common. But you need to understand that does not make them *normal*. (Car-jacking is common. That doesn't make it normal, either—except in L.A.).

## Boob-ology

After months of talking to experts in what my husband refers to as *boob-ology* (the field is called *lactation*, honey, if you're listening), I finally learned all the things it would have been nice to know as a breastfeeding novice, things that would have made breastfeeding pleasant from the beginning. I could have avoided a lot of the problems that seemed inevitable (except for the impertinent questions from strangers) if I'd known more. And I wasn't totally ignorant. I'd read the pamphlets I was handed. I'd gone to a childbirth preparation class. But watching someone drive and driving yourself are worlds apart. (At least you don't have to learn breastfeeding in "Breast-Ed" with three sniggering peers in the back seat). I'd decided early on it had to be easy or else how could humans have survived for thousands of years? So I reasoned that I really didn't have to pay close attention when we reviewed breastfeeding at our last Lamaze class. And hey, if it didn't work out, I had other options. Right?

Wrong. What many new mothers don't realize—because their doctors don't tell them, their baby books don't tell them, and their friends and relatives don't tell them—is that choosing between breastmilk and formula is like asking "Would you rather have perfectly created, sterile, chemical-free organic, nutritious food—or I.V. fluid?"

"I look parents in the eye and tell them that formula is not good for kids," says pediatrician Robert Hamilton. "But formula is not dangerous." Still, Dr. Hamilton says he is frequently met with resistance. "When I tell parents that a year of breastfeeding is best, they look at me like I'm some sort of radical and say, 'But I thought you were a Republican!'"

He is. But whether you're a Democrat or a Republican, breastmilk is better for your baby than formula. Breastmilk is a substance that is so unique and so precious, nothing factory-made comes close.

We can't make blood, hearts, kidneys, livers, eyes, or anything else that human beings need, in a factory. We have kidney dialysis and temporary hearts. But only human beings make the perfect parts. And only human beings make perfect milk for their offspring.

## "Why Didn't My Mother Breastfeed?"

Maybe your mom breastfed. Maybe she didn't. Even though almost 60 percent of new mothers try breastfeeding today, the generation that mothered us was brainwashed by formula companies and medical literature to believe that breastfeeding was crass and unsanitary and that formula was modern and healthy (incidentally, so was smoking at that time). Only a small percentage—less than 20 percent—of our mothers breastfed. Like lace making, breastfeeding became a lost art (I think we can live without handmade lace, however).

About fifteen years ago, when researchers really got serious about studying breastmilk, their astonishing findings turned everybody's myths about breastmilk upside down. Formula, that "modern miracle," was finally put to the test—and fell way, way short of mother's milk. Many diseases, some annoying, some chronic, and some even fatal, seem to be tied to the absence of breastmilk. About four out of one thousand babies in the United States alone dies every year as a direct result of not getting breastmilk.

Breastfed babies on average are healthier, leaner, even smarter (!) than their formula-fed counterparts. These conclusions are not based in fanaticism—they are based in science. As more information comes out, more women are getting educated about this miracle substance that's also darned convenient, inexpensive, and "modern" again.

## "Madge, I Just Love My New Freezer!"

But as a culture, we really messed things up. Remember in the '50s when everyone thought frozen dinners were the only way to eat? That's what formula was to our mothers. It was a way of cleaning up nature, improving, packaging, freeze-drying, and processing the world. A medical text published in 1964 heralded the "new formula," calling it "better" than breastmilk.

As a result, women in this country forgot how to breastfeed. We got a little weird about breasts, too. They were no longer needed to feed babies, so they went out and got jobs in commercials and appeared in *Playboy*. Now, we're so used to seeing breasts tap dancing and lounging around, we have a hard time remembering what they were for in the first place! But the way we feel about breasts is simply our perception of their function.

To prove this point, an American doctor tells a story about walking through the wards of a Muslim hospital in Saudi Arabia. He walked in on a group of new mothers who were sitting around talking and breastfeeding their newborns. When they saw a Western male, they freaked. Fabric flew everywhere as the embarrassed women rushed to cover—their heads. Not one of them covered their breasts. In their country, it was their heads and faces that strange men weren't supposed to see. Not their breasts. Heck, those were just like feet and hands to these women.

## "Why Aren't Doctors on the Bandwagon?"

Ninety percent of doctors polled in a recent study agreed that they should be involved in breastfeeding promotion. But if your experience during prenatal check-up visits is like that of most women, you've probably found that the choice of deciding between breastmilk and formula seems to be of as much interest to your doctor as whether you'll paint the nursery yellow or green.

In a poll conducted by the *Journal of the American Medical Association*, 55 percent of the doctors most likely to attend to you postnatally in the hospital admitted they don't know enough about breastfeeding.

About the same number couldn't answer a simple series of questions asking them how they'd treat some common problems. While doctors do want their patients to breastfeed, they can't make you do it, and most of them won't stress it unless you ask.

We are only just past the days when medical schools had professors who taught the way one prominent professor did into the 1970s. This was his lecture to his medical students about breastfeeding (here in its entirety):

"What's baby's is baby's and what's Daddy's is Daddy's." His lecture on formula took days to deliver.

Even today your chances of finding a doctor who is knowledgeable, helpful, and supportive of breastfeeding are less than one out of three, according to the *Journal of the American Medical Association*. (If you've chosen a certified nurse midwife, you will have better luck; these nurses have usually had some kind of lactation training and often refer patients directly to lactation consultants.)

I tell you this about doctors not to beat up on them, because some of my best friends are doctors (were, anyway). But you need to know that breastfeeding is not a hot topic in medicine because it usually doesn't involve the skill of the physician. It is a seemingly small thing that accomplishes big things.

And unfortunately, there is another reason why doctors and nurses in this country are largely ignorant about assisting breastfeeding mothers and helping them resolve breastfeeding problems. Formula companies have a vested interest in keeping doctors' shelves stocked with formula (to the tune of about $5 to $6 billion a year). So most of the information about infant feeding (including breastfeeding) is put out by, you guessed it, formula companies! These companies also give away samples and prizes to doctors, like pens, writing pads, posters, and even pricier items like cash and trips. Mothers who make breastmilk don't hand out free goodies. That means even nice, conscientious doctors will probably hand you the same can or packet of formula a pharmaceutical company marketing representative just handed them.

## The Influence of Formula Companies

This happens in hospitals, too. Formula companies supply hospitals with free formula, along with bottles and sterile water. They even get the hospitals to sign exclusive contracts to accept only their donated brand, and they give hospitals cash, sometimes in the six-figure range, for that privilege.

When you get a formula sample handed to you by your doctor or a hospital, you're probably not getting that particular brand of formula because your doctor prefers it. You're simply getting access to the formula-marketing machine in the form of a freebie that you'll later pay for if you formula-feed—to the tune of $1,000 to $1,500 a year per baby. If you've noticed, nothing else at the hospital is free, because they don't expect you to go out and spend $1,500 on brand-name gauze bandages or thermometers over the course of a year. The companies who bring you formula also propagate the myth that the ability to breastfeed is something you either have or you don't, like whether you can touch your tongue to your nose or not. The message is: try to do it, but if it doesn't work, there's always this lovely canned food.

## "Everybody Uses Bottles"

But let's say you aren't influenced by the discharge packs or the formula advertising. The sheer prevalence of formula and bottles in this country may be the biggest hindrance to breastfeeding. Every baby doll comes with a bottle. Television shows either make fun of breastfeeding or show a woman propping a bottle of formula. We are immune to these images—so immune that they seem normal and breastfeeding seems a little "out there."

Dorinda is breastfeeding her four-month-old. But her husband Andy said he would support whatever she wanted to do. He says, "I think it's great that there's a choice." Andy was breastfed as a baby while Dorinda was not. Andy says he knows many of breastfeeding's health benefits, but because he grew up also seeing bottles and formula, like most of us, he perceives breastmilk and formula as simply different means to accomplish the same thing.

The problem is that comparing breastmilk and formula is like comparing a real leg and a prosthesis. Dr. Paul Fleiss, a well-known California pediatrician and breastfeeding expert, says, "We think formula is a good second choice. But it's not even a good third or fourth choice." If you have it in your head that breastmilk and formula are the same, you're like the jury that goes into the trial already convinced of the defendant's innocence. No evidence to the contrary is going to sway you.

## Guilt

I have had long discussions with people who insist that they know "a lot of women who couldn't do it," so "it's great if you can, but if you can't you shouldn't be made to feel guilty." Guilt is something people usually feel because they think they've let somebody else down. It's uncomfortable to feel guilty, and no mother wants to think she hasn't done the best for her child. But consider that the guilt you feel over the choice you make about feeding may last a long time. Some things you'll be unable to prevent, like the nice blue ding my daughter got on her cheekbone when she waved around a metal rattle some nincompoop (me) had given her. But in nearly all cases, breastfeeding is something all mothers can do.

"In my experience, the guilt comes later," says Dr. Jay Gordon, a nationally recognized pediatrician and breastfeeding expert, who often finds the mother of a sick child weeping in his office when she finds out breastmilk might have prevented or minimized the illness. "Women say, 'Why didn't somebody tell me?', or 'I wish I'd gotten a second opinion because my doctor never told me how important it was.'"

"Many doctors and nurses don't want to get into this with women because they don't want to make them feel guilty," says Marsha Walker, a nurse and lactation consultant. "But at what other time do we not give people information because we're afraid of making them feel guilty? We don't worry about making a cardiac patient feel guilty when we inform him that smoking and drinking will kill him."

On the other hand, Dr. Gordon says women who've "tried hard" and because of some unforeseen, complicated problem that's usually physiological, can't breastfeed, "shouldn't be made to feel guilty." But after helping thousands of women get it right, Dr. Gordon is quite specific about what it means to "try hard."

"It means make a lot of phone calls. And it means exhausting *all* of the available resources." (And there are plenty. Check the Appendix).

## You Won't Be Able to Breastfeed If You Don't Know How

Katherine is seven months pregnant with her first baby. When asked whether she will breastfeed, she says, "Oh yes. At least I'm going to try to." That's a natural answer. Katherine has never had a baby, and she has no idea what to expect. Her friends have told her breastfeeding is hard and her sister told her it hurts.

Everybody's anatomy is different. With breastfeeding, it's anatomy times two: yours and your baby's. It's possible you may need more knowledge to get over certain anatomical hurdles so that you can breastfeed with your particular set of circumstances. As a culture we do not yet value breastfeeding enough. So when it doesn't work, those who should be supporting you—hospital staff, doctors, friends, relatives—may not know that breastfeeding is possible for more than 95 percent of new mothers (many experts believe it's even higher than that). In Davis, California, for example, 97 percent of mothers breastfeed, thanks to many support services.

## The Rest of the World

In Sweden and in other developed countries, it's considered unethical not to breastfeed. Of course, many of those same developed countries are also topless bikini states. Gary lived and worked in Europe for three years, and admits he got rather blasé about naked breasts. He was much more open to breastfeeding than his wife Wanda. "She wouldn't do it in public, but I'd seen topless women buying groceries near the beaches in France, so I thought it was not a big deal. But she did."

The fact that breasts are not a big deal in other parts of the world may help to explain why the worldwide average age of weaning is 4.2 years, though recently, some have challenged those numbers and say it's closer to age 2. There is new research that suggests humans are physiologically intended to be given breastmilk until they are 7 or 8. Years, not months. I hope your bottom is okay after falling off your chair. I'm not suggesting that you breastfeed until your child begins college. All good things must come to an end, preferably before your child figures out computers.

## "Okay, I'm Ready. Now What?"

Time for a reality check. The smooth transition from breast-as-ornament to breast-as-thermos works great in theory—we've all seen the idyllic paintings of mother and child. What you may not fully understand until you are a breastfeeding mother (or father of a breastfeeding baby) is that breastfeeding is still sometimes considered a private matter. And unless you like hiding in dirty bathroom stalls, you'll soon discover that public breastfeeding is sometimes viewed in about the same way as . . . hmmm . . . let's find a good parallel . . . passing gas in a crowded room of strangers.

I'm not saying you have to love the idea of using your breasts as your child's first refrigerator. I'm not saying you have to commit to breastfeeding until your child is old enough to sing along with Bert and Ernie. I'm not even saying you have to trade in your sling-back pumps for Birkenstocks. Breastfeeding isn't about being the perfect mother (however, it does bring you inches closer to the title). But before you make up your mind not to do it, make sure you're making an educated decision. Chele Marmet puts it this way: "People need to understand that when they're deciding between breastmilk and formula, they're not deciding between Coke and Pepsi . . . . They're choosing between a live, pure substance and a dead substance made with the cheapest oils available."

## Chapter 2

# Breastmilk vs. Artificial Baby Milk: The Fizzled Great Debate

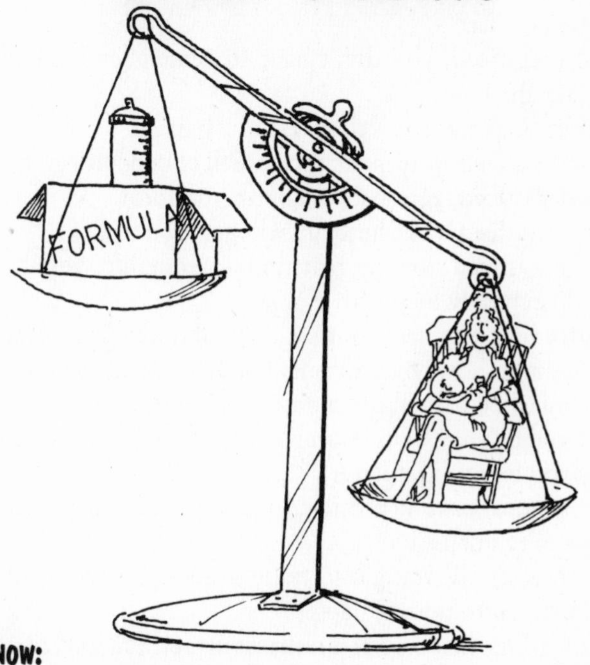


**Did You Know:**

1. Breastfeeding improves your cleavage.
2. Breastfeeding encourages bonding (it's an incredibly warm, comforting feeling for both of you).
3. Breastmilk provides nutrients not found anywhere else.
4. Breastmilk staves off allergic reactions and potentially lifelong allergies and asthma.

5. Breastmilk protects your baby and makes him less likely to get sick; formula-fed babies see the doctor almost twice as often as breastfed babies.
6. Breastfeeding dramatically lowers rates of serious illness. Breastfed babies are four times less likely to be hospitalized for bacterial infections; less likely to suffer from SIDS, cancer, dermatitis, ear infections, diarrhea, diabetes, liver diseases, and other afflictions.
7. If you breastfeed, you're less likely to have to stay home with a sick infant.
8. Breastmilk is cheaper than formula.
9. Breastmilk is easier to prepare and digest than formula.
10. Breastmilk is always the right temperature.
11. Breastmilk is always clean.
12. Breastmilk is free.
13. If you breastfeed, you don't have to remember food every time you leave the house.
14. Breastfeeding makes traveling less of a hassle.
15. If you breastfeed, your pediatrician will commend you for it.
16. If you breastfeed, your baby will love you for it.
17. If you breastfeed, your husband will get used to it.
18. If you breastfeed, for the first time in your life, you'll be a 42D (and it'll certainly help with #17).
19. Breastfeeding may help your child avoid a weight problem later in life (research shows that formula-fed babies gain too much weight, while breastfed babies gain a normal amount).
20. Breastfeeding may help you avoid a weight problem later in life (helps you lose weight faster).
21. Breast pumps make it possible to give your baby breastmilk even when you're not around.
22. If you breastfeed, you get to trade in sacky maternity clothes for shirts with button-down flaps.
23. Breastfeeding helps your uterus contract and return to its old shape faster.
24. Breastfeeding represents a style of parenting: right off the bat, you're willing to adjust your life to your baby's and give a lot of love. You might save your child a lot of time and money he'd have spent in therapy.
25. Studies show breastmilk is the perfect brain food during the first year of life and may increase your child's I.Q. by as many as 5–10 points (think how smart you'd be if you'd been breastfed).

26. Breastfed babies are 40 percent less likely to have misaligned teeth (maybe you can forget saving for braces).
27. Breastfed babies have better eyesight.
28. Breastmilk is environmentally sound (and you don't even have to recycle it!).
29. And the best reason to breastfeed? "Enzymatically hydrolyzed reduced minerals, whey protein concentrate, palm olein, soy, coconut, high-oleic safflower oils, lactose, maltodextrin, potassium citrate, calcium phosphate, calcium chloride, salt, potassium chloride, magnesium chloride, ferrous sulfate, zinc sulfate, copper sulfate, manganese sulfate, potassium iodide, soy lecithin, mono and diglycerides, inositol, choline bitartrate, sodium ascorbate, alpha tocopheryl acetate, niacinamide, calcium pantothenate, vitamin A acetate, riboflavin, pyridoxine hydrochloride, thiamine mononitrate, folic acid, phylloquinone, biotin, vitamin D3, vitamin B12, taurine, L-carnitine."

*That's what's in formula.*

## "What's Wrong with Formula? I Know Lots of People Who Had Formula, and They're Just Fine"

Babies will still grow, prosper, and maybe even go to an Ivy League college if they're fed formula. But there's a reason why researchers call breastmilk "white blood." Breastmilk isn't just food. It's actually closer to unstructured, living tissue (like blood) than it is to food. Because breastmilk is full of white blood cells, antibodies, vitamins, water, protein, hormones, growth factors, and even ingredients that kill bacteria and viruses, breastmilk is capable of doing for babies on the outside what nutrients fed through the placenta do on the inside. It offers the perfect balance of everything a baby needs to develop physically and neurologically.

Babies are immature when they're born (that's why they act like babies). Human babies are the most immature of all of nature's babies, and do most of their maturing outside the womb in the months after birth. The brains of human infants are only one-quarter complete at birth. The other three-quarters of that growth begins at birth and is most accelerated during the first few years, though the brain will keep growing until the baby is a teenager. Much of that growth is due to emotional, physical, and neurological stimulation they get from you. You are what you eat, says the old proverb—but are babies also what they eat? Science says, "Yes." Keep in mind good nutrition is most significant in the very young.

## IQ and Your Flame-Proof Suit

Could your baby's IQ even be influenced by breastmilk? Researchers say "yes." Consider this: In a study published in 1993 in the British medial journal *Lancet*, eight-year-olds who were given breastmilk in the first month of life scored 8.3 IQ points higher than another group fed formula.

In another study published in 1996 in the *Journal of Human Lactation*, 4-month-old babies exclusively fed breastmilk were compared to another group of four-month-olds fed formula or breastmilk supplemented by formula. The researchers found that babies fed only breastmilk "differed significantly" from the other groups, including the group fed a combination of mother's milk and formula. Exclusive breastfeeders were ahead in both physical and behavioral development, keeping up with all of those "what your baby may be doing" charts and even exceeding many of the developmental milestones, unlike many in the other group. They were checked and compared again at a year and the differences still held up.

Another study looked at the mental and motor development of eighteen-month-olds. Even after controlling for things that are decidedly hard to control for (how smart the babies' moms and dads are, how much stimulation there is for baby, how many other kids in the family are competing for mom's and dad's attention, etc.), the researchers still found a "robust statistical association between type of feeding and child intelligence." One more thing: Some follow-up work suggests there are long-term developmental differences.

This is upsetting news for those who weren't breastfed (including me, since I myself was minimally breastfed) and those who don't breastfeed their own children. I tell you this because each time I've talked about a link between breastmilk and IQ, I've needed a flame-proof suit. Some will say the IQ differences are "small" or "insignificant," but the studies taken together suggest the boost to IQ could be as low as one point, but may be in the range of five to ten points. I'll let you be the judge of what seems "small" or "insignificant" to you.

But breastmilk doesn't just make babies smarter. Scientists have identified more than three hundred components in breastmilk, and that's just a fraction of what's in it. They believe the combination of all that's in breastmilk strongly influences a baby's brain, behavior, and growth. It is also a big boon to babies' and children's immune systems, lessening the severity of some illnesses and even preventing others.

Scientists don't call formula by its nice, euphemistic name. They call it artificial baby milk or ABM, because that's what it is—a dead, manufactured, artificial substance.

Since artificial milk first became available, it's been recognized that babies fed formula suffer more illnesses. Breastfed babies have half the number of doctor visits and one-tenth the number of hospitalizations that bottle-fed babies have. Bottle-fed babies have more gastrointestinal and urinary tract infections. And if genetics have conspired to make your baby a more likely candidate for allergies, asthma, or diabetes, breastmilk has been shown to actually block these genetic factors or at least minimize their effects. New research is even pointing a finger at the high quantities of manganese in formula as a possible link to Attention Deficit Disorder. One recent study seems to suggest that breastfeeding for more than three months could protect a child against appendicitis. Another study by a nutritional epidemiologist found that women who were breastfed as infants had a 30 percent decrease in risk for developing breast cancer.

Breastfeeding your baby is good for you, too. Women who don't breastfeed are more likely to develop osteoporosis, premenopausal breast cancer, and ovarian cancer. Women who breastfeed for longer than three months significantly cut their risk for those diseases. Yet another study reports that new mothers who breastfeed produce lower levels of stress-related hormones return to pre-pregnancy weight faster, and when you're an old lady, make you less likely to fracture your hip, thanks to improved bone remineralization.

## Call It What You Like, but It's Still Artificial Milk

If you can think about formula not as some wonderful human invention but as what it really is, *artificial* baby milk, you might have an easier time entertaining the idea of breastfeeding. Watch formula commercials with a new eye: syrupy music and a much-too-thin model who looks about twenty grinning with her best Maybelline smile (at the camera, not the infant). Then the quick look at the baby, who'll coo on cue. Then cut to a product shot, and that reassuringly warm voice-over: "Why trust anything but the most gentle of formulas for your baby's delicate system? [whispered] Breastfeeding is best, but only [fill in the brand name] comes in a vacuum-sealed can with a handy measuring spoon. When you can't give your baby [whispered] breastmilk, give your baby [fill in the brand name] in a can."

Formula companies aren't even supposed to be advertising as widely as they are. The United States signed a World Health Organization (W.H.O.)

agreement promising to follow the W.H.O. code that bans formula advertising and distributing free samples. Since there has been no public pressure for the United States to enforce the ban, formula companies have essentially ignored the mandate.

## Who Thought of Formula?

During World War II bottle feeding was a handy invention for women who had to pitch in for the war effort—and take their breasts with them to factory jobs. They used homemade formulas, usually made from cow's milk. Women in the '30s and '40s used a mixture of Pet evaporated milk and Karo corn syrup (there was even a recipe for baby formula on the back of the milk can). But because baby humans have much more delicate systems than baby cows, baby humans have a hard time digesting cow's milk.

Formula companies have driven themselves crazy trying to manufacture a rough approximation of a substance that already exists! Do you know how they came up with the recipe for formula? Years of research? Scientific grants to come up with the perfect food for babies? A team of Nobel Prize winners working together to concoct a formula?

No. Dairy farmers were trying to figure out what to do with a by-product of milk, butter, and cheese production, the thing that was left over after everything else was processed and sold. That by-product is called *whey*. At the same time, to maximize profit, industrious men were trying to figure out how to market a food for babies to compete with homemade formula and breastmilk. These businessmen figured out that if they mixed whey with oil and water, they could feed it to babies without killing them (bad idea if you're trying to establish a market for your product). So the very first ingredient after water in most formula is essentially a waste product of dairy production. Then the manufacturers added vitamins and either palm, soy, or coconut oil—which are among the cheapest oils available—and voilà, they created formula. These oils are the very same ones used in the movie theater popcorn that people are passing up for health reasons!

## So Why All the Rubber Nipples?

Many people have still another problem with breastfeeding. If feeding a baby involved any other part of your anatomy—say fingers or elbows—no one would hesitate. But you have to use your *breasts*. And because everybody in our culture is so much more comfortable seeing breasts used to sell toilet cleaner and cheese puffs, it's hard for them to see what have evolved into favorite sex objects taken out of context. Bottles, rubber nipples, and formula are very far removed from breasts, and most people are much more comfortable looking at rubber nipples than they are with the possibility of eyeballing the real thing.

Yes, there will be pressure not to breastfeed. Yes, unless you live in a cloister, there will be times when you'll have to do it in public. But it isn't mandatory K.P. duty. Like pregnancy, it is for a finite period of your life. And it is mostly a pleasant duty. The good you do in this early period will last a lifetime for your child. (And no, they'll probably never thank you for it.) Plus, there are ways around your own modesty, variations you will learn in this book so that you *can* feel comfortable.

### Your Own Prejudices

Marge, a Long Island mother, found the whole concept "disgusting" and had nearly decided not to breastfeed when she mentioned to her friend June that she was taking a cross-country car trip soon after the baby's birth. June, who'd breastfed, pointed out how convenient breastfeeding was. Marge wasn't sold on the idea until June also pointed out the size of Marge's Volkswagen Bug trunk and then went through the list of things she'd need if she bottle fed. Just for starters, she'd need bottles, pots for boiling water to sterilize the bottles, and a supply of formula.

During delivery, the doctor misread Marge's chart and mistakenly gave her a shot to dry up her milk. But Marge was now committed to the idea and told him to get her milk back or else. The problem for her was that only a mother with a pump or a mother with a baby can restore a milk supply. So Marge did both. When her baby wasn't breastfeeding, she was pumping. She was almost too effective—her milk came in in such huge quantities, she fed the excess to the dog. Marge went on to have two more children and normal rations of milk. (Too bad for the dog.)

### Bonding

More so than bottle feeding, breastfeeding helps the natural process of bonding between mother and child. Mothers who've done both with different children admit they bonded much faster with the baby that was breastfed. Breastfeeding is something neither of you will ever forget. (Your grown-up baby will store the "memory" in his physiology and in the way he relates to the world.) This does not mean that women who feed their babies formula aren't good, loving mothers. Some are, some aren't. Just like some breastfeeding mothers are good, some are so-so, and some are, well, let's be politically correct, "maternally challenged."

You can't help but establish an incredible bond with your baby through the unavoidable closeness of breastfeeding. In addition, nature provides a whole slew of new hormones that are released into your body while you're breastfeeding your child—kind of like the endorphins you get from a good workout. Prolactin, one of the hormones released, is called the *mothering hormone*. Nature provides it for you so that physiologically, at least, you feel like a mommy. You'll experience a calming, relaxing sensation when your milk starts to eject. And it might be the only time you feel calm for a while!

## Keep an Open Mind

If anyone comes on too strong in favor of breastfeeding, try to keep an open mind. Once you're educated about this miraculous substance called breastmilk, you may find it hard not to proselytize also. Women who encourage you to breastfeed do so because they care about children, not because they're trying to force their way of parenting on you. If you breastfeed for three days instead of not at all, I commend you. If you do it for three minutes, you get a handshake. However, if you do it for more than six months, or better yet, closer to a year, you'll receive a fabulous cubic zirconium—and far fewer pediatric bills because your child will likely be far healthier. (I was kidding about the fake diamond, though not about the doctor bills.)

Yeah, yeah, yeah, you're saying. You're even possibly having what we journalists call the "MEAGO" reaction: "My-eyes-are-glazing-over." We all know there are plenty of good reasons to floss our teeth, drink carrot juice, and wear SPF 30 sunscreen. Just knowing something is good for us doesn't make us want to do it. But consider this: that little alien being who spent nine months growing inside of you, giving you indigestion, flabby arms, and a waist the size of Aunt Bea's, is a pretty powerful motivator. Breastfeeding is *really* good for your baby. And it's for a limited time only. Keep this in mind on the days when you really don't feel like wearing bras with drop fronts, shirts with flaps—or that perfect accessory that goes with everything and leaves white patches on any shoulder it touches: your baby. You just might even miss that incredible closeness when your child is thirteen and pretending he doesn't know you on a family outing.

## How Common Is It?

The most recently completed study showed that 59.4 percent of women initiate breastfeeding by the time they leave the hospital. That means they've tried it. Some women give it up in the first few days and weeks because they don't have enough information, because they don't have anyone to help them, or because they're encountering problems that in most cases could easily be fixed. You've heard various reasons from friends and relatives who told you they couldn't breastfeed. Just so you don't wind up thinking this is an innate ability only special people have, like being able to wiggle your ears, most women who "couldn't" actually could have. They may not have known this, and you probably can't convince them otherwise, but to be blunt, they didn't know what they were doing because they just didn't have enough information, and whoever tried to help didn't know enough either.

## Hey, It's Hip

Breastfeeding is now the trend, it's true. But just because it's hip doesn't mean it's a passing trend. The percentage of breastfeeding mothers has been climbing steadily every year. Doctors and scientists now freely admit that artificial baby milk is at best a very crude approximation of breastmilk. New facts make it harder and harder to ignore the amazing health benefits for both baby and mother. Artificial baby milk manufacturers have even been forced to, in effect, advertise their products with the notice "breastmilk is best" or "breastmilk is the preferred feeding for infants." (Check the cans. They really say this.)

A lot of people find it uncomfortable to face the fact that breastmilk *is* best. Bottle feeding has been considered the normal way of feeding a child, and before this moment, you probably never thought about it. Now, you might be wondering, "If real breastmilk is so much better, why does anyone choose to feed an infant artificial baby milk?" Good question.

# Chapter 3

# If It's So Great, How Come Everybody Doesn't Do It?

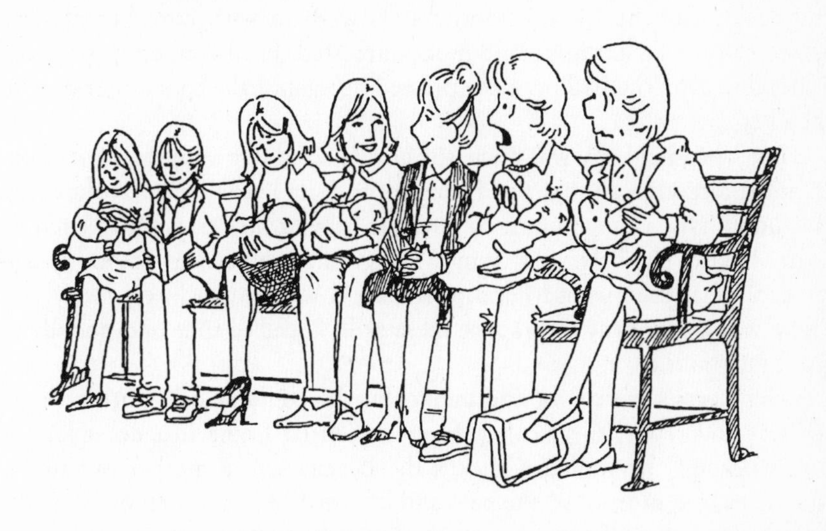

At an Ohio zoo, a female gorilla lived by herself. It's hard to breed gorillas in captivity, but eventually this gorilla was courted, won over, and impregnated by a visiting male. When her baby was born, the gorilla did a terrible thing that mother gorillas do if they haven't been taught a particular skill. She killed her baby.

She killed the baby because she didn't know how to feed him. Gorillas will do one of three things after they give birth. Their first choice is to breastfeed. If they don't know how to breastfeed, the gorilla world gives them only two other options: let their offspring starve, or kill them. This mother gorilla had lived her life in captivity and had never seen another gorilla breastfeed. Even though we think some things come naturally for every mammal but us, it seems that most primates, even gorillas, need help to learn how to feed their young. When this gorilla became pregnant again, her keeper knew she needed help to avoid a repeat performance. Somehow, he had to teach her how to breastfeed her baby so that number two wouldn't suffer the same fate as number one. But how?

Somebody told him to call La Leche League, the organization founded in 1956 that is a mother-to-mother (human mother, that is) support group for breastfeeding women. Of course! Why hadn't he thought of that before? The League agreed to help, and each day a volunteer who was a nursing mother came to the zoo and fed her baby in front of the gorilla. For days, the gorilla couldn't have been less interested. She fished fleas off her fur, scratched her behind, made faces. But as day after day went by, and new La Leche League mothers showed up with bare breasts and babies, the gorilla got more and more interested. Finally, when it was close to her due date, she had her nose pressed up against the bars of her cage to get a better look.

But when her baby was born, the gorilla acted like a typical new mother. She'd forgotten all that she'd learned from La Leche League volunteers. She didn't have a clue on how to hold the baby or how to get it to latch on to her breast. The baby was crying. The gorilla mother was obviously agitated. She had seen what to do; in fact, she'd watched it closely for weeks. There was just no way to practice these skills ahead of time and nobody to grunt questions to.

Her keeper feared for the infant, but he couldn't call Gorilla Social Services and report the mother. So he called La Leche League again. "It isn't working!" he wailed. Quickly, the League sent a mother out to the zoo. She stood in front of the bars and attached her baby step by step. She brought her baby's chest to her chest, slowly cradled the baby's head in her left arm, held her breast with her right hand, and tickled the baby's lips with the nipple to get the baby to open his mouth. Then she pulled the open-mouthed baby toward her breast and with one rapid arm motion, got the cooperative baby quickly onto her breast. The gorilla watched, mimicking the moves step by step until, with a nearly audible sigh of relief, the gorilla looked down at her chest and saw her baby feeding happily for the first time. When she had another baby, she didn't need any help from the La Leche League.

So, you see, breastfeeding is not always easy, unless you've grown up seeing it done. Like gorillas taken out of their normal habitat, humans also have to be taught how to do it. But even if it isn't an innate skill for us, it might be for our babies. Pioneering research in Sweden unveiled a stunning sight:

left on their own, without a lot of interference after an unmedicated non-problematic delivery, babies who were placed naked on their mother's abdomens for one hour were able to get to their mother's breasts and latch on without assistance. The average time it took these newborns was forty-five minutes. Babies who were left with their mothers for twenty minutes, then removed for baths and measurements before being returned to their mothers, no longer seemed to possess this instinctual sense of direction or latch-on skill. That's why new AAP guidelines say get the baby on within the first hour after birth.

So now I've contradicted myself. I said breastfeeding was hard, then I said babies can do it themselves. Because we live in a bottle-feeding culture, because a great number of us give birth with the help of pain medication, epidurals, or C-sections, and because most hospitals in this country want to turn over their beds as quickly as possible and won't give you forty-five minutes of peace and quiet right after birth, expecting a newborn to crawl to a waiting breast is a pretty tall order. But even if you can't avoid an episiotomy, an epidural, or a C-section, you can still avoid formula. The problem is, we're nearly as isolated as that gorilla mother because as a culture, we know so little about the hidden powers in our mammary glands.

## "Why Doesn't Mom Encourage Me to Breastfeed?"

My mother's generation (think pillbox hats and bouffant hairdos) considered breastfeeding vulgar and low-class, sort of like applying baby-blue frosted shadow to the brow line or carrying a pink teasing comb in your back pocket. When Dorinda told her mother she planned to breastfeed, her mother said, "Ugh! Why?"

My mother happened to find a pediatrician from Yale who was one of the pioneers in breastfeeding in this country. She was encouraged to breastfeed all four of us, so she did. But she was considered a freak in our suburban Connecticut neighborhood. And I learned nothing about it from her because she was (and is) very modest. I didn't even know I had been breastfed until I asked her.

Laura's mother Louise had breastfed her three children but never discussed it with her daughter. In the 1960s, Louise lived in one of those neighborhoods where all the women had Tupperware parties and bought Mary Kay cosmetics. She breastfed with her Jackie Kennedy suit discreetly undone. When the neighbors found out, there was a line of little kids outside of Louise's house. The mothers had decided a field trip to Louise's house would be nearly as educational as a trip to a museum—a lesson in anthropology and primitive human behavior. The only kids on the block who knew nothing about it were her own growing children.

### "It's Just Not Done, Dear"

Don't be too hard on your mom if she wasn't part of that small minority. But what this means for you is that the best source of information—Mom—may not exist for you. In fact, it's more likely your well-meaning mother or mother-in-law will pass along the same information her pediatrician gave her decades ago—something similar to this gem I found in a 1964 textbook titled *The Fear of Being a Woman* written by a Harvard professor: "[Mothers] should be told that the child will not be deprived, that in fact, artificial feeding is better for the infant . . . . Considering the hazards [of breastfeeding], it might be well that no mother nursed her child." And that from a doctor! This may be the information your mother or mother-in-law still has pasted somewhere in her brain, so be tolerant of her even if she isn't of you.

### "Psst! Hey, You, I'm Over Here!"

Plus, there's all that free formula hospitals give away. The problem with free formula is that there may be a day when you feel insecure about your supply of breastmilk. And winking in the cupboard will be that handy container of artificial baby milk. "Ah-hah!" you'll think. "This will tide us over!" But this is the same reason why mothers don't like their three-year-olds to eat birthday cake right before dinner. Two things will happen: One is that if your baby fills up on formula, he won't be sending the signal to your body to keep producing lots of milk. You'll stop making as much as he needs if you supplement. The other thing is that he might decide it's easier to just glug from a bottle. Next time you offer the breast, he'll want the bottle. (By the way, his "preference" is meaningless. Your toddler will "prefer" artificially colored, flavored, sugared candy over broccoli.)

### The Bottom Line

None of these reasons explain why some women try breastfeeding and quit and why others are adamant about not wanting to do it at all. Here's when we finally get to the bottom line: to breastfeed, you have to be kind of comfortable with your body or at least willing to try to *get* comfortable, and, something that surprised me, you have to be a little bit assertive, too.

You have to be pretty convinced that you're doing the right thing to withstand the subtle and not-so-subtle comments from other people. We live in a culture that isn't always supportive of breastfeeding mothers, and you'll run into pressure from a lot of women who bottle fed and think you should, too.

If your mother, sister, neighbor, grocer, or best friend's brother's wife's mah-jongg partner didn't breastfeed, they're likely to be less than enthused about your decision to do it. Actually, they'll probably feel a little threatened, which is understandable. You're doing something they didn't do and maybe deep down, think they should have.

Here's where your partner, mother, sister, and friends come in handy. Make them read this, too. They've all got the time. You're the one who's up all night and running to the bathroom every ten minutes.

Your husband or partner especially needs to understand the benefits of breastfeeding, so that he's not at your elbow with a bottle. Start by telling him that Michael Jordan was a breastfed baby and Michael Jackson was not. Your partner will turn out to be your biggest ally—or saboteur—depending on his feelings about the subject. Expect, even from the most highly evolved man (you know, the one who's several evolutionary leaps beyond the Cro-Magnon), to still get some resistance. It usually comes in the form of those "Mine!" looks. Though my husband rarely said anything, he was given to long, possessive glances at my breasts. He finally broke down at my daughter's first birthday party and asked me if he could have "them" back. Just think: your baby and your husband will both be learning how to share at the same time.

Pam, the mother of three, gave up breastfeeding her first two children after a week of frustration each time. Her husband, who liked his sleep and wasn't a particularly helpful dad to begin with, would grumble, "Oh Geez, just give 'im a bottle! I can't stand all this commotion!" Each time, Pam gave in. But when number three came along, she decided to put up with her husband's griping, her newborn's attempt to figure out the sucking technique, and her own engorged condition. When her husband once again suggested she just "plug him up with a bottle," she got out of bed, found a leftover pair of wax lips from her childrens' Halloween bags, and got back into bed. "Honey, will you kiss me?" she said demurely. When he turned over and planted a big sleepy kiss on the waxy surface, he yelped in surprise. "Get it now?" Pam said. "Which do you like better? Real lips or wax ones?" Then she pointed at her infant, who was trying to suckle at her breasts. "Which do you think he prefers?" Her husband never gave her a hard time again.

## "How Long Do I Have to Do This?"

A lot of women want to know before they've even started how long they "have" to breastfeed. Because they haven't yet done it or because they're in the most unpleasant, beginning stages, they pose the question the way you'd ask your physical therapist "How much longer do you have to contort my knee into that painful position?" Most of the time, child-rearing is a pretty pleasant occupation, or nobody would procreate. And most of the time, breastfeeding is a pleasant occupation, too. Sure, there are bare minimums if you want to pass along immunities, prevent allergies, or "bond" with your baby. But try to get past this maddening need to have a goal or a deadline. Kristine took her baby Addison to see her in-laws, and says her mother-in-law kept coming in the room when she was breastfeeding and asking her when she planned to stop. "She was nuts about it. She kept saying, 'You need to set a deadline.'" Kristine says it was as though "my breasts had a date stamped on them, and the milk would go sour after a particular date." Babies don't have much use for deadlines, especially arbitrary ones.

By the year 2000, the U.S. Department of Public Health had hoped to increase mothers who breastfed to at least 75 percent and get at least half of all new mothers to continue breastfeeding for six months, with the hope of many breastfeeding for a year (and beyond). It hasn't happened, though there's still hope for the new millennium. That's because the American Academy of Pediatrics (AAP) now recommends six months of nothing but breastmilk, then breastmilk along with other foods for a *minimum* of one year. And sit down, this will shock you: science is still on your side if you continue into or past your child's second year of life. The World Health Organization (WHO) recommends exclusive breastfeeding for six months or longer, then breastfeeding and supplementing with food to age one. WHO encourages mothers to continue up to and beyond age two. This recommendation doesn't change for developed countries. Contrary to a lot of information that is out there in baby books, your child will get nutritional and disease-fighting advantages for the length of his breastfeeding. Your milk will constantly change to meet his needs, and scientists are just beginning to start research on babies who were fed breastmilk long-term. (You do not have to breastfeed for as long as the AAP or WHO recommend. It's simply a guideline that may help you if people give you a hard time. Remember: *any* time at all spent breastfeeding, even if it's just a few weeks, is much better than none at all.)

Okay, okay, you still want an answer to "How long do I have to do this?" "I tell people, 'six months is a very good beginning,'" says Dr.

Gordon. Nine months will give your baby some basic protections, including guarding him against severe allergies later in life, the onset of juvenile diabetes, and even appendicitis.

Remember when you were seven, and your best friend told you how babies were made? It sounded disgusting, didn't it? "I'll never do that!" Now it sounds strange to breastfeed for a long period of time. You might think you're prepared to breastfeed for a month, maybe two. That's fine. Give yourself a goal if you need to, though try not to see it as set in stone. When you're doing it for *your* baby, it'll look different and feel different. It *is* different when it's your child. (Think of what you put up with from your husband or partner that you'd never tolerate from a stranger, a salesclerk, a colleague, or a friend.)

You'll do things as a parent that you *never* thought you'd do. You'll think it's cute when your toddler offers you a bite of a gnawed, soggy Zwieback, and you'll probably even take a bite instead of recoiling in disgust. Even if you feel a little weird about breastfeeding right now, you will gradually come to feel differently. Give yourself time. Even if you've been exposed to someone breastfeeding and thought it was distasteful or it made you feel like you wished you were in another room, it will be different when you are intimately connected to that little person on your breast.

Don't pressure yourself or feel pressure from anyone else to decide ahead of time. You will have plenty of time to think about weaning later. Once you begin, you can always stop. But if you don't start, it can be very difficult, if not impossible, to change your mind later.

## A Trial Period

Allow yourself the possibility of getting to know your child and working out together what is most logical and comfortable for both of you. It might be that you feel most secure with a breastfeeding trial period of three to six weeks, at the end of which you'll decide if it's for you. Dorinda, whose baby is now four months, said she had to keep telling herself, "Just get to two weeks." Then when she got to two weeks, she told herself, "Just get to four weeks." By six weeks, she didn't need the steady coaching anymore. "I forgot that I ever wanted to quit."

Try to make it through your first month without basing your decision on this particular time period. The first month is the worst month. Once you're through this, the experience will radically change.

You may set out to make it to three months. Breastfeeding is considered well-established by that time. By three months, many women decide that it isn't such a big deal anymore and feel better about doing it indefinitely. If people are peppering you with questions, be vague and change the subject, because only two people really have a say in how long you breastfeed. You are one, and your baby has a voice in it, too, a very loud one. In addition to telling new parents that six months is a good beginning, Dr. Gordon advises people to wait until the baby is seven to eight months, "and then decide whether you're going to be a medium-term or a long-term breastfeeder."

## "You Mean Cigarettes Aren't Good for You?"

Along with all of their prejudices, many people are misinformed or uninformed about breastfeeding. That's a problem. When the facts about cigarettes and secondhand smoke became inescapably grim, it gradually became politically incorrect to smoke and blow carbon monoxide, tar, and nicotine on other people. Eventually, the same pressure might be brought to bear against artificial baby milk, which currently masquerades as the norm. Right now, a shocking number of people still think formula and breastmilk are equal or close in value. (Then again, 40 percent of Americans believe they've spoken to an extraterrestrial). It's upsetting to hear people tell you that "it's the same" or "we turned out okay, and we weren't breastfed" or explain why they didn't do it, with the number-one favorite reason: "I couldn't make enough milk."

## Excuses, Excuses

I'd like to call these *excuses*, but we all have dear friends who will tell us these *reasons* stood in the way of their breastfeeding. You will hear them over and over, so let's take seven of them, including these three, one at a time. Incidentally, you don't need to lecture everyone who has an opinion about this on what the facts are; just keep them in mind so that it'll be easier to withstand the comments you're bound to hear.

### Excuse One: Formula Is Practically the Same as Breastmilk.

It's not the same or even close, as we saw in Chapter 2.

### Excuse Two: I Wasn't Breastfed, and I Turned Out Okay.

No, our generation wasn't breastfed, and we lived. But we have allergies, asthma, eczema, diabetes, childhood ear infections, cancer, attention deficit disorder—and high psychological bills. There's no way to know what effect breastfeeding might have had on our generation. I'm not saying that we wouldn't have any ailments if we'd all been breastfed. But many doctors say the full effects of breastfeeding last a lifetime. And no question about it, breastfeeding definitely limits the number of serious illnesses seen in children.

The reasoning behind this excuse says "It was good enough for me so it's good enough for you." We started breastfeeding in greater numbers when new information came out. Don't close off your mind to that new information.

### Excuse Three: He'll Get Attached to You, and It'll Make Him Dependent.

You're most likely to hear this from your elders, because the people who raised us worried about spoiling their children. People who practiced "attachment parenting" (i.e., they picked up their crying kid and tried to figure out what was wrong) were "hippies." But a lot of research ground has been covered since then, and there is ample science (and I don't mean psycho-babble pseudo-science) to back up the conclusion that a strong attachment between parents and babies leads to healthy children.

There's ongoing research in this area, which is fascinating. It includes a book titled *The Mystery of the Infant-Mother Bond and Its Impact on Later Life: Becoming Attached* by Robert Karen. Karen's research, which was begun by Dr. John Bowlby on orphans, says that classic insecure attachment problems manifest themselves in sleeping and eating problems, tantrums, trouble separating, and clinginess. Children who have insecure attachments with their parents are often the ones who become very aggressive later in life.

This means that people who are ignorant of this research will tell you you'll have more problems if you form a strong attachment to your child by soothing him, holding him, feeding him, maybe even letting him sleep in your bed. They are wrong. If you do the opposite of what they're telling you, you'll avoid the fearful problems they're warning you about. I've seen this in action over and over. It's not just theory. It really does work in practice. There will be people who may even tell you you're spoiling your baby by attending to his needs, including his need to suck frequently. Rebecca's mother told her that she was spoiling Jacob by letting him suck even after he was clearly satiated. "He's just trying to get you to hold him," she said. Exactly.

### Excuse Four: If You're Tense, You'll Make the Baby Tense, So It's Better to Bottle Feed.

Carolyn loathed the idea of breastfeeding. A self-admitted high-strung person, she was not the least bit enchanted with the idea of using her breasts as a food source. "It was just a complete turn-off to me," she says. Carolyn's best friend told her *she'd* tried to breastfeed for a month and hated it, and offered Carolyn one more dire piece of information. "She told me it was really painful to wean the baby. Her breasts were hard as rocks." (Carolyn's friend used the cold turkey weaning method, which is never recommended. More about weaning in Chapter 14.)

So when Carolyn's daughter Julia was born five years ago, Carolyn immediately opted for formula. Her pediatrician supported her decision. "He thought I was really uptight, and he said if I was that tense about it, I'd make the baby tense." But this idea doesn't make sense if you think about a woman's biology. Breastfeeding mothers actually produce *fewer* stress-related hormones, and the hormones stimulated during breastfeeding are a natural relaxant.

Baby Julia was always sick and developed serious allergies, a problem Carolyn shared. "I kept thinking, 'What if I'd breastfed? Would she be so sick? Would she have allergies?" Carolyn remembers.

When Carolyn got pregnant a second time, she bought a book on breastfeeding and for the first time seriously considered it. And then she did it. Carolyn wasn't tense after the first few days. In fact, she says she "loves" breastfeeding. And better still, her second daughter is healthy and, so far, free from allergies.

### Excuse Five: You're Only Doing It for Yourself.

There will be people who will suggest that you are breastfeeding to get your own ya-yahs .... Miriam's pediatrician (now ex-pediatrician) actually said as much. "He said, 'You need to stop cold turkey. You are only doing this for yourself.' My son was just turning one. Breastfeeding was always a neutral activity for me. I was definitely not doing it for myself."

The most likely candidates who will suggest that breastfeeding is for your pleasure alone are those who were born without breasts, namely men. But other women might also try to discourage you with this incredibly negative and naive criticism. Katie was persuaded to stop breastfeeding her son after a relative told her she was harming her son because she "liked" breastfeeding him.

Sometimes I rocked my baby for myself. Sometimes I think I had my baby for myself. Sometimes I hug and kiss her—for myself. Getting pleasure out of your child for all of the positive, good things you are doing for him shouldn't make you feel guilty. It should make you feel good.

### Excuse Six: My Friends Say It Hurts.

Severe pain when breastfeeding indicates an underlying glitch; and no, it's not an indication that you have a low pain threshold. "Common" pain, or pain that may be a little startling at first but is bearable, is reportedly experienced by 80 percent of mothers and usually lessens within the first few days and disappears in the first few weeks. One of the worst things about pain isn't always the pain itself; it's the *anticipation* of pain. You want to do everything you can to avoid getting into this vicious cycle. When your baby first takes your breast into his mouth, it is likely your eyes will open wide, very wide. It is a surprising feeling the first time. During the first few days when you are producing colostrum, it is your baby's job to bring your milk in, and he may be sucking hard. Your nipples may sting a little. But there are many ways around pain that we'll get to later. And that initial pain doesn't last very long.

### Excuse Seven: I Can't Make Enough Milk.

This is probably the number one concern of new mothers. Let's put it this way: if you don't shop for food, it's unlikely groceries will magically appear in your cupboards. If you don't breastfeed regularly and on demand when you're getting a milk supply going, guess what? You won't make enough milk. Your body is smart; it will make as much milk as your child (or children) need. Women can feed twins, even triplets on their own breasts. I even know of one set of quintuplets in southern California who are being breastfed by their mother. Five babies, two breasts, and one mother are doing fine.

Although you're not alone if you worry that you can't or aren't making enough milk to feed your baby, very few women are biologically incapable of lactating and making plenty of milk. That's why they named us *mammals*—because we have mammary glands (you'll be so much fun at the next cocktail party or Trivial Pursuit game!). Most of us can produce enough milk to feed our own children. And if we wanted to become wet nurses, we could theoretically make enough to feed a small play group.

The worry over milk supply is due in part to our need for concrete measurements, but there just are no ounce markings on our breasts. There are things, however, that can get in the way of establishing a good milk supply, and we'll talk about them in the next chapter.

A very small number of women (experts disagree but it's in the neighborhood of 2 to 5 percent) actually do have problems making enough milk. During the early nineties, the health issue that became the number-one scare story on breastfeeding was something called *insufficient milk syndrome*. Insufficient milk syndrome got big play in reputable newspapers and on major newsmagazine television shows. But not one of the experts interviewed mentioned that although dehydration is a possible consequence of breastfeeding, *death* is a possible consequence of formula feeding.

Experts disagree over whether or not there even is such a thing as insufficient milk syndrome. The term was reportedly coined by a scientist being paid by a formula company. In many cases, mothers were breastfeeding their babies according to bottle-feeding directions, meaning they weren't breastfeeding often enough. Remember that formula takes longer to digest and babies take in more at each feeding, so bottle-feeding babies have fewer meals than breastfeeding babies.

Breastfeeding babies who don't get fed frequently enough can get dehydrated. Another consequence of too widely spaced feedings is a drop in a mother's milk supply, which can also lead to dehydration.

There *were* a handful of cases of babies who suffered severe dehydration and ended up permanently damaged. Though this is rare, it made for a dramatic story—so scary that women were quoted saying they felt "safer" using formula, which is the height of irony. In countries where formula and bottles aren't available, there is no such thing as insufficient milk syndrome, and mothers have nearly a 100 percent success rate with breastfeeding.

Almost all supply problems can be fixed with the help of an expert. Jill Dieteker, a registered nurse who became a lactation consultant, makes house visits to four women a day, five days a week (that's twenty women a week, over a thousand a year). She has yet to find a woman whose body is physically incapable of making enough milk. "The ones who aren't committed to breastfeeding are the ones who have the most problems," she says. "They're the ones who quit because they weren't doing it enough and 'there wasn't enough milk.'"

But Chele Marmet, director of the Lactation Institute, disagrees that commitment is the problem. "We've found that it isn't a lack of commitment. Mothers are very committed. Some are just having a lot of problems and need help, not commitment." That means, if you need help, even for something small, get it. Being a beginner at something is always a challenge. You're allowed to feel confusion, particularly when the stakes are as high as they are with new babies. You're allowed to wish that your breasts were transparent so that you could see how much milk you're making. But you can easily learn how to know if your child is getting enough. The more you know, the more confident you can be that you're doing the right thing and that your child is thriving because of your effort, and the easier it'll be to integrate breastfeeding into your life—until you do it the way you do every other thing you're comfortable doing. You know, like breathing, eating, sleeping . . . well, maybe not sleeping, now that you have a newborn.

## Get Rid of Your Calendar or Organizer

One last obstacle may stand in the way of your breastfeeding: trying to maintain a schedule. If an infant teaches you one thing, it's to dump your organizer for the first year. Babies have their own schedules, and trying to force them to adapt to a feeding schedule that's convenient for you is about as sensitive as regulating the number of diaper changes.

## Be True to Your Feelings

It's important that you don't feel that the breastfeeding police will arrest you if you vary from what some overenthusiasts have decided is the only correct way to go about breastfeeding. Each woman has her own individual situation, problems, extenuating circumstances, and so on. Mothers are already so polarized as it is. We spend a lot of our energy pointing out all the "bad" mothers we know. Try not to play this game with breastfeeding. If you want to do it, and your best friend doesn't, truth be told, you will have less in common with each other. You may eventually even come to feel less connected to women who choose not to breastfeed. You don't need to beat 'em or join 'em. Nadine says, "When I talk to my best friend, she doesn't exactly know why I wanted to do it. She bottle fed because she thinks breastfeeding is gross. She actually said, 'How can you let your daughter suck on your breast?'" Nadine says the friendship cooled not because of her friend's squeamish comments but because Nadine says her friend just didn't understand the closeness and the bonding that breastfeeding facilitates. "I'm not saying she doesn't love her son. But I really don't think the bond is the same." Easiest way to deal with this? You can let the friendship cool until the children are older, then try again. Or you can just be low-key about breastfeeding and hope that maybe your friend will open up to the idea of breastfeeding future children.

## It Isn't a New Religion

It is possible to take reverence of breastfeeding a little too far. I tried to interview a woman who is a mother and a birthing consultant. She told me she found "nothing humorous" about breastfeeding and that if I wanted "cute anecdotes," she was the wrong person to talk to. "I approach breastfeeding as a spiritual thing," she told me in a none-too-warm tone. "It is not funny. It is spiritual."

Okay, so it's spiritual. But it can also be hilarious. I'm all for treating that wondrous bond with reverence, but I think that consultant could afford to lighten up. Some women will look upon breastfeeding simply as the best way to feed their infant. But it does encourage the fusing of a powerful bond. And it is perhaps the purest form of human connection there is. That's why many great artists have some sort of ode to breastfeeding mothers, in the form of the Madonna-and-child-at-the-breast paintings and statues. But for all of us regular moms who are just trying to provide eight to twelve square meals a day, it's a little off-putting to feel as though breastfeeding must be discussed in reverential tones.

## Do It Your Way

You may not be able to face the idea of breastfeeding for as long as six months or a year. You may want to breastfeed only in the morning before work and at night when you get home. You might want to pump and give your baby pumped milk in public. You may decide to breastfeed exclusively for three months, then supplement after that. These are all okay alternatives. No, they aren't perfect alternatives. But your goal is to do what you feel comfortable doing, not to reject breastfeeding completely because you can't measure up to what feels to you an impossible standard. No one parents "perfectly." Frankly, I don't believe that anyone breastfeeds perfectly, either. You have to figure out what works under your set of circumstances. But you need to know what the ideals are. Doctors and exercise physiologists will tell you what the best diet and exercise regimen is. You may not always hit the mark, but there's no point in withholding information. You need to know what that ideal is. And remember: Nutritional advantages are most significant when you're a baby.

# Part II
# Mine Didn't Come with a Manual

## Chapter 4

# Getting Ready for the Big Arrival

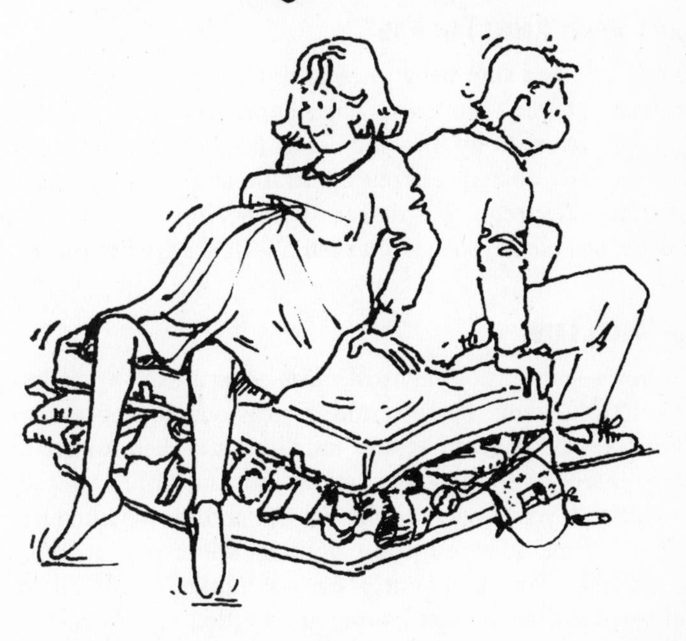

So now that you're committed to the idea, it's time to tell you the nitty-gritty truth: expect a learning curve. Before I had a baby, I *really* thought, "How hard could breastfeeding be?" Heck, I learned how to program my VCR—and women throughout history with no formal education have breastfed with ease.

What I failed to understand is that I wasn't the only one learning. Your baby will be new at everything, including breastfeeding. What I also failed to understand is that women throughout history had expert teachers helping them learn: their own mothers, who lived with them under one thatched roof (I didn't say it was a perfect arrangement). And one more thing: women throughout history didn't have what at first glance seems like an easy out: formula.

Since "breastfeeding is a confidence game," according to Dr. Derrick Jelliffe, one of the foremost authorities on children's nutrition, it'd be nice if your doctor or hospital could impart a little confidence. Successful breastfeeding requires practice. Along the way, you'll develop confidence. But don't count on a doctor or nurse holding your hand while you get confident.

## "I Can't Worry About This Now"

If you haven't had your baby yet, you're probably so consumed with other worries as "D-Day" (your due date) approaches that you don't want to add to your worries by thinking about how or whether to breastfeed. I myself was busy obsessing about my irrational fear of an episiotomy. Do a cross-hatch cesarean, I'll deliver on the floor of the Commodities Exchange, just please, *please* don't put a scalpel anywhere near that area!

## A Few Weeks Later

Good news—no episiotomy. Bad news—that wasn't what I should have been worrying about. For me, and it turns out, for most women, breastfeeding takes time, practice, and usually a little help to get to the point where you are comfortably loaning this intimate part of your anatomy to a tiny infant that you'll swear could suck the chrome off a bumper.

First, let me give you a few pointers while you're calm and not in labor screaming your lungs out. (That was a little joke. You'll be fine. I didn't scream one time, though I swore just a little.)

## Preparing Your Home: Concentrate on Your Freezer

Try to plan ahead. Stock up your refrigerator and freezer. If you hate to cook, try to find nutritious frozen meals. If you don't mind cooking, from now until you give birth, every time you cook, make a double portion and freeze half of it. While your baby is breastfeeding, you need to try to stay conscious of what your hand is stuffing into your mouth. You'll likely be so tired that you'll open the refrigerator and put whatever your fingers first touch into your mouth. Forget paring, peeling, boiling, and sautéing.

## Finding a Pediatrician

As you may already know, you need to line up a pediatrician while you're still pregnant. There is still no perfect, foolproof way to find the ideal doctor. Most people either use the Yellow Pages or rely on the recommendations of friends. Take recommendations, but know that people are at heart a tad lazy and don't relish change. Breanna stayed with her baby's doctor even though she didn't like him because it was "easier than finding a new one."

Call local hospitals where pediatricians have privileges and get some names. Nurses are great sources of information. Local lactation centers usually know all the pediatricians in town who are good *and* who support breastfeeding, and La Leche League can give you names, too. Once you have a few names, make appointments to interview the doctors on your list. Most doctors won't charge for this, but some do, so make sure you ask in advance. Helen was surprised to be presented with a bill for $100 for a consultation. Most pediatricians are used to being interviewed ahead of time. If you find one who doesn't do this, cross him or her off your list.

Find out the doctor's academic credentials and whether the doctor is board-certified. Is this doctor a member of any professional organizations? Does he or she teach at any local academic institution? But also trust your gut instincts. Would you feel comfortable "bothering" this person on a Saturday or after office hours? Solo practitioners can be fine, as long as they have someone who covers for them when they're not available. No matter whom you chose, make sure there's always a doctor available by phone and after hours. Babies have this uncanny sense of timing and usually pick weekends and after-business-hours to get sick.

Does the doctor encourage you to call with questions? Will he or she actually take your call? Will he or she see you promptly if you sense a problem? Look for a doctor who is gentle, makes eye contact, and spends some time with you during your interview. He or she should answer all of your questions patiently. If the doctor seems impatient with your questions, this is likely how you'll be treated during office visits with your child. Going to the doctor does have some of the feel of a three-ring circus. You'll be distracted, and it's hard enough to take care of your child and get your questions in, let alone remember the answers. If the doctor barely disguises his or her annoyance at the amount of time you're taking up, move on. You want a doctor who will talk to your child and give you thorough, understandable explanations.

## Does This Pediatrician Really Support Breastfeeding?

One of the most important things you can find out is whether this doctor is supportive of breastfeeding. You can simply ask, though 90 percent of doctors are initially supportive of breastfeeding. A few further questions will clue you in immediately as to how much he or she really knows about breastfeeding and whether he or she will be able to help you if you run into difficulty. If it's a male doctor with children, ask him if his wife breastfed their children and for how long. For a woman with children, ask her if she breastfed and for how long. (The longer the better, particularly if they make it to one year or more.) Ask him or her what percentage of the mothers in his practice breastfeed and what percentage are still breastfeeding at their baby's first birthday. Ask him or her: "What is important about breastfeeding?" "How much breastfeeding education do you have?" "Is anyone in your practice board-certified in lactation?" "To whom do you refer breastfeeding difficulties?"

If the doctor says, "Breastfeeding isn't for everyone," this is not a good sign. Nor is ambivalence, as in the case of Lynn's doctor, who said, "It's six of one, half a dozen of the other." This is not the doctor you want treating your child when there's a serious medical question. "Take off the leg? Oh, I dunno. Six of one, half a dozen of the other. Walking isn't for everyone. Sure, take it off."

But many excellent pediatricians don't know much about breastfeeding simply because it still isn't a part of their medical training. Just the same, any doctor who gives you the impression that the decision you make about breastfeeding is not important is doing you a terrible disservice. A doctor who's doing his or her reading will know that breastfeeding is as important—if not more important—than anything else you could do for your baby that first year of life. Unless you have a medical problem that prohibits you from breastfeeding (such as cancer), you'll want a doctor who'll help you all along the way.

Some pediatricians end up learning a thing or two from their patients. Karen had bad allergies, and preventing allergies was the only reason she wanted to breastfeed her unborn son. But at a consultation, Karen's pediatrician told her he thought she was "too uptight" to breastfeed. She *was* tense about it, and she really didn't want to do it. He sensed this, and during their ninety-second interview, he steered her toward formula. Karen knew it was better to breastfeed and she'd told the doctor about her own history of allergies. But she didn't know how much better; and the doctor didn't help. So when he said, "just use formula," she assumed he knew best and would have told her "if it was a big deal or that much better to breastfeed," she says. "But I didn't make an informed 'choice.'" Her baby Jason had massive allergies and so many ear infections that he eventually needed surgery to put in a ventilation tube. Both problems are far less prevalent in breastfed babies.

Karen was pregnant with her second child when she asked the doctor if her second baby would be in for the same kinds of illnesses. He surprised her by saying, "Breastfeeding seems to make a big difference." "I was so angry," says Karen. "I kept thinking, 'Why didn't you tell me that before?'"

Karen stayed with the same doctor because he was good at everything else. When he saw how well her second son was doing on breastmilk, he did some more breastfeeding research and now explains to his patients what they're choosing between. "If he'd told me the first time what he told me the second time, I never would have bottle fed," Karen says. "I still look at all that Jason went through, and think, 'What if?'"

### Why You Want a Pediatrician Who Likes Breastfeeding Mothers

Your pediatrician doesn't have to make you feel like a hero. You won't even need applause. You'll just need someone who understands the medical value of breastfeeding. If you start out with a pediatrician who truly supports breastfeeding, you'll have your own personal medical expert and advocate in your corner before you even enter the hospital. This person is more likely to be able to recommend a lactation consultant if you need one and can probably answer more questions about breastfeeding, such as which foods to avoid if your baby is fussy or which drugs are dangerous when you're breastfeeding. A doctor who doesn't believe in handing out cans will be more likely to help keep you breastfeeding instead of turning you on to artificial milk at the first sign of any problem that will take him more than two seconds and five words— "Why don't you try formula?"—to solve. At the very least, you want a doctor who doesn't give you outdated, inaccurate information. Many experts say that doctors who give you the impression that it doesn't matter how you choose to feed your baby are giving you advice that probably qualifies as malpractice. "This seems to be the one area where you can practice medicine in the 1990s—with 1960s know-how—and not get sued," Dr. Jay Gordon says. "Yes, I think it borders on malpractice. I think it's genuinely unintelligent for a doctor not to promote breastfeeding vigorously." (Don't bother suing, though. It's considered standard care to offer a "choice.") It's easier for a doctor to tell you by phone to try formula than it is to have you come in for a visit, assess your baby, figure out your breastfeeding problem, or refer you to a lactation consultant.

### Does This Pediatrician Actually Like Children, or Is He Sorry He Didn't Go into Radiology?

Make sure the doctor truly likes children and likes what he or she does. You don't want to shortchange your child in the warmth department. You want good medicine, but you also want good children skills. It's possible to find both in one person. Doctors who grab, prod, poke, and roll children around like they're objects without saying so much as a word to them don't have great children skills. Adults have these experiences, too. I had to have a lump removed from my breast and a doctor walked into my hospital room and wordlessly began squeezing and probing my breast, maintaining eye contact with my nipple. "My name is Janet," I said acidly. "That's my breast. And you are?????" He got the message, let go of my breast, and introduced himself before continuing. Your baby is even more vulnerable than you because nearly every experience is a new experience—and he doesn't know a doctor from a serial killer.

The doctor who sounds menacing, but does everything with a big, phony smile and a handful of lollipops, is just as bad. Even with the promise of a lollipop, your child will still hate this doctor.

You can learn a lot by seeing the way a doctor relates to children. If the doctor will permit it, stay at the office and watch his or her bedside manner with a patient. Explain to a friendly parent that you're checking out pediatricians and you like this doctor. Ask the parent if she or he would let you observe part of the child's doctor visit. Most mothers and fathers are happy to impart what they know and may let you watch from the door for a minute or two. Your observations will tell you volumes about this practitioner.

## Nurses Count, Too

Don't forget about the doctor's nurse, either. The nurse will likely be the person easiest to reach by phone. He or she can let you know the best times to come for a physical (when the doctor isn't crazed), sneak you in for the shot you forgot at your last visit, or answer simple questions. Your child's nurse is also the person you will spend the most time with when you are at your doctor's office.

### "What's the Big Deal?"

You may see your own doctor once every two years, but keep in mind that by the end of your baby's first year, you will likely have seen the pediatrician at least eight times—at three days, two weeks, one month, two months, four months, six months, nine months, and twelve months. If this seems like a lot, remember that formula-fed babies see the doctor almost twice as often as breastfed babies. And if it's a doctor who has a busy practice and requires a six-month advance appointment, this may not be the doctor for you, even if he or she is the best in town. What good is the best if you can't get in?

### "What If I Don't Have a Choice?"

In most towns and cities, you'll have a choice of pediatricians, even on a restricted insurance plan. If you have no choice and your pediatrician isn't supportive but you think his or her other medical skills are intact, keep this pediatrician but find another person to whom you can address questions about breastfeeding (see the Appendix).

## Personal Prebirth Preparations: How to Toughen Your Breasts

In previous decades, doctors and books used to tell women to rub their breasts with terry cloth to "toughen" the skin. They were also told to pull and twist their nipples. I even found an old magazine that told women to "file" their breasts with an emery board. But after those breasts had been toweled, pummeled, twisted, yanked, and filed and the first layer or two of skin had been removed, who'd want to use them to breastfeed? Doctors later learned what mothers already knew: this not only was painful, but also didn't accomplish anything except to turn women off breastfeeding.

### "But I Have to Do Something!"

If you're the kind of person who has to try something, here's what you can do. In the weeks leading up to delivery, start wearing a T-shirt without a bra. You're not doing this to make a feminist statement, but because the friction created between your breasts and the cotton will toughen your breasts. If you're uncomfortable without a bra, take an old bra and cut out small circles in the middle of each cup so that your nipples will be exposed to your shirts. Your goal is not to produce calluses. Your breast tissue is soft and sensitive and even just exposing your breasts to air will help toughen them. You can also expose your breasts to sunlight, but *do not get burned.*

Unless you're from the south of France, your breasts have probably never seen the sun, so be very careful. Stop using soaps or astringents on your nipples and areolas in the months before birth. If you wash the natural oils away, you'll make your breasts more sensitive. As I said, twisting your nipples or rubbing them with anything harder than a feather is *not* recommended. Leave your poor breasts alone.

## Don't Pump Ahead of Time

Some doctors used to recommend pumping before the baby is born in an effort to avoid engorgement (swollen breasts). But early pumping not only does nothing for engorgement, it also does two things that are dangerous: it can encourage uterine contractions, because hormone production is stimulated, and it can drain your breasts of colostrum, the first milk you make, which is full of immunities to anything you've ever had, been exposed to, or been immunized for.

## Nursing Bras

Since you won't fit into those nice little lacy things you used to wear anyway, you might as well get used to your "mother bras." Heck, you've probably already broken the lingerie fashion barrier with maternity underpants that look like pup tents.

Get a few nursing bras before you deliver (two is good). When you're buying these bras, don't get your old size. Maternity bra cup sizes go up to H. Kristine, who suddenly found herself a D-cup (still letters away from H), thought "it looked like I'd swallowed two footballs." The best time to buy a nursing bra is a month before your due date. Go to a maternity store and buy a bra that fits you now. If you can put the bra on and it's comfortable on the second to last hook, without binding or pulling, you should be fine. The nursing bras you're looking for are the ones with the friendly little drop fronts that open up like long underwear and snap or clasp closed. You don't have to spend the money on these, but they're more convenient to use than regular bras. Your breasts may be tender during the first few weeks of breastfeeding, and you will probably find it less painful to drop the flaps than to hike tight elastic up over your breasts or reach around behind and unhook your bra.

Buy all-cotton bras. Even if you're big-breasted, don't get bras with underwires. Those can put pressure on your mammary ducts and cause breast infections. (Some women buy them anyway and report they had no problems. But these bras are more likely to cause problems, so why take a chance?) The reason you want all cotton is so that air keeps moving, your breasts stay dry, and you avoid nipple soreness. If you don't want to wear a bra, don't. Though a lot of literature tells you to, there's no evidence that a bra does anything other than make you feel more comfortable physically. If a bra makes you uncomfortable, don't wear one.

## Nursing Shirts

Most maternity stores and lactation centers that rent or sell breast pumps also carry a lot of clever nursing shirts. That's right, you'll also have to put away the slinky silk blouses for a while and be prepared to look like Dolly Parton in a rugby shirt. What's great about these shirts is that unless someone knows what they are, they're unlikely to notice the carefully camouflaged flaps. You can get by with two or three of these shirts, though you'll be darned sick of them in just weeks. Buy these before you deliver too, because you'll be most awkward breastfeeding in the beginning. "I was afraid I'd never be able to go out of the house," Jennifer says. "I wore nursing shirts at home, then practiced in front of friends. I was just paranoid. After a few weeks, I thought, 'Oh heck, if they see a boob, they see a boob.'"

Check the Appendix at the back of the book if you're having trouble finding these shirts. You can order them through the mail. (You can also hint around to friends who want to give the baby a gift.)

### Expecting Twins?

If you're expecting twins, triplets, or more, the breastfeeding clothing on the market probably won't help you. It's designed to expose one breast at a time (once you open one slit, the other slit slides across your chest so that you can't feed two babies at the same time). Mindy had twins, a boy and a girl, and was always able to wear a T-shirt. In public, she usually fed the children one at a time, beginning with the twin who was making the most noise. At home, she fed the two babies at the same time. Each had his own breast.

### Dressing to Undo

When you get good at it, you won't even need nursing shirts. Some women never buy them, particularly women who've nursed more than one child. Theresa fed Dominic, her third child, while wearing regular clothes, though she advises women to "always wear two pieces." That means a loose shirt and pants or a skirt. Anything that buttons up the front will work; you can simply unbutton from the bottom. A large T-shirt that the baby can fit partially under works, too. The baby's body will cover the minimal bare skin that shows. It'll take you a few months before you can breastfeed while waiting in line at the grocery store, while sipping cappuccino at a counter, while talking to an old friend at a party (I did this), even while doing sit-ups in a postnatal exercise class (I did this, too). Your only fear need be that some stranger, who wants a better look at your "sleeping" baby, will alert your infant, who'll pick that moment to release your breast and give a big grin.

### Do Not Go Near Your Prepregnancy Wardrobe for a While

One lactation consultant advises women to go out and buy "two nice outfits that [they] feel pretty in" after they've given birth. If your husband balks, tell him you have a prescription from a medical expert: these clothes are for your mental health. None of your old clothes will fit yet, and you will hate wearing your maternity clothes once you're no longer pregnant. If you try to squeeze into your jeans, you'll likely end up in the emergency room with surgeons trying to get you out of them. (And by the way, nursing shirts don't count as part of these two outfits.)

## What to Take to the Hospital

For my first baby, I had my bag packed for weeks, which was dumb because I eventually delivered two weeks past my due date. By the time we were on our way to the hospital, everything I needed had been fished out of my bag. You don't need anything special to breastfeed except pillows.

Put your spare pillows in your own pillowcases. Use those dumb rainbow-striped ones that your mother gave you when you went off to college. That way, your pillows from home can be distinguished from the hospital pillows, so an orderly doesn't kidnap yours and take them to geriatrics. Buy cheap new ones if you don't have a lot at home. Hint: use the cheap pillows until your baby stops spitting up and pooping on everything. Take as many to the hospital (they'll go in a large trash bag) as your husband or partner can comfortably carry, but try to take at least four. Most hospital beds come equipped with one poor excuse for a pillow. If you have a nurse who responds when you press that red emergency button, you might get two pillows. But remember, hospitals are not hotels. They do not run scurrying with extra pillows and blankets when you complain to "housekeeping." You'll need five or six pillows (especially if you end up having a C-section). When you're first learning to breastfeed, the pillows are your training wheels. They'll help you hold the baby, keep you from getting a sore back, and help you get in the right position so your baby can breastfeed correctly.

### SLINKY NIGHTGOWNS

If your grandma gave you a nice nightgown with those two slits in front for breastfeeding, obviously, take it with you. But if you don't have this kind of a breastfeeding nightgown and don't want to buy one, you can use an old extra-large T-shirt and cut slits down the front where your breasts are. If you can't squeeze into a T-shirt with your big belly now, don't worry, your belly will soon be smaller. (Unfortunately, you'll still look about five months pregnant after you've delivered. I hope I'm not the first one telling you this. I hate being the bearer of bad news.) You can wear your robe or the hospital gown over the T-shirt after you've delivered. I personally preferred to let my daughter lie on my mostly bare chest. New babies need warmth and skin-to-skin contact. If you deliver in a hospital where you have some privacy and no intern barging in on you every five minutes to practice his bedside manner, this might work for you.

## AT THE HOSPITAL

### THE GOOD OL' DAYS

When you were born, your father probably paced the hallways, and your mother was so drugged, she didn't recognize you for days after the birth. Things are different in most hospitals now.

### SOME THINGS YOU NEED TO KNOW ABOUT HOSPITALS

Some hospitals are "baby-friendly" and some are not. Shop around if you can. The goal of the Baby-Friendly Hospital Initiative is to eventually award the truly baby-friendly hospitals with certificates. Some of the certification criteria include not handing out formula, keeping mother and baby together after birth, and having policies that support breastfeeding.

You may not have a choice of hospitals because there's only one in your town or for insurance reasons. But in any case, try to take a tour of the place where you plan to give birth so that you're not walking in blind (and in hard labor).

### About Nurses

Be forewarned that the economic crunch in the last five or so years has affected hospitals. They may not be as well staffed as they used to be during your time in labor, delivery, and postpartum recovery. Nursery nurses used to be responsible for about five mother-and-baby couples. Now they may have fifteen or more. This is the reason why they want all of the babies in one place so that they don't have to keep running from room to room. Even if your hospital advertises rooming-in, in which the baby stays in your room, you'll need to ask if it is a twenty-four-hour service or just a nine-to-five thing, when the hospital is better staffed.

Since hospitals have cut costs, there may only be two people on duty at night: one to watch babies, one to watch mothers. One nurse will stay with the babies in the nursery while the other nurse stays "on the floor" to help mothers.

### About Policies

Nurses tell me that many hospitals will say they don't have "policies." That's their way of diplomatically getting around answering your question if you ask, "What are the hospital's policies?" Better to ask what the "environment" is like, particularly after hours. Can the baby stay with you at night? Inform yourself about the hospital's rooming-in rules because it's important to keep your baby with you. If you know your hospital's environment beforehand, you can be prepared if you need to let them know what *your* policies are. They'll deliver thousands of babies. You may only have one.

### Hospitals Are Businesses

Keep in mind, you are purchasing a service. (Just wait until you get your bill.) Do not forget that medical care is not free, even if hospital staff sometimes act like they're doing you a big favor (where else can you drop $5,000 to $10,000 in a day and still get surly service?). Hospitals will do things as efficiently as they can because they are trying to make a profit, and who can blame them? And that means they will do things that are convenient for them, not necessarily for you.

## Your Hospital Etiquette Affects Your Breastfeeding Success

When women have just given birth, I think it's fair to say they are at their worst. Many don't have the energy to be polite. "I felt like saying to the nurses, 'I'm sure you'd like me—if I hadn't just been in labor for thirty-seven hours!'" says Jill.

Some women intend to breastfeed but feel so rotten, they are past the point of caring how the baby gets fed. If the mother doesn't initiate breastfeeding, the hospital has to do something. No one will force you to breastfeed, any more than someone (other than a drill sergeant) can force you to exercise. Ultimately, it is your decision. The nurses and doctors are harried. The baby is tired. You're tired. Those assigned to care for you (and for twenty other mothers and babies) may be thinking, "Aw heck, it's too much trouble to answer your questions, work with you to get your baby on your breast, *and* listen to you complain. Since it's all the same to you, I'm going on my break. Here's a bottle."

Unless you're adamant about what you want, you may find that nurses, relatives, and friends won't know enough or care enough to make sure you breastfeed. In the beginning, a bottle seems easier. But before you're in shape, so is sitting on your couch and eating cheese doodles. Everything worth doing (well, almost everything) takes some time, effort, and concentration. And this time, you're not doing it for just yourself.

## "Don't They Know How to Do This, Either?"

Many hospitals have stopped employing lactation consultants as a way of trying to cut costs. You may get little or no help from the nurses because many don't know how to get you started or how to fix breastfeeding problems. And the nurses who might have been able to help you in the past are now simply too busy to stay with you for as long as you'll need the help. "My nurse was really frustrated with me," Janine remembers. "She was practically tapping her foot and saying, 'C'mon! C'mon!'" Finally, Janine told the nurse to leave and called a friend who was breastfeeding a six-month-old. "It was much calmer with my friend." Since Janine had no real problems, she only needed support from her friend, who talked her through it and encouraged her while she learned how to breastfeed.

Corky Harvey, a nurse and lactation consultant, spends two hours a day trying to help new mothers in hospitals. She functions mostly out of the goodness of her heart, because many hospitals still won't pay for the services of a lactation consultant. Though Corky inevitably ends up staying at the hospital longer trying to help everyone who needs it, she never has enough time. The day I followed her around at a Los Angeles hospital, she saw six woman-and-baby couples. She had exactly twenty minutes for each woman, and every woman she saw could have used three times that amount of time.

## Some Tips to Make Your Hospital Stay More Pleasant

### Try to Be Nice

It always helps if you ask for things in a nice way. "I don't mind people who know what they want," says one postpartum nurse. "I'll do it for them, but it's much easier when they are nice about it instead of rude and demanding." Always start by being nice and assuming you'll get what you ask for. Be as calm and patient as you have it in you to be. My husband taught me this. He can talk anybody into anything. Before I met him, I spent a lot of time with various people in service industries, not getting anything accomplished except exercise for my lungs. You can always rattle cages later. Most medical personnel are nice people. They are in their profession because they care about people. They may want to help you but have their hands full because they're understaffed. Keep this in mind if the service stinks.

### Take a Number

That's one of the reasons why you should bring along the number of a lactation consultant in your area. You may not need to call her, but it's good to know you can get some help in a hurry if you need it. Check the Appendix in the back of the book for breastfeeding organizations that could recommend a consultant.

### When You Arrive

When you get to the hospital, make sure you or your husband lets the nurses know in advance that you have decided to breastfeed. In general, hospitals are reasonably supportive of breastfeeding mothers. But you need to sound confident when you say you will be breastfeeding. I've seen mothers say, "I'd like to try breastfeeding, though I don't know if I can do it." That leaves nurses the opening to say, "Well, we'll have to see. You can *try*." Start out knowing that you can breastfeed. That is not in question, like whether or not you'll need an emergency C-section. Ask that the nurses attach a small sign to your baby's bassinet signaling that no pacifiers or bottles be offered to your baby (gifts, checks, cash—but no rubber). The sign, which lets the staff know the baby is being breastfed, is important only if the baby spends any time away from you, and will ensure that no one gives him a pacifier or a bottle of glucose water or formula. You want to avoid nipple confusion (more on that later).

## Labor and Drugs

For my first delivery, I found the Lamaze classes I'd taken to be almost no help when I was in heavy labor (maybe I was just a bad student). My memory of that B.E. ( which does not stand for blessed event—it stands for "before epidural") was of me trying to keep from twisting my husband's head off each time he'd gaily announce, 'Okay, let's count, honey." Maybe that's why for my second delivery, I chose to show up at the hospital fully dilated at 10 centimeters, though I didn't get a discount for the 30 minutes I actually used their labor and delivery room.

I had two different experiences of labor: one with drugs, and one without. Though this is obviously anecdotal, baby number two (no drugs) was slightly more interested in breastfeeding and a little livelier at birth than number one was.

Most doctors and anesthesiologists will tell you epidurals are safe, and they likely are. However, that said, many nurses, doctors, and lactation consultants report anecdotal evidence—though no hard data—that epidurals do affect newborns. The liberal use of epidurals may be responsible for some of the breastfeeding problems babies encounter. I tell you this not to make you feel guilty if you have an epidural, but so that you are forewarned. Babies born to women who've had drugs during their labor may be more sluggish than those born to mothers who did not have drugs. They also may have sucking problems. (But try telling a woman in the worst pain of her life that an epidural is not an option. It's like suggesting a root canal without anesthesia. Some women really don't have tremendously painful deliveries. Some are in a lot of pain. Some, like me, turn into the Exorcist until it's all over.)

"I do see a difference between epidural babies and nonepidural babies," one labor and delivery nurse says. "Epidural babies are sleepier, less interested in the breast and have a harder time latching on than nonepidural babies." But not all doctors agree. "I don't think it's a big deal," says Dr. Gordon. If you've had an epidural and breastfeeding does not seem to be working, get a lactation consultant to help you.

## Your First Hours with Your Baby: "How Soon Can I Breastfeed?"

The general rule is the sooner you get your baby on your breast, the better. If not immediately, then in the first twenty minutes after birth and before more than one hour goes by, according to AAP guidelines. (But all is not lost if there's some medical need to separate you from your baby even for some time. In fact, lactation is still possible, although not as easy to start up, months after you've had your baby. But don't count on this because it is a lot of work.)

Newborns typically have an alert period immediately after they're born. If you wait even an hour, they're usually so exhausted, they fall asleep. If you take advantage of that window of wakefulness, your baby will probably be far more interested in your breast. Let your husband and the nurses know that it's very important to you.

## The First Thing Your Baby Wants Is You

Remember the groundbreaking research in Sweden where newborns moved by themselves from their mothers' abdomens to their mothers' breasts and latched on unassisted? If I hadn't seen this, I would never have believed it. In the Swedish research, newborns who got to spend a little time with their mothers' breasts were far less likely to have breastfeeding problems weeks later. Those who'd been separated from their mothers were often still having trouble weeks after birth.

Newborn babies seem to come with an instinctive treasure map that only works for the first hour after birth. Your breast will be the first thing your baby's going to want to see anyway (after he's seen you and your husband, of course). The more time you have right after the baby is born to hold, soothe, and cuddle him and introduce him to your breast, the better it'll be for him. His innate skills will stay intact if he gets to your breast sooner rather than later.

## "Where Are You Going with That Baby?"

Make sure you ask why your baby is being taken away. Some "urgent" medical needs are sometimes nothing more than hospital procedure. Nurses can delay weighing the baby, though they will probably insist on giving an Apgar test at one minute and again at five minutes. The Apgar test is your child's first S.A.T., so make sure he brushes up for it. No, actually it is a test developed by Dr. Virginia Apgar to evaluate your newborn's general condition. Most babies pass.

## Don't Be Disappointed If He Doesn't Start Guzzling

Some newborns will latch on immediately; some might just want to play with your nipple (not hockey or catch, just a little get-to-know-you session). Either is okay because at least they're getting familiar with their new home.

If you feel cramping or pain in your uterus the first few times you breastfeed, don't worry, you're not going into labor again. Breastfeeding stimulates uterine contractions, which is a good thing. After you give birth, your uterus is big enough to carry a bag of groceries in. You want it to shrink back to its old size (or close at least), and breastfeeding speeds up this process.

### "I Thought He'd Be Hungry after Months of Nothin' but Amniotic Fluid"

Full term newborns have an inborn reflex to suck. They will do this after birth, but not because they are hungry. Most full-term babies have packed on a layer of fat and water in preparation for birth. Their birth weight can be deceptive, particularly if you had a lot of fluids during labor. Some of that fluid will come off, so your baby will lose some weight—up to 10 percent of his newborn weight. You don't need to worry. In fact, after an earthquake in Mexico that demolished a maternity hospital, one newborn was found alive after eight days under the rubble. Newborns typically lose between 5 and 10 percent of their birth weight during the days after birth, then begin to gain again. By the end of two weeks, most of them are back to their birth weight or close to it.

### The Bonding

Ahh, yes, that all-important bond. You will probably have mixed feelings when your baby is born. You may think you know this baby, but it's actually going to take some time before your bond with him is cemented. Bonding is a process, not an event. Don't feel strange if it's not love at first sight when you first hold your baby. When you look back, you'll be convinced that it was. You will gradually fall in love with him. We're programmed to love whatever comes out. As your baby starts getting bigger and responding to your face and your voice, your emotions will naturally deepen. All that diapering and feeding and holding and rocking and breastfeeding will strengthen your maternal instincts. (This applies to deepening paternal instincts, too—minus the breastfeeding.)

### What Comes Out First?

When doctors talk about liquid gold, they are referring to colostrum. It's also sometimes called *super milk*, though I always feel the need to add,

"Dunh-dunh-dunh-daaah!" every time I hear it called that. "Faster than a speeding breast, it's Supermilk!"

Once your newborn latches on, he'll get his first shot of colostrum, which is like his first immunization. You are passing along all of your immunities to him in liquid form. Colostrum will also get your baby's bowels moving so that he can pass the meconium in his system. This black, tarry looking substance is his first poop, though you probably won't want to save it. (One nurse told me the story of a woman who was having trouble naming her baby because she liked "unusual" names. When she heard the nurses talking about meconium—because her son was two weeks overdue and had passed meconium in utero—her ears perked up. "'Meconium.' I like that name." Then she looked into the unsuspecting eyes of her baby boy and said, "I'm going to call you 'Meconium.'" The nurse swears this is a true story.)

Don't worry about the meconium. It is not a sample of the poops you'll have to change for the next two to three years. Michael describes changing son Jared's diaper the first time. "It was like scraping road tar off of a marshmallow." You (or your partner, though it'd be fairer to rotate) will only get a day or so of meconium before your breastfeeding baby's poop turns into a nice, nearly sweet-smelling substance (I'm not kidding).

Colostrum has a laxative property that gets the meconium moving out of your baby. Frequent nips at your breast will mean the meconium will move faster out of his delicate system, and he's a lot less likely to end up with other problems like jaundice.

"I tell my patients to breastfeed around the clock from the beginning," says Dr. Gordon. This means feeding your baby every hour and a half to two hours. And that means you may have to wake him and get him to breastfeed. "I see people so happy to have a baby that sleeps that the baby isn't getting colostrum," says Gordon. "The baby can cycle down very quickly, and then you've got a mess."

Also, getting your baby on your breast soon after his birth will be a first practice session. You'll need to get good at breastfeeding, and it'll stimulate your breasts to begin to produce milk. Most importantly, frequent, on-demand feedings from the beginning—generally every two hours, or a minimum of eight and hopefully closer to twelve times in a twenty-four-hour period—will ensure a strong milk supply, keep your baby hydrated, and give him the full benefits of colostrum. Frequent breastfeeding has some real benefits for you, too. It can relieve the pain of engorgement and possibly even prevent it.

## Five Hospital Breastfeeding Tips

Laura is a La Leche League Leader who counsels new breastfeeding parents. She says she tells parents five main things, because they don't seem capable of absorbing much information (due to a syndrome called "Preparenting Traumatic Stress Disorder" and no, insurance doesn't cover it). She tells them, "No pacifiers, no bottles, baby rooms-in with you at hospital, feed on demand, and call for help if you think you need it." Laura says that if mothers follow these five rules, "it's hard to mess up."

## That's Why They Call Them Babies

Newborn human babies are born with characteristics that resemble those of the fetuses of many other mammals. They cannot yet survive on their own (sorry for stating the obvious). After the first few months, they spend the bulk of the remaining first year straining and struggling to get away from you. But in the beginning, it's as though their new womb is your breast. Dr. Gordon gives women who are about to deliver one golden piece of advice: "Don't let go of your baby." That means, *you* need to babysit, not the hospital. Being separated from you puts stress on your baby. He's been with you his whole life, and his first look at the world will be much easier if you're there to comfort him and he's not in a room filled with other babies and heavy machinery.

Your baby doesn't know where he ends and where you begin. The breast becomes his source of comfort and nourishment—it's an all-purpose filling station. You do not have to teach him this. He comes out with this knowledge.

"It was the closest I could come to replicating the womb," Wanda, the mother of Taylor, says. "Taylor was two weeks early, and I just kept her on my chest, kind of like a little marsupial. It was a more natural transition." Wanda says her husband Gary was so proud of his new daughter, he took a packet of pictures to the office. Wanda finally got a look at the photos. "I said, 'Gary, have you been showing these around?' Every one of the pictures showed me, the kangaroo mother, with Taylor hanging on and my breasts hanging out!"

## "What's Exclusive Breastfeeding?"

*Exclusive breastfeeding* means just that. No bottles, vitamins, pacifiers or thumb sucking. I know. Sounds like overkill. But that's the definition, and in truth, your baby doesn't need anything else. The reason everybody says avoid all the manufactured sucking tools for a while (bottles and pacifiers), is because studies have shown that in addition to confusing your baby, they also lead to early weaning and decreased milk supply.

## "Doesn't He Need Water?"

Breastmilk is 88 percent water, so don't give your baby water or juice because you're afraid he isn't getting enough to drink. The U.S. Centers for Disease Control issued a warning in 1997 not to give young babies water because it can, in fact, be dangerous. Check with your pediatrician, but most doctors say wait until the baby is at least six months before you offer water. Theresa's mother-in-law kept bringing in bottles of water to give to Theresa's baby. Finally in exasperation, Theresa said, "You want him to have water?" She unscrewed the bottle and drank the water herself. "There. Now he has water."

That's how you'll supply vitamins and minerals too—by ingesting them yourself. The American Academy of Pediatrics says you do not need to give vitamin supplements if you have a normal diet and no extenuating problems, but if your pediatrician prescribes vitamins for your baby, they aren't harmful. Strict vegetarians may need to give their babies vitamins, so check with your pediatrician.

## The Importance of Rooming-in

Even if you're exhausted, try not to get talked into having your baby spend his or her first night in the nursery so that you can get your rest. You had your rest. Consider the last 16 to 48 years of your life, depending on how old you are, your rest. Your baby needs you. He or she has spent his entire life safely squashed inside of you. Glass, chrome, and fluorescent lighting aren't quite as comforting as the warm, gushy space next to mom. If your baby goes to the baby nursery, he will be "wrapped up like a mummy, placed in a plastic box by himself, and turned to face a wall," says Marsha Walker, a registered nurse and lactation consultant. "That's called abuse if you do it to prisoners."

Hospitals cannot force your baby to sleep by himself in the nursery (unless he has some kind of medical problem that needs to be monitored). Nurse Walker, who has cared for many newborns, says that even if a mother is not breastfeeding, having the baby sleep with her is preferable. "It stabilizes vital signs much faster." The hospital might tell you that they're afraid the baby will get cold. A newborn's body temperature will regulate itself perfectly if it's placed skin to skin next to one of its parents, not in a hospital bassinet.

### "But It's Our Procedure!"

The hospital that I delivered at encourages mothers and babies to stay together. But other hospitals have other policies . . . excuse me, environments. It may be normal procedure in your hospital's environment to separate new mothers and their babies, but if you tell them that *your* normal procedure is to keep your baby with you, they will eventually back off. Your baby can sleep in your bed with you. Nurses will frequently just put up the bars on the sides of the beds and wrap towels or blankets around them. The baby isn't going anywhere anyway, but everybody feels better if they do this.

### "There's Not Enough Room!"

If the hospital tells you that there is not enough square footage, and you will be in violation of state law if the baby stays with you overnight, ask them why you weren't in violation of state law during the day. And if they have designated maternity rooms that can't handle having mothers and babies in them together, then *they're* the ones in violation of the law.

### "He Might Get Kidnapped!"

The other argument they might throw at you is that they're responsible for the baby's safety while you're at the hospital, and the baby might get kidnapped! "That never happens," says Nurse Walker, "but it sure scares parents." Reason through this argument: do you think the baby is more likely to disappear while one person who isn't related to him is taking care of him and fifteen other newborns, or while he is snuggled up next to you? By the way, you are now responsible for that baby. The hospital can't do anything to your child without your permission, so ask them whether that means they're responsible or you are.

### "I'm Being Nice, and They Still Want to Take the Baby"

If you're too tired and it looks like it's going to be a battle, have your husband, partner, friend, or relative take care of the matter out of earshot. Your last resort is, of course, to leave. No one can make you stay at a hospital, and if you threaten to leave, you'll probably get to keep your baby in bed with you. (If you do leave, the hospital will ask you to sign a consent form that indicates you understand the hospital isn't taking responsibility for your decision to leave "against medical advice.")

## Keep Him Away from Pacifiers, Glucose, and Formula

I didn't want my daughters out of our sight once I'd had them. More irrational fears, perhaps, but I have an active imagination and I could envision tired nurses handling them like chickens on a conveyor belt. But that wasn't the main reason why I didn't want them in the baby nursery. Aside from the delicious comfort of being next to his mother, another reason to keep your baby with you and your partner is to keep away anyone who might be tempted to stick a pacifier or bottle of glucose water into your baby's mouth. What he needs to eat is in your breasts. Giving your baby glucose water or formula from a bottle or a pacifier to suck on will set you back in breastfeeding, do nothing for your baby, and create problems. When Ben was a newborn, he was given a bottle by his nurse. Ben was born with a poor suck, but, even if he hadn't been, he did what all babies who drink from a bottle do: he just closed his mouth around a hard nipple and pulled his tongue back. The milk dripped in. When he wanted to stop the flow, he pushed on the nipple hole to slow the flow of milk, so that he could swallow. A totally different activity from breastfeeding. Ben wasn't lazy. He just needed help learning how to breastfeed. When a child has a lazy eye, the good eye is covered with a patch to strengthen the muscles of the weak eye. When a baby is learning how to breastfeed, you don't encourage the weaker behavior by strengthening it.

## "I'm With You in Theory, but How Do I Sleep?"

Now that you've won one battle, what about the war? The war for the next six months will consist of nightly battles to get sleep. Trying to get some sleep is by far the hardest part of being a new parent. That incredible fatigue will go away . . . in about eighteen years when he starts college. But in the hospital at least, studies have shown that women who keep their babies with them get about as much sleep as those who don't.

Dealing with sleep deprivation is harder if you've had a difficult delivery. Any woman who has been through a hellish and tiring birth does need sleep. Even though your partner's been through it with you, he's probably not in physical pain. And I'd bet money he had a dog or cat when he was little that he was up with at night nursing back to health. Have him take his shirt off and let the baby sleep on his chest, if there's another bed in your hospital room. That way, the baby is with you.

## C-Sections

Although every woman wants a healthy baby no matter how he gets out of her, many women who've had C-sections feel bad that they "missed the moment." But not half as bad as they feel from the physical trauma of a cesarean birth. Even though it leaves a small scar, it is still major surgery, and for many women who are exhausted and sick from delivery, breastfeeding is the last thing on their minds.

"By the time I had an emergency C-section, I'd been up for two days," says Miriam. "Your instinct when you're that sick and that tired is to tell everybody to go away—including the baby." In fact, when Miriam's husband brought son Lucas to her, she was so ill, she quickly said, "Take him!," pushed her new bundle of joy into her husband's arms, and promptly vomited. "I don't know if I'll ever be able to tell him that the first time I saw him, I threw up," Miriam says. This does not mean that if you have a C-section, you won't be able to breastfeed. It simply means that if you've had a cesarean birth, you will need even more help getting your baby positioned and latched on than someone who's delivered vaginally, because a huge section of your body will be in pain. But some mothers have no problems, thanks to their babies. Jane had a C-section, and her baby was brought to her hours after birth. "Little Alyx knew just what to do. She started the hunt-and-peck mission and found exactly what she was looking for. Our first meeting, and she was already teaching me," Jane says.

Most hospitals will allow your partner to stay overnight with you. If you have had a C-section, the nurses probably won't allow the baby to stay in your room with you alone because you'll need help. If your partner, friend, or relative is willing to stay with you, you should be able to keep the baby in your room. During the night, your partner can take care of the baby while you get two to three hours of sleep, and he can bring the baby to you for breastfeeding. That way, you will not have to wait for an overwhelmed nurse to bring you your baby hours after he's signaled he wants to be fed.

## What If the Unexpected Happens?

If for some reason your baby can't go right to your breast, don't despair and assume that your chance to breastfeed is gone. Most women who end up with a C-section or some other labor complication had no preparation for it and did not expect anything to go wrong. I brought along cassettes, board games, and a new bathrobe to wear in the halls of the hospital during my first labor. But when I got there, I was forced to spend the next thirteen hours flat on my back with my feet up in stirrups. My daughter was in some weird position, and every time I sat up, her heart rate promptly dropped from 160 to 40 beats per minute.

You may panic if things don't go as planned. How do you bond if the baby isn't delivered to your breasts seconds after birth? What if you end up with general anesthesia as Michelle did? "When the nurse brought me Jenna, I was so groggy, I thought she was trying to hand me a bunch of blankets, so I handed her back." Miriam was still throwing up hours after giving birth and was in no shape to breastfeed Lucas until the next day.

Your baby might be premature, have neurological problems, Down Syndrome, a cleft palate, or some other unforeseen problem. Or the baby may just have a minor problem and now you are worrying that all is lost with breastfeeding because you didn't do it the "right" way, and your baby had a few bottles and didn't make it to your chest until the next day.

Sure, it would've been nice if you'd had a twenty-minute labor, no drugs, and a baby who didn't look like a Conehead when he finally came out. But that rarely happens. You need to concentrate on whatever hand (or head shape) you've been dealt. If you're having problems and can't get the baby to latch on when you're finally ready to try, don't fall apart. If the baby needs to be fed, then feed him. If what you have is glucose water or formula, then give him that until you can give him colostrum. Ask the nurses to bring you a breast pump. (Most hospitals have the super-duper, heavy-duty expensive machines.) If your baby is not starting up your milk supply, the pump will have to be the stand-in. You will probably not get much at first. In fact, you might not get anything. But don't be discouraged. Make sure first of all that you're using the breast pump correctly (check Chapter 11). If you're pumping one-quarter of a teaspoon of colostrum, mix it with whatever else your baby's drinking and give it to him. In the beginning, even a few drops is wonderful. He doesn't need a lot to reap the benefits.

## "Everybody's Telling Me I'm Doing It Wrong"

If the people closest to you—your mother, your husband or your partner—are not informed and supportive about breastfeeding, they may say things such as: "Are you sure he's getting enough to eat?" or "Look, if it's causing you that much pain, just give him a bottle."

Nadine toughed it out after her unexpected C-section, only to have the nurse, her husband, and her mother-in-law continually undermining her by insisting that what daughter Chanel really needed was a bottle. "We're from a bottle-feeding culture," she said. "Bottles and babies have become synonymous." In fact, bottles are so much a part of babies to us that bottles are seen as a necessity. Even breastfeeding mothers have dozens of bottles. Bottle motifs are everywhere. Can you imagine your shower gifts wrapped in paper decorated with breasts?

Nadine said even the nurse was half-hearted in her efforts to help Nadine get Chanel on her breast. "I just don't think she was that supportive of breastfeeding, and she got really tense with me—as if I should know how to do it." Nadine also noticed that Chanel was sluggish, most likely suffering from the effects of anesthesia. "She didn't seem interested, and I couldn't get her latched on. But she did seem hungry."

Nadine's husband, mother-in-law, and the nurse finally ganged up on her and actually took the baby away to give her a bottle. But Nadine didn't give up. It took two days—and several dozen tries at it—before Chanel got the hang of it. She eventually did, and all the relatives backed off. "They just weren't educated, and didn't understand how much better breastmilk is," Nadine said. Chanel is now six months old and had no other breastfeeding problems past the first week.

## Check-out Time Is 11 A.M.

The biggest problem with hospitals is you can't stay in them long enough. Thanks to dwindling medical resources and the cost of care, many insurance policies will push you out of bed less than twenty-four hours after you've given birth, if you've had a normal (not a cesarean) delivery. In some states, only legislation ensures a woman a forty-eight-hour hospital stay. You may just be beginning to learn how to breastfeed when a nurse is pointing at her watch and an attendant is standing around waiting to change the bed like a grumpy motel maid. In the good ol' days, which must have been from about A.D. 1410 to 1503, you were allowed to lie around for more than a week with constant attention. People would check up on you regularly and help you through any small problems that cropped up.

Most breastfeeding problems take a few days to develop. By the time you're having trouble, there's no one around to help. And sometimes, you may be having a problem that you aren't even seeing, one that a nurse might have picked up on during her rounds.

Some insurance policies will cover a follow-up visit from a lactation consultant or a nurse. Some will even pay for a home visit a few days after birth to see if your milk has come in and to make sure the baby is okay. See if this is the case for you. The two-week wait before your first visit to your pediatrician is way too long if your baby isn't getting enough milk. (Not all pediatricians routinely see newborns at three days.) So how do you know if you're doing it right in a world full of professionals who aren't around when you really need them? Read on.

# Chapter 5

# Directions: Inserting Breast A into Mouth B

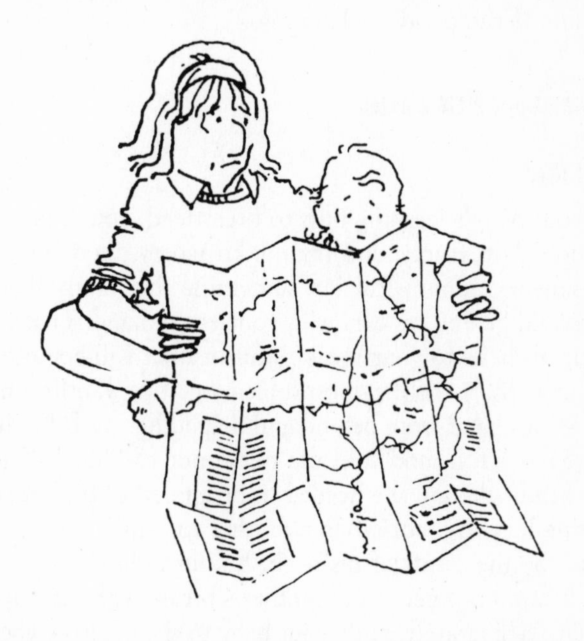

Did you know that your body will eventually make a quart of milk or more every day to feed your baby? Did you know that your baby is the most effective suction machine there is? Did you know that your sex life will change?

When you're learning to breastfeed, you've just been pregnant for nine months, been hospitalized, and had an object the size of a sack of potatoes wend its way through a tube formerly the diameter of your index finger. Or you've had a C-section, no picnic either. You have no idea which way the circus animals should face on the disposable diapers or how to keep poop from leaking out of the leg holes of the diaper wrap; how to get this delicate, slippery, thrashing set of arms and legs in and out of the kitchen sink for a bath and whether to alert 911 when that sweet-smelling, teeny-tiny bundle bellows louder than Roseanne.

But your most immediate problem is how to turn your breasts into drinking fountains. Getting this right will take some time, and you'll be under pressure because somebody might be screaming at the top of his lungs while you work on your technique. Deep breathing helps here. Try not to get frantic. "It was harder than I thought," says Julia. "When the nurse handed me my baby, it was like saying, 'Here's a needle. Now give yourself a shot.' I had no idea what to do."

## A Few Things about New Babies

### Hold on Tight

While your baby's learning how to breastfeed, you're going to have to help him, hold him firmly, and try not to worry about hurting him (or dropping him—a common fear but something that rarely happens). Hold his head low and behind his ears with your entire hand. That way you'll be able to guide his head to your breast. Your instinct will be not to force him to do anything. Mira was having problems getting Kaitlin on. When the nurse held Mira's hand from behind and helped her push Kaitlin's head on her breast, Mira let go and told the nurse not to "hurt" Kaitlin. Kaitlin needed her head held and she needed to be guided to the breast. The push wasn't hurting her, any more than a mother cat hurts her kitten when she picks him up by the scruff of his neck. Kaitlin didn't have control of her head yet and could not get to her mother's breast without help. You won't always need to deliberately guide your baby to the breast—when babies get control of their heads, they'll pop right on their mark. But in the first few weeks, you'll have to guide them.

### Rooting

Your baby's brain is wired to signal him to open his mouth in preparation for his mommy's breast if his lips are brushed, the sides of his cheeks are stroked, or his head is touched above his ears. You can get him to "root" or open his mouth by holding your breast and brushing your nipple against his lips. A healthy newborn will open his mouth if any part of his face is touched.

### "Why Do Babies Like to Suck?"

Like sleeping, sucking when you're young is a physical need, not a whim. So in addition to satisfying the feeding needs of your child, you need to also satisfy the comfort needs. If you can share your breasts with your baby, you will be able to share other important things like your time and attention. Having somebody who loves you and holds you and kisses your boo-boos is important for healthy psychological, emotional, and intellectual development. Skin-to-skin contact is particularly important for newborns and babies. They need to be close. They need to be held and stroked and talked to. You may have heard the famous story of the scientist who kept his newborn daughter in a box and fed her without ever exposing her to human touch. Gee, big surprise, she grew up disturbed.

### "Can I Spoil Him?"

Marian was worrying that holding her son all the time, getting up at night to feed him, and responding every time he cried was spoiling him. At least that's what her mother said. She was fretting over this when her husband said, "Marian, he's just a baby." Tell yourself that a few times. "He is just a baby. He is just a baby." Babies can't do calculus, and they really aren't capable of manipulating you until they're in their teens—you know, thir-teen months, four-teen months, and so on. You can't spoil him until much, much later. Right now, he's making noise because he needs something.

## A Few Things About You

### Your Breasts

Since we've all been in locker rooms, we know that all breasts do not look alike. There are millions of variations on breasts. Before your baby is born, you might want to take a closer look at your own. You may have inverted nipples, flat nipples, short nipples, or extra-large nipples. If you do, you're not deformed, and you probably have never noticed any of these characteristics. But you should be aware of how your nipples are shaped so that you understand how they could make breastfeeding harder for your baby.

### A Test for Inverted or Flat Nipples

A quick test to see if you have flat or inverted nipples is to cup your breast and press the tissue together. Position your fingers one and one-half inches behind your nipple. Your thumb should be at about 12:00 on your breast and the rest of your fingers at 6:00. Gently compress the tissue (this is what the baby will do, too). Watch what the nipple does. If it flattens against the breast tissue or inverts, you have inverted nipples. (Check Chapter 9 for information on breastfeeding with inverted nipples.)

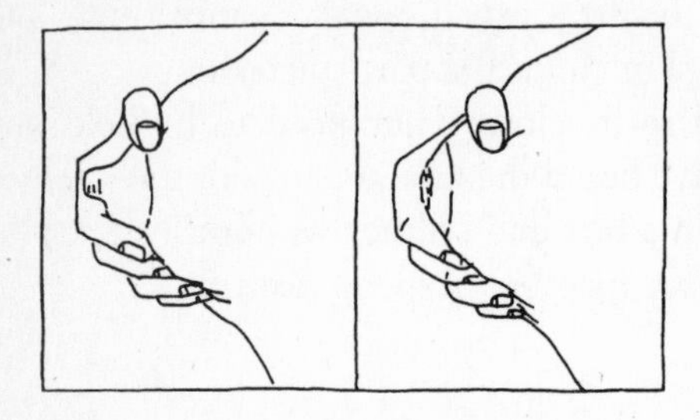

Test for inverted nipples: You won't be able to tell if your nipples are flat or inverted unless you try this test. Place your hand behind your areola, and pinch your breast as if your fingers were to meet through the skin (left). If your nipple stays even with the breast tissue, or pushes inward, you have flat or inverted nipples.

## A Test for Being Tongue-tied

One more thing to check. Stick out your tongue and have the baby's father do the same. If either one of you notices that the underside of your frenulum (the short tag of tissue under your tongue) is keeping your tongue from lifting or sticking out of your mouth, you have a short frenulum. Beware. Your baby may inherit the same tongue-tied condition, and he may need expert help in order to breastfeed. And even if you aren't tongue-tied, your baby could still be, so store that little piece of information in the back of your head. If you have sore nipples and there is no other cause, this could be it.

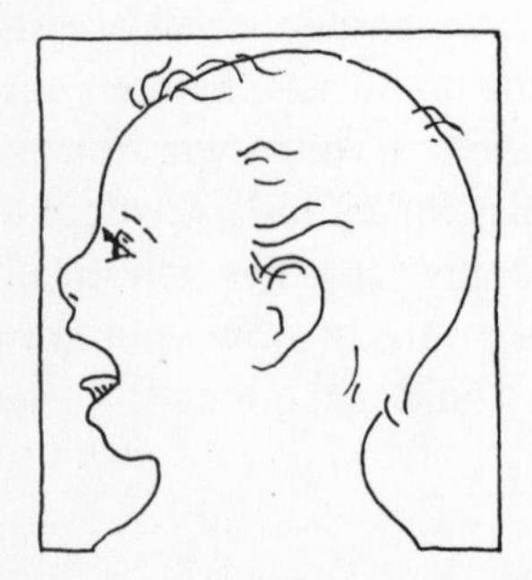

A bunched tongue (also called a "short frenulum"): See how the tongue is tacked down to the bottom of the mouth by a short piece of tissue? If your baby has problems sticking out his tongue, his suck will be off and you will have sore nipples.

### Ready for the Directions?

I hope you are reading this section before your water has broken. Otherwise, read fast, really fast. It might help if you have something to practice on—a doll or a teddy bear or even a paper bag filled with newspaper with a face drawn on it.

### Your Baby Does Not Get Milk by Sucking on Your Nipples

Are you surprised? "Ninety-five percent of the women in my breastfeeding class thought this," says Sasha, a first-time mom. Don't feel silly. Many women who've never seen a baby breastfeed think this is what he's supposed to do. I did.

### "Okay, So What's He Supposed to Suck on Then?"

Your baby gets milk by sucking on your areola tissue, the darkened area behind your nipple. My daughter was sucking on my nipples instead of the areola tissue for a few days. If your baby does this too, he'll get minimal food and you'll get sores in a spot for which Dr. Scholl's makes no remedy. Most of those stories you've heard about how painful breastfeeding is begin with this extremely common error. Mothers don't get their babies' mouths far enough onto their breast.

### First, Pretend Your Breast Is a Dartboard

Look at your breast in a mirror. You have breast tissue, then an areola, then a nipple: light tissue (BREAST), a circle of darker tissue (AREOLA), then the nipple (NIPP . . .) in the center. Most women have an areola that's about one to one and one-half inches in diameter. Some have bigger areolas.

If your entire breast is a dartboard, then the areola is a ring on the target and the nipple is the bullseye. There is a reason why most women's areola tissue is darker than their breast tissue. The areolar margin, or the line where your areola stops and your breast tissue begins, is the baby's mark. Since all breasts were not built alike, and areolas are different sizes, the Lactation Institute tells mothers, "your nipple plus an inch," so get out your measuring tools. That's what you're aiming to get his mouth around.

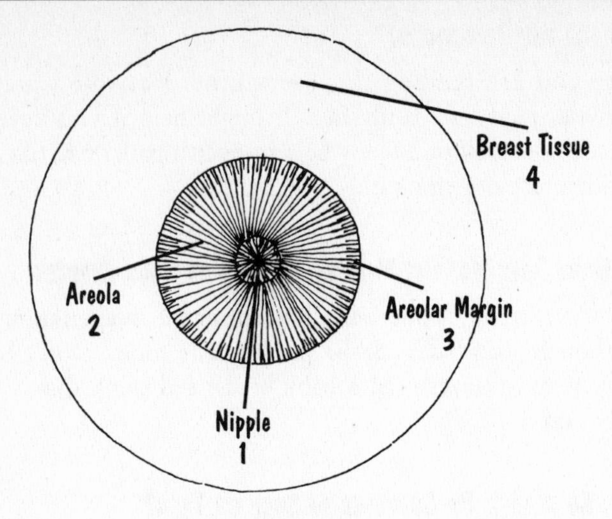


The breast "dartboard"

## Now, Pretend You're a House

Think of your breast as a house with a lot of internal plumbing. Let's say you want water. Some of the water is stored in the pipes, some of it comes from a larger water supply. You signal the pipes that you want water when you turn on the faucet. Water pressure will push the water through the pipes, and you'll keep getting water until you signal that you've got enough by turning off the faucet.

Scientists used to think women didn't store milk like cows, but that thinking is rapidly changing based on new research. Milk production goes on at all hours in your "house" by a cluster of milk-producing cells deep inside your breast called *alveoli*. Depending on how much storage capacity you have in your breasts (roughly determined by their size, but not always), you may be able to store a lot or a little.

That means if you have breasts that can store a lot of milk, your baby may take more milk at each feed and feed less frequently. Similarly, if you don't have a big refrigerator/freezer in your "house," your baby will probably feed more often to take in as much milk as his friend gets from his big-breasted mother. Don't worry about running out of food if you're breastfeeding your baby on demand. Scientists have found there's always more where that came from. Your breast is never truly "empty." The baby decides how hungry he is, but mother nature always leaves some extra in the breast.

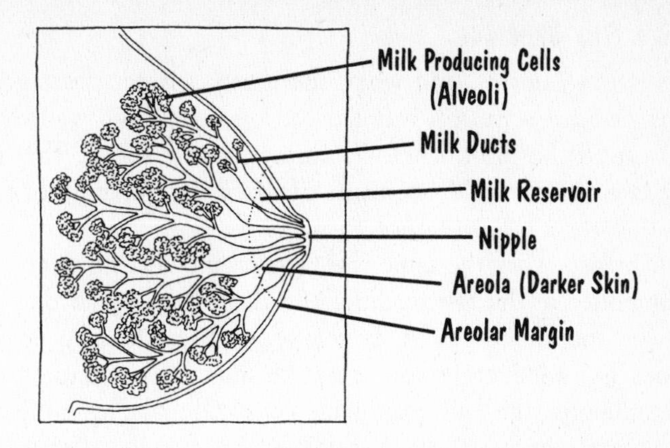


Internal plumbing: This is the production mechanism for breast milk.

## WHAT'S THE SIGNAL TO MAKE MILK?

Your baby is probably largely responsible for sending the cue to your body for how much milk he wants. His sucking and draining of the breast is the signal to your house that the faucet has been turned on and to keep it comin'. The water pressure is the air-tight seal he forms with his mouth around your areola. Once the faucet is on and the water pressure is correct, your body will release hormone number one, prolactin. This hormone sends a signal to the milk-producing cells that their break is over. It's time for them to punch the time clock and get to work making milk. Then a second hormone, oxytocin, is released. This hormone tells the milk-producing cells to send the milk stored through the milk ducts. As the baby sucks, the milk travels along the milk ducts to milk sinuses under the areola tissue. When the baby compresses your breast tissue and the sinuses that lie underneath, the milk is ejected into your baby's mouth through the openings in your nipple. Isn't that cool?

This is a harmonious process when the baby is doing his job correctly. But if, say, your baby isn't latched on well and isn't compressing the milk sinuses properly, the milk-producing cells will get backed up and, just as though you'd turned off the faucet, the whole system shuts down. The milk-producing cells will think their job is done because the "faucet" is off—and they'll punch off the clock. The alveoli also learn from each feeding. If they're left with a lot of extra milk, they will not donate it to charity. They will think, "Oh dear. We made too much. Better not do that again."

## Avoiding a Milk Shortage

We live in Los Angeles, and when there was a water shortage, the water company decided to ration water based on how much water each household had used the month before. Unfortunately for us, the month they chose was a month we'd been out of town, so our monthly ration was enough to bathe a mouse—once.

Your breasts work the same way. They remember how much milk your baby demanded at the last feeding, and that's how much they're thinking you'll need this time around. If you aren't breastfeeding enough or the baby does not adequately compress the milk sinuses and stimulate hormone production, the milk-producing cells will make less milk. If this happens frequently enough, those lazy milk-producing cells will just spend their days reading the paper, and you may find yourself without milk. This is the reason why it is not a good idea to supplement with artificial baby milk. Your body won't get the signal to make milk if formula is taking its place. What usually happens is you make less and less milk while supplementing more and more until you've unintentionally weaned your baby. You'll hear friends say, "I wasn't making enough milk, so I had to switch to formula" or "My milk just suddenly dried up." Now you know why.

One more thing that can happen. The hormones oxytocin and prolactin are produced in your pituitary gland. This gland doesn't do its job well if you are releasing adrenaline because of fear, tension, fatigue, or pain. That's why you need to relax when you're trying to breastfeed or pump.

## Increasing Your Milk Supply

If something happens and you aren't breastfeeding enough, you can easily increase your supply over the course of a few days by turning on the faucet (letting your baby breastfeed) more often. Have confidence in your body's amazing ability to balance your milk supply with your baby's demand for milk. Check in Chapter 9 for other ways of increasing milk supply if your milk is low for more complicated reasons.

## One of the Two Biggest Mistakes: Positioning

The first mistake you can make is positioning yourself and your baby incorrectly. Your second biggest mistake can be if your baby "latches" his mouth onto your breast incorrectly. We'll get to that in a minute. But if you don't hold the baby properly and get yourself situated, then you have no hope of getting the opening in mouth "A" to line up with the tabs on breast "B."

## Pillows

Remember all of those pillows you were planning to take with you to the hospital? Here's when they come in handy. First thing to do is position your body before somebody hands you the baby (or if you're practicing, the doll). If you are able to sit up after you've delivered, you should have someone help you arrange your pillows. Put a pillow behind your lower back and one behind your head, one under each of your forearms, and one across your lap. If you use pillows to prop your arms and your arms to prop the baby, nobody should be uncomfortable. And all this preparation will likely save you from back pain and sore nipples.

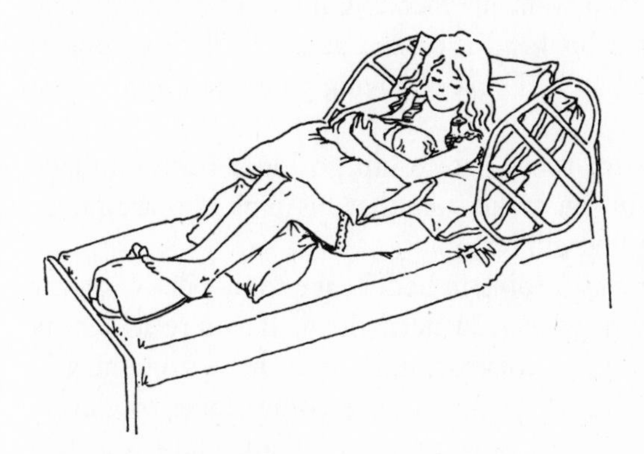

Pillows are your training wheels. Check out where to place all five of them: behind your head, under each arm, on your lap, and under your knees (this reclining position with all of the pillows is great after a C-section).

## Get Comfortable

Make sure, first and foremost, that you are in a position you care to hold for anywhere from fifteen minutes to an hour or more. Remember your junior high gym teacher? "Ladies, back straight, shoulders down, stomachs in." You don't want to feed your baby with your back slumped over, your butt in a weird position, or your neck crunched. Once you've settled yourself into position, you're ready for the baby. The idea is for you to move him onto your breast, not for you to lean your breast into him.

## Nothing Is Fun the First Time

The problem is, the first few times you try to get your baby attached, you'll be awkward. Your baby will probably be squirming and hungry. And oh, god, he will cry! That sound! Anything to stop that sound! You'll be fumbling and upset, unless you're an incredibly calm person. Try not to panic if your baby cries. The crying will stop soon, very soon. But if you don't get him on right and he ends up sucking on any part of your nipple, the next person crying will be you. According to experts, 95 percent of breastfeeding problems are the result of incorrect positioning and latch-on.

### Simple Positioning Rules

Experts offer a few simple rules. You and your baby need to face each other. And no matter what position you choose, his head and mouth need to be even with your nipple so he's not pulling on your breast tissue. Since his mouth is open WIDE, his chin should be right up against your breast. If he is facing you so that your chests are facing each other or touching, he'll be in a better position to get a good grip on your breast. You don't want his face looking up at you. You want his face FACING your breast. He'll still be able to see you. But if his head is turned at all, he'll be pulling at your breast instead of pressed on it. Think of having your chest to his chest and his chin to your breast.

Another thing to check for is the baby's hip position. Babies initially move as one big piece. So if you make sure that his hips also are facing you, then you know that his lips will be too.

You will not always be breastfeeding in bed. Leave some pillows on the rocking chair, so they're there when you need them. If you're under six feet, you may want to invest in a footstool, unless you have something in your house that'll pass for one. It is much more comfortable to elevate your feet while you breastfeed. It gives you more of a lap, keeps your legs from getting sore, keeps you from crossing your legs and cutting off circulation, and helps keep your baby from hanging off of you.

## Avoiding the Second Biggest Mistake: Latching-on

Once you're in the right position and your baby's in the right position, it's time to try to get him latched-on. The most important thing you can do is MAKE SURE YOUR BABY LATCHES ON correctly. That's in BIG letters for a REASON. This is the key thing in breastfeeding to make sure your baby always gets milk and you don't get sore. I put my daughter Olivia to my breast about ten minutes after she was born. And she started sucking. I thought that was it. I remember thinking, "My God, it works!" (No, that's a lie. First, I thought, "Isn't she smart?" Yeah, I know sucking is a reflex, but she was very, well, reflexive.) But once she'd found my nipple, she wasn't about to let it go, and that was the problem. I let her get on any way she wanted to, and that meant she tried to suck on my nipples. The first few times you put your baby on your breast remember that just because your baby's mouth is *on* your breast does not mean he's breastfeeding. He may not be latched-on.

Shelly complained to her nurse that breastfeeding "didn't work" because Kayla screamed each time she was put to Shelly's breast, and the pediatrician was concerned because Kayla was losing way too much weight. Kayla was in contact with Shelly's breast, but she was not latched-on correctly. Kayla had only Shelly's nipple in her mouth. Remember all of that internal plumbing and the hormones that need to be flowing in order to make milk? If the baby doesn't latch on properly, then the whole thing won't work.

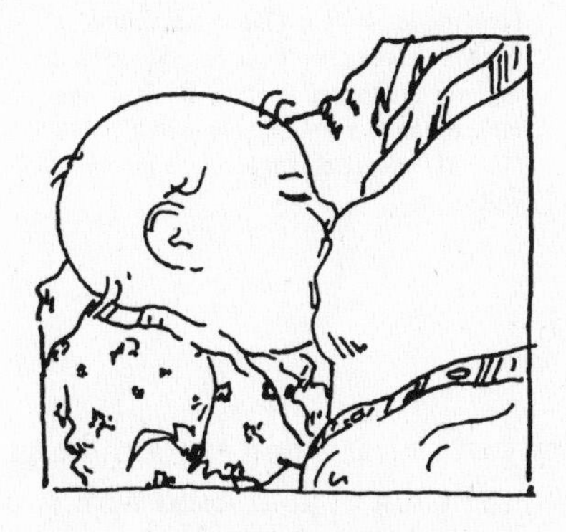

A good latch-on: Look carefully at the baby's mouth. See how his lips peel back ("flange"), and how wide open his mouth is? Also notice how much breast tissue he's taken in: the entire areola is in the baby's mouth.

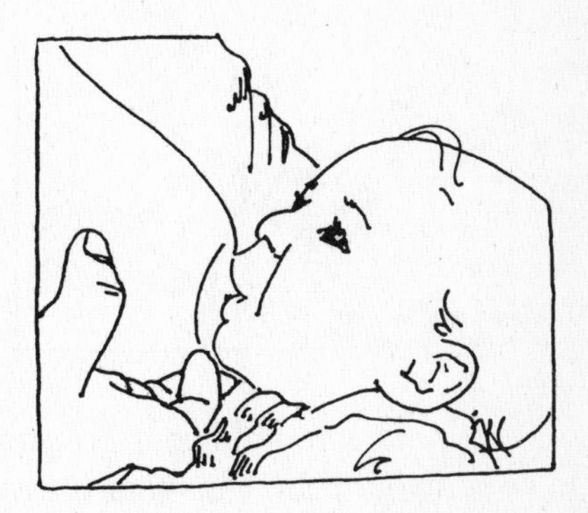

A bad latch-on: The baby is pursing his lips and taking in only the nipple. If your baby looks like he's whistling, forming an "O" with his lips, or making any kind of clicking noises, take him off and try again, or be prepared for sore nipples.

## Getting Him on Your Breast

To avoid pain and make milk, remember your baby needs to take your nipple plus one inch of areola tissue into his mouth. That means he may put your nipple and your areola in all the way up to the line of the regular skin. (If you have huge areolas this may not apply to you. The baby only needs to take one to one and one-half inches of tissue into his mouth.) Getting his mouth around all of this is latching-on.

## How to Hold Your Breast

If you do what I did and hold your breast with your hand by gripping it anywhere near the areola tissue, you'll end up with "chewed-up nipples," according to Chele Marmet, director of the Lactation Institute. Instead, hold your breast well behind the areola tissue so that you're offering more than just a pinched nipple to your baby. You're only holding your breast to support it and to guide it into your baby's mouth. Depending on the size of your breasts, you may be holding your breast halfway from your nipple to your chest wall if your breasts are large, or all the way against your chest if your breasts are small.

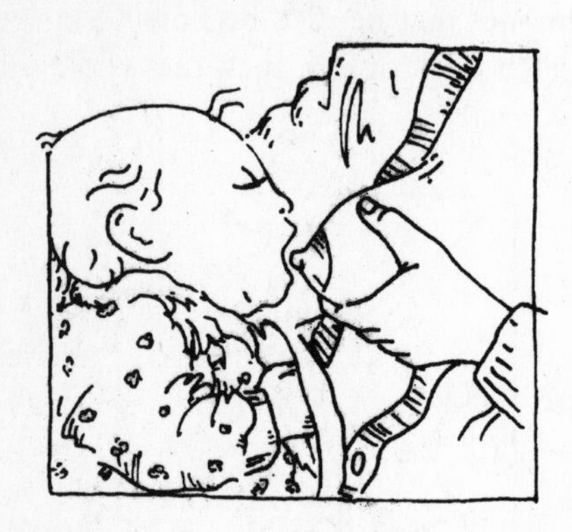

Holding the breast: Place your thumb at twelve o'clock, and your fingers cupped under your breast at six o'clock. Using either hand, your fingers will form a "C." Make sure that the baby's mouth is wide open.

Practice how to hold your breast and put it near a doll's mouth before you've had your baby. Cup your breast in the palm of your hand with your thumb on top at twelve o'clock and the rest of your fingers helping support your breast at six o'clock. But don't cup your breast with your palm. Instead, use your fingers to control your breast. Avoid holding your breast like a cigarette, using only your forefinger and middle finger. That's a good way to get sore nipples, too, because your baby won't get far enough onto your breast.

### How to Hold His Head

When you're new at breastfeeding, it's best to hold your baby's head with one hand and your breast with the other. But where you put your hand is important. Hold your newborn's head directly behind his ears when you're getting him latched on. If you move your hand up and touch your baby above his ears, you'll drive him crazy because you'll be messing with his rooting reflex.

### Open Wide

Once he's facing your breast, you need to understand just how wide your baby needs to open his mouth in order to latch on to your breast correctly. Look at yourself in a mirror and open your mouth all the way, as wide as you can to see your molars in the back. That's how wide you want your baby's mouth to be when you put him on your breast. I know you won't believe this, but babies CAN open their mouths that wide. Your baby may not open his mouth that wide the first time he gets a chance at your breast. But you need to be patient and reinforce the idea that he won't go on your breast until his mouth is wide open. He will learn. He wants your breast and will play by your rules. Nature has intended for the baby to do this, so even if it takes you a few tries, do not let your baby latch on with a "little" mouth. This process could take you a few tries, maybe even a few days, before you both get the hang of it.

Since your nipple is simply the centerpiece, the baby should not be placing any direct pressure on it. Once your areola and nipple are in your baby's mouth, your nipple will be pulled out about three times its normal resting length. Don't worry. It was made to stretch. That's because the baby needs to form the areola tissue into a teat. If he's taking in enough breast tissue, your nipple will be back in his throat in what lactation experts call the S spot, or sucking spot, where his hard palate meets his soft palate. Unlike that famous "G" spot, the S spot is not hard to find—and you'll feel much better in the long run if he gets it right.

Don't worry about the baby biting your nipples. Your baby's tongue will always be covering his gums and later his teeth when he breastfeeds so that those glistening, sharp little things cannot come into contact with your breast tissue. He can't breastfeed and bite at the same time. Whew, eh?

### Open Mouth Game

If your baby is like my second baby Julia, opening her mouth *wide* wasn't something she always felt like doing. The Lactation Institute tells mothers to play the "open mouth" game. When your baby is alert and not hungry, hold him so he faces you. Then say "open" and open your own mouth wide. You'll look silly, so do this without an audience. Keep doing it. Eventually, even a newborn will start to mimic what you're doing, (and both of you will get the chance to play fish in the school play). Getting them to *open wide* should eventually be easy with just the verbal cue, "open."

### The Process

It helps if you can understand what's going on inside your baby's mouth, since you obviously can't see what's happening. Though breastfeeding babies are described as "sucking" when they're at the breast, that's not really what they're doing. They're not sucking the way you would through a straw. Inside of his mouth, your baby is keeping your areolar tissue between his tongue and the roof of his mouth. To get milk, he'll press his tongue from front to back against your breast, compressing the milk sinuses with his tongue and pressure from his jaw. His mouth, which is tightly sealed around your breast, provides the suction so that the milk is ejected.

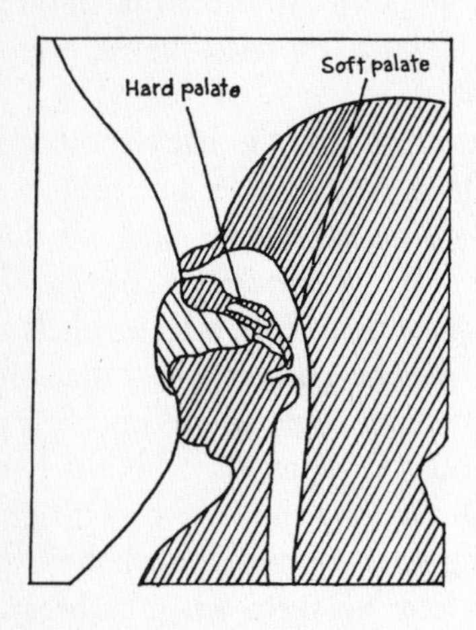


What's going on inside: The entire areola and nipple form a "teat" inside the baby's mouth, reaching all the way back toward his throat.

## Time for Lab Work

Try this experiment. Get a glass of liquid. (Or if you're too tired, yell for your husband to get it.) Now, drink some of it and pay attention to what your tongue is doing while you're swallowing. Feel how your tongue presses against the roof of your mouth in a wavelike motion? That's what the baby's tongue should be doing in his mouth. What he does when he's drawing out milk and swallowing is really not much different from what you do when you swallow. But he may have to work a little harder since he's just learning these skills.

## Prying Your Baby Off Your Breast

If he doesn't open his mouth wide enough, you'll need to start again. But first you'll have to extricate your breast from the jaws of life.

To break the baby's suction on your breast, stick your clean little finger into the side of your baby's mouth, sliding your finger until you can feel the suction is broken. Then gently pull his mouth off your breast. Detaching cleanly is tricky at first, and I don't advise pulling even a preemie off without first breaking the suction. Your nipple won't come off in his mouth (I promise), but it'll feel like it did.

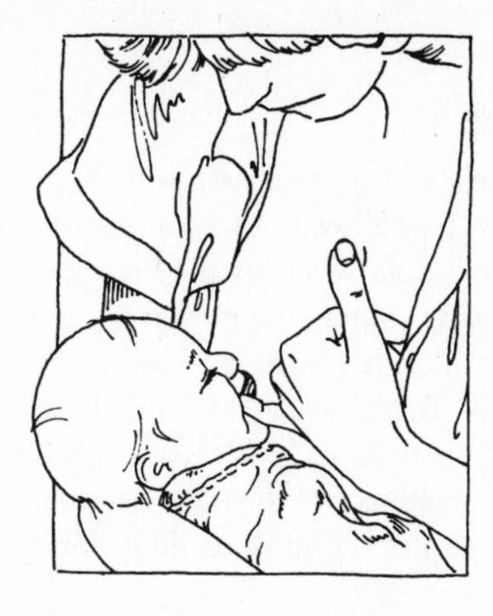

Breaking the seal: To remove your baby from your breast, slide your clean little finger into his mouth and onto his gums until the suction breaks. Keep your finger in his mouth until he's completely off your nipple.

## Milk Ejection

### It's Ejected, Not Let-down

Although the actual process of milk being expelled is frequently called a *let-down*, its clinical name is *milk-ejection reflex*. Milk is ejected into the baby's mouth—or squirted, if you will. It doesn't dribble out the way it would from a bottle. Think of a cow's udder. You massage, squeeze, and press and milk comes out. Pause, repeat.

## "What Does Milk Ejection Feel Like?"

The sensation of your milk ejecting (or letting down) feels almost like the mild tingling of a limb that has just begun to go to sleep. (Not everybody has this sensation.) It can tingle or stinge so intensely that it's nearly painful. This feeling goes away after a few weeks, but it's still a very definite sensation. You will also actually see your breasts shrink from Anna Nicole Smith size down to your normal size. Somewhere between week six and week twelve or so, your body will have figured everything out, and the size of your breasts will be much more normal. You also won't be able to feel the milk in your breasts. This does not mean you're not making enough milk. It means your body has now graduated to the next level. This is important to remember. Some women think the lack of sensation means they aren't making milk. What you were feeling in your early breastfeeding days was fluid, blood, and swelling, oh yes, and milk. When all of that calms down, you really won't be able to "feel" your breasts making milk, unless you miss a feeding.

## What Your Baby Sounds and Looks Like

The sound your baby will make if he's getting milk is a soft, "Ugh, ugh, ugh," like the sound you make when you swallow with a sore throat. You'll see a slight movement where his jaw is following his tongue movement, and then you may hear a faint swallowing sound. You may also see his ears move. Don't be concerned if it looks like he's working hard to get your milk. That's how it's supposed to look. Babies suck in what experts call a burst-pause pattern. That means they'll suck, suck, suck, swallow, pause, then suck, suck, suck again. Until you begin to feel the milk-ejection reflex, your baby will be working diligently to get the milk to flow. Sometimes, this can take a few minutes.

If your baby's lips are pursed tightly together, or if he looks like he's whistling and you can only see his mouth moving, he's not sucking correctly. If you hear little clicking or smacking sounds, he hasn't got it right, either. He'll look kind of like he has fish lips, what experts call *flanged.* "I never had sore nipples because I wouldn't put my breast into Francesca's mouth until her mouth was open wide. Sometimes, she was wailing when this happened," remembers Suzan. Take advantage of a wide-open mouth, whatever the reason. If you don't get the baby on right, you'll need to take him off and start again.

## Madam, Your Choice of Positions

Now that you've mastered the basics of positioning and latching-on, here are some of the various ways you can hold your baby for breastfeeding. When you're in the hospital, you'll likely be propped into a sitting position to breastfeed. If you've had a C-section, you'll need some assistance getting into a position that causes you the least pain possible. (Positions that are comfortable for those of you who've had C-sections will be noted. *Comfortable* is a relative term here.)

## Cradle Position

The most popular position is called the cradle. This is probably the position you'll graduate to. Get in a sitting position, supported by pillows. Put one pillow behind your head, one on your lap, and one under each of your forearms. To feed your baby from your left breast, you will cradle him in your left arm, putting his head in the crook of that same arm. He'll be lying on his right side, and his chest will be facing your chest. Your other hand will be free to guide your breast. Remember to keep your hand way back on your breast so that you are offering nipple, areola, and tissue. Look down at your nipple, and aim it straight for your baby's mouth instead of up to the ceiling or down to the floor. Try to maintain control of your baby's head by keeping your elbow flexed.

If your baby's mouth isn't open, brush any part of his face, particularly his lips, with your breast so he'll open his mouth. Once your baby's mouth is open WIDE, use RAM (rapid arm motion) to quickly pull him on to your breast. Because those incredibly powerful little jaws will clench tightly closed, you'll want to be fast enough to get the entire breast right up to the areolar margin into his mouth.

Even though you want to be decisive and firm in your efforts to get him on, you also want to be gentle or you'll scare him. One nurse told me that she had watched a lactation consultant force a baby's head onto his mother's breast in an abrupt, almost brutal way. The baby was so startled at being treated roughly that when the mother tried to get him on for his next feed, he arched his back and cried. Gentle but firm is the ticket.

Also, as with all positions, make sure the baby's arm is along his side and not pinned in an uncomfortable position. This will also keep him from pushing his arm against your body, something that can cause sore nipples.

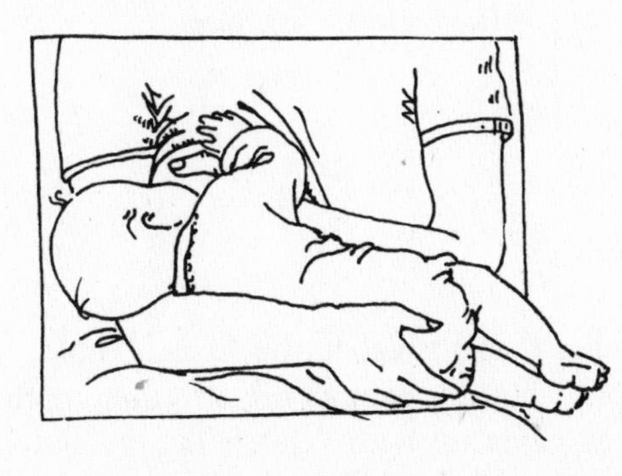

The cradle position: One hand holds your opposite breast, while your other elbow and forearm support the baby's head (usually used when baby is older, and you're both pros).

Don't skimp on pillows. Even if he feels very light when you first get him on your breast, your arms will begin to ache soon if you don't have pillows to support them. Also, as you start to get tired, your arms will loosen their hold on the baby, and he could slip from his hold on the areola tissue down to the nipple. Even a fraction of an inch can make a difference when you're trying to avoid sore nipples.

Nurses know the cradle, and that's what they'll probably try to show you, but it's not the easiest hold when you're inexperienced. You won't have good control over your newborn's head using your elbow as a support. As he gets more control on his own, it will become easier for you.

## Transition Position

When you're breastfeeding a newborn, this position (or the "clutch" position) is probably your best choice. The same hand holds the same breast, so if your baby is feeding from the left breast, your left hand holds your breast. Your baby's feet are down by your right elbow, his chest is against your chest and your right arm supports his back. Your right hand is free to hold the back part of his head, low and behind his ears.

The down side to this position is it's darned uncomfortable to hold onto your breast for half an hour, and you will not have any hands free to do anything else, like scratch an itch.

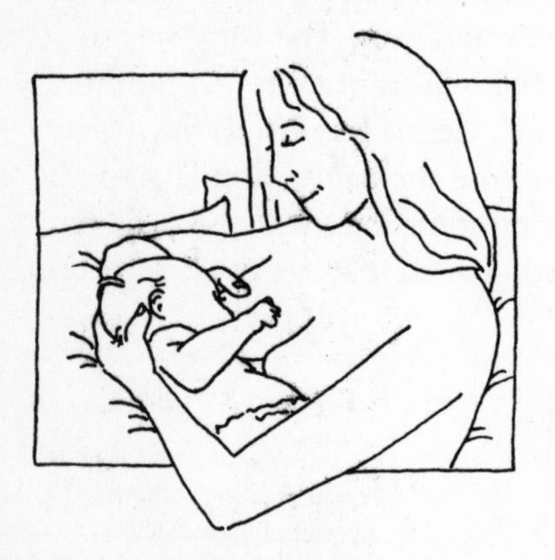

The transition position: The hand on the same side holds your breast. The opposite arm supports the baby's body, and the hand holds and controls the baby's head (an especially good position for when baby is very young).

## Clutch or Football Position

Next position (this feels like a ballet class!) is called the "clutch" hold. It used to be called the "football hold," but not enough breastfeeding mothers had played that game, so they came up with "clutch" as in "clutch purse." And like a clutch purse, your baby will be lying on his back clutched between your side and your flexed arm. For feeding on your left side, use your left arm to support the baby's body, and your left hand to support his head. Your opposite hand will hold and guide your breast. Your baby will be flexed at the hips and his bottom will be against whatever you're leaning against. Even though he looks like a contortionist, remember that new babies still like being in the fetal position. It'll be years before he'll need to stretch out his legs—and hog the entire couch. But as he gets bigger, make sure his feet are up in the air or near his body so he can't push against you with his feet. (Otherwise, your nipples are in for big trouble if he gets a good hold and does a blast-off with his legs.)

Lactation consultants teach this hold to mothers who've had C-sections. It's also a good hold if you're having latch-on problems or your baby is having sucking problems.

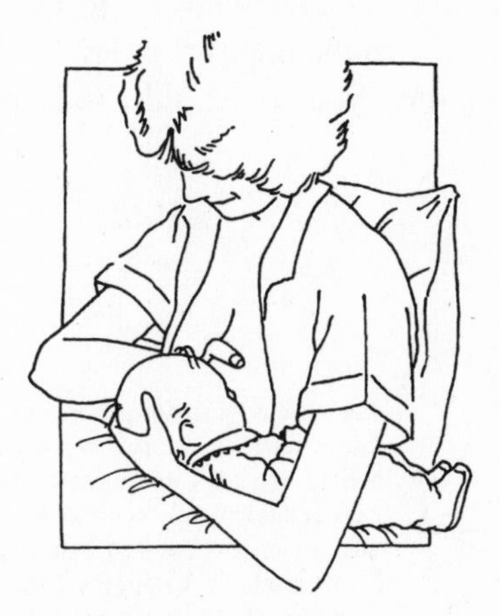

The clutch (or "football") position: The baby's head is supported by your hand, but instead of lying along your chest, his body rests between your side and your arm, clutched like a purse or football. His feet protrude from under your arm, while the opposite hand holds your breast (great position for beginners and for C-Sections).

### Cradle Lying-Down Position

This was my favorite position because I was usually sleeping while doing it. If you can manage this one in the hospital, it's a great way to get some rest. Once again, left side directions go like this: you'll be lying on your side with a pillow between your legs. (See? We're getting trickier and trickier. Soon you'll be feeding him standing on your head.) Put one or two pillows behind your head, a pillow between your legs to prevent backache, and, especially important for your back, a pillow behind it for support. (If it's bedtime for your mate, he can be the pillow substitute.) Put your baby on the pillow that's under your forearm. If you're on your left side, your left arm will cradle the baby, who will be on his side, facing you. His head needs to be elevated by your arm to avoid having milk flow into his Eustachian tubes, a recipe for an ear infection. If your baby is very young, put a rolled-up receiving blanket behind his back so that he stays propped on his side. You want to make sure that if he gags on any milk or spits up, it spills out of his mouth (another good reason to have a towel under him).

Don't put your arm over your head. That's a good way to get a painful shoulder (or even bursitis in the future). You might have to move your arm around to figure out what's comfortable for you, but resist that urge to put your arm over your head. Since you are lying down, even if it's the middle of the day, you'll probably fall asleep. Leaving your arm above your head is like falling asleep in the sun slathered in baby oil for a few hours beginning at high noon. You'll be in pain when you wake up.

As you get good at this position, you will eventually get to the point where you will be able to switch your baby to the opposite breast by bringing him across your chest and flipping onto your other side, still holding the pillow between your legs.

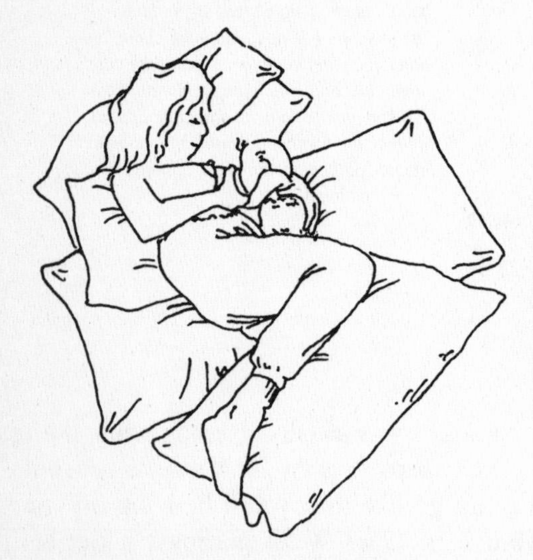

The cradle lying-down position: Your knees squeeze one pillow, another is behind you for back support, and you have additional pillows under your head and under the baby to bring him to breast level. Your opposite hand holds your breast, and your same arm and hand support the baby (a great position for fatigued beginners and for C-sections).

## Alternate Lying-Down Position

I had my right shoulder reconstructed. I know, fascinating, eh? There's a reason why I'm telling you this, though. Because it's painful to lie on my right side, I often fed my daughters from both breasts while lying on my left side only. This position is very similar to the cradle lying-down hold. The difference is that once you've fed your baby from the lower breast, you might want to feed him from the top breast without turning onto your opposite side.

If you do what I did and simply lean forward, you will not only increase the odds of getting sore nipples, you will also increase your odds of needing a visit to the chiropractor.

Instead, turn your chest so that it's at a 45-degree angle to the bed. All you need to do is lean forward, take the pillow out from between your legs, and support the weight of your body by flexing your top leg and crossing it over the lower leg. Your bent knee will be almost at hip level, resting on the mattress.

Once you've gotten your body into a comfortable position, you should be within centimeters of your baby's open mouth. You'll have the baby cradled on the pillow. You may need to take the arm you're lying on and move it around until you're comfortable again.

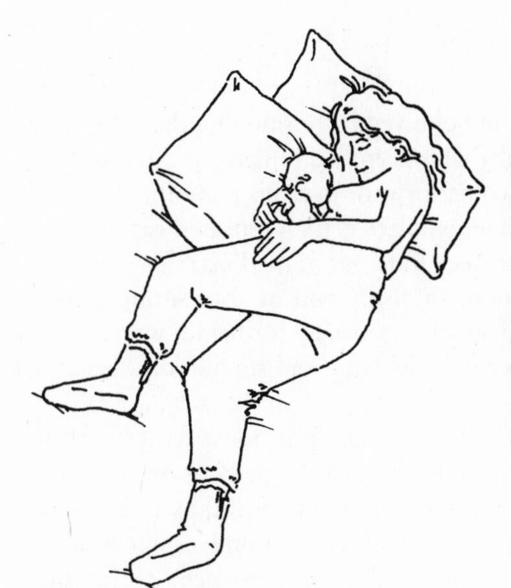

The alternate lying-down position: Use this one if you want to feed your baby on both breasts without rolling over and changing sides. After feeding the baby from the breast closest to the bed in the cradle lying-down position, brace your top leg on bed to support your back, and shift baby to the top breast (a great position if you can't lie comfortably on both sides, and at night if you breastfeed while sleeping).

### Cross-Cradle Position

If you have twins, it's possible to modify both the cradle and the clutch hold so that you can feed both babies at once. You can feed each baby individually, but it's faster and quieter to feed both together (since one twin won't be howling while he waits his turn, though most mothers will offer a soothing finger to suck on for the odd man out). In the cross-cradle hold, each baby is held in the cradle hold in separate arms of the mother. The twins' bodies "cross" each other at the waist, with one twin on the outside and one on the inside. You can also do a double-clutch hold with each twin in the clutch hold or mix and match the cradle and the clutch, depending on the babies' and your preference.

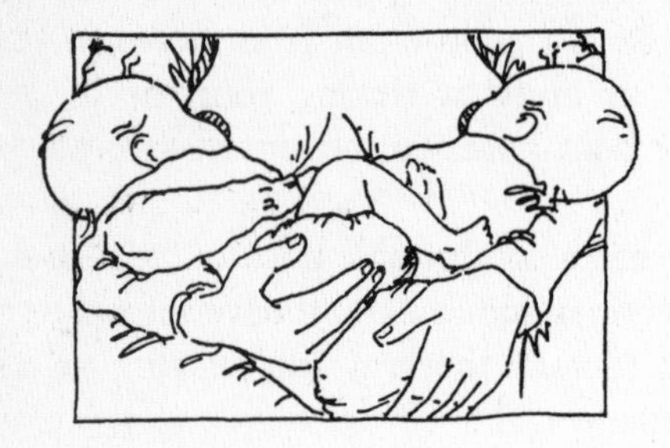

The cross-cradle position: Both babies are held in cradle holds on separate breasts (used for twins or multiples, so you can feed two at a time).

## Special Positions

Many breastfeeding problems can be solved by positioning the baby differently. Small problems, like a baby who keeps his tongue on the roof of his mouth or curls it so it doesn't come forward over his gum line, can easily be helped with gravity. Also, babies who are getting repeated ear infections can be fed in a sitting position to keep milk out of the Eustachian tubes.

In "side straddle sit" position, the baby will be in a sitting position straddling one of the mother's legs (this is usually for babies who are over ten pounds). One of your arms holds the baby and supports his head and the other holds your breast.

There are other positions called "prone" positions: either with the baby sitting, kneeling, or lying in a "lateral prone" position on your chest. (The lateral prone is one of the most comfortable positions to breastfeed in.) For all prone positions, you have pillow support under your head and knees and are lying on your back. Your baby is either placed on his knees (if he's a newborn, it looks like he's curled face down in a fetal position on your chest) or sitting if he's a little bigger. These are good positions for babies with receding chins.

## Other Concerns: Large Breasts

"They look like the breasts that ate Toledo," moans Wanda. I've seen them. She's not exaggerating by much. "When Taylor breastfeeds, it looks like she's blowing up a big balloon. They're about three times the size of her head." If you have very big breasts, you'll probably want to support them if you breastfeed while lying down. Take a rolled-up towel and put it under your breast for support to keep it from listing into the space between your body and the bed.

## "Can He Breathe?"

Don't worry about smothering your baby when he's breastfeeding (if you hear him rasping for breath, then, yes, do worry about smothering him). Babies have those cute little button noses with wide round nostrils for a reason: so they can get air while they're sucking. You can always use your free hand to create a little airhole if your breast is blocking his breathing passage. But babies won't choose food over air. If they aren't getting enough air, they'll come off the breast and scream at you. That's your clue. Also, be sure not to put too much space between your breast and his mouth to create an airway, because your baby will either come off your breast or end up sucking just your nipples.

## Remain Calm (*!#$#!@#$#!!!)

Your baby may get frustrated, but you can help him by calmly talking him through it. I've seen babies scream in frustration as their mothers get more and more upset. Those same babies will painstakingly try again and again when their mothers are calm. It's the difference between somebody yelling, "Faster, you idiot!" and a soft, "You can do it! That's it. Wonderful!" If you find yourself coming apart, have somebody else hold the baby and comfort him by giving him a finger to suck on. Walk around for a minute or two until you're ready to try again. If you're upset *and* trying to teach your baby a new skill, he will react to your stress level.

Women who pretend to be calm and try not to lose it when the baby cries eventually get their babies on their breasts. This is why some doctors will tell you that if you get agitated and stressed out, your baby is better off if you don't breastfeed. But remember that nature has thought of this and figured out a way around it by providing hormones that help nursing mothers relax. If you can get breastfeeding going, you will eventually feel *less* stressed out. When your hormones are working, breastfeeding is a very calming experience.

# Chapter 6

# The First Few Days: Tackling Common Obstacles

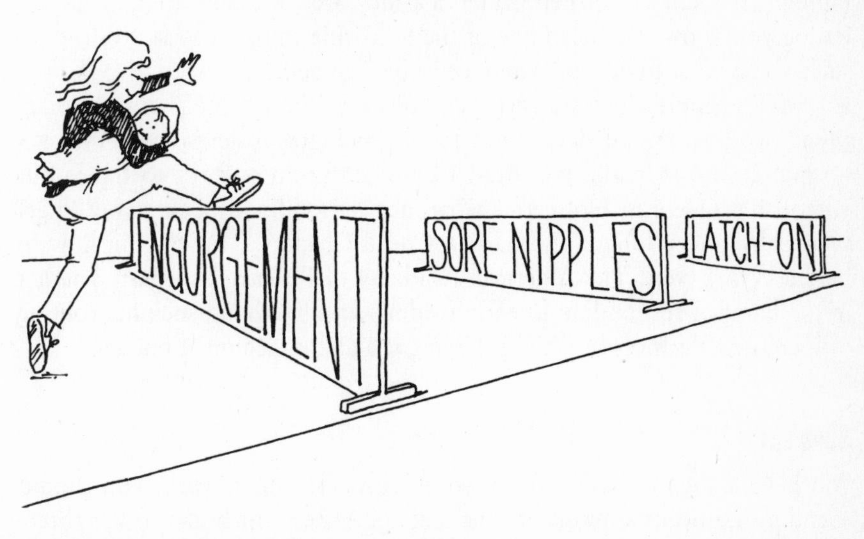


Hooray! You're home from the hospital! "I couldn't wait to leave," Geraldine says of her hospital stay. "I think the only one who got any sleep was my husband. My daughter and I were too busy looking at each other".

## "Who Put Me in Charge?"

You're normal if you're worried. It's a shock to find out that you're the person in charge of your baby. "Everybody kept asking me what to do," Miriam says. "I kept thinking, 'How the heck should I know? I never did this before.'" Contrary to popular belief, aliens do not swoop down the night you give birth and implant the mom chip in your brain. You will not automatically know what to do. Getting to know your baby and figuring out how to help him is a learning process. Try not to forget that. You are not a bad mommy if you're feeling depressed, overwhelmed, or even unhappy. Motherhood is a big adjustment.

## Crying: "Who Turned the Switch On?"

If your baby slept peacefully through his first few days, you are in for a big surprise. Babies cry. Nice babies, difficult babies, active babies, passive babies. Oh, you knew that? An average baby cries about ninety minutes a day. That may seem like a lot, but add up the amount of time you talk during the day. String all of your talking together and it'd be at least ninety minutes, wouldn't it? When babies cry, they are communicating. They are letting you know they need one of the following things: to eat, to sleep, to suck, to be held, to be stimulated, or to be changed.

Many people chalk up crying to colic (an often dubious and misdiagnosed syndrome) and decide not to respond. Regardless of whether it's normal crying or colic, you need to pay attention and try to figure out what the problem is. No matter what, not responding is a sure way to get your baby to cry longer and harder. Check Chapter 7 for tips on how to help a crying baby. The American Academy of Pediatrics suggests you get in the habit of responding to early feeding cues like hand-sucking, rooting or increased alertness or activity. Crying is a *late* indicator of hunger.

## Survival

You have a lot to recover from, so go slow. The first week, you should spend a significant amount of time resting. Anne went home to her three-year-old twins, who were so happy Mommy was home, they put her to work making them sandwiches and reading stories. When they noticed their new sister was hanging around a lot on Mom's breast, the twins started to sulk. "How come she has to come along?" they wanted to know. "Can't you just make her a sandwich and leave it for her in her crib?"

If you have other children, you're probably laughing at the idea of putting your feet up for a week. If you don't have other children, take advantage of your "lack of responsibilities," and lie around as much as your baby will let you. Try to take a nap when he takes a nap, even if you're someone who doesn't sleep during the day. Your body will recover quicker, and you'll be better able to withstand nighttime waking to feed your newborn.

### "Help!"

Even if you're someone who is so self-sufficient you stitched up your own episiotomy, now is the time to take any help that's offered from friends, relatives, and your partner. Your postdelivery objective should be giving yourself a minimum of two weeks during which your only job is caring for your baby. That's it. That's your only responsibility. Forget the thank-you notes, dishes, laundry, phone calls. If the cousins want to visit and you want the company, fine. Let them bring dinner.

### I Hope You Made Extra Casseroles

These first few weeks are the reason why everyone tells you to make double meals for three weeks before you deliver and to put the second dinner in the freezer. (I have never been that organized. The only thing in our freezer was melting ice cream and some chicken with freezer burn.)

### Set Up a Breastfeeding Station

It helps to set up a breastfeeding station. Some women like to feed their baby in the same place every time, such as on the couch, on the bed, or in the baby's room. I liked all three of these places and, depending on my mood, I'd move from place to place. If I wanted to watch television, it was the couch. If I wanted to sleep or read, it was my bed. If I wanted to just hold my daughter and stroke her hair and watch her eat, it was the gliding chair in her room. Consequently, I was forever trying to locate all of the things I needed for each feeding, which quickly got out of hand. (When number two came along, she was lucky to be fed with Mommy in a sitting position. Most of the time, she got fed while I made a peanut butter and jelly sandwich for her sister with my free hand.)

Having one breastfeeding station, perhaps initially in your bedroom, works best. Get a table that you can put right next to where you're sitting so that everything is within arm's reach. Here's what you'll need: the phone (unless you've unplugged it, turned on your answering machine, or can stand to listen to it ring); reading material (if you have a hearty baby who can nurse for as long as your breasts hold out); and the remote control. Babies like to suck for long periods of time, particularly in the early weeks, and you probably will enjoy a certain amount of cooing, holding, and caressing your baby. But a lot of babies don't like to be stroked when they're nursing. They've got a job to do, darn it, and you're interrupting! If you're spending a few hours a day breastfeeding, though, you'll want some entertainment. Chele Marmet tells new mothers in her lectures, "Connect the baby to the boob and connect the mother to the boob tube." I liked to rent movies that I knew I'd never get my husband to watch with me. That included sappy romantic love stories and anything else he'd never agree to watch. I rarely watched an entire movie at a sitting. I'd watch them in twenty- to thirty-minute increments. At first, I felt incredibly guilty because I wasn't "doing anything." But I *was* doing something. I was holding and feeding my baby; and you can always pause a video to attend to whatever your baby needs instead of saying, "Shhhh! Wait until the next commercial!" (If you have other children, this advice is out the window.)

I'd also suggest you never sit down unless you have fresh water near you. I never remembered to bring water with me because when babies want to eat, they want to eat *now*—not in a millisecond—now! My daughters would begin to breastfeed, gulping and swallowing, and I'd curse myself for forgetting the water again. When someone else is drinking, particularly when you're the source of all that liquid, you'll be thirsty. Nine times out of ten, I'd have to rely on the kindness of my husband to get me a drink. He started to keep track after a while, and I still owe him about 432 trips to the refrigerator to get him a drink while he watches motorcycle racing. I could easily have put paper cups and one of those pump dispenser thermoses at my breastfeeding station. Or you can leave a bottle of water out, so that you don't have to always remember to bring a glass with you. If you cover any water that you leave out, you won't find dust bunnies floating around in your drink. Drink frequently, but don't force fluids. Pay attention to thirst. If you over-hydrate yourself, you can actually reduce your milk supply.

## "Honey? Would You Do Something for Me?"

Your husband or partner can help you, even if he leaves for work early and you're home with the baby. Ask him nicely to put out nutritious snacks for you every morning at your breastfeeding station. If he doesn't do this, it's likely you'll put whatever is closest to you into your mouth. He can put out a bowl of fresh fruit, nuts, whole-grain bread—something nutritious that can stay out all day. (You can also get a cooler. I even know one husband who bought a mini-refrigerator for the bedroom.)

## More about Colostrum

For a few days after you get home, your body is probably still producing colostrum. This will go on for anywhere from two to four days after the birth. Colostrum is full of immune-boosting properties, and it's all your newborn needs until your milk comes in. Justine, a first-time mother, worried that baby Chloe wasn't getting enough to eat because colostrum didn't look that great to her. It may not look that appetizing or plentiful to you, but your baby will think it's a four-star meal. New babies are not ready for catcher's mitts—or a lot of food. In fact, a healthy, full-term newborn could survive several days without anything. (Don't try testing this at home.) All they need the first few days is a few squirts of colostrum every few hours. (They're taking in between one-half teaspoon and one teaspoon a feeding, and that's plenty.) Expect to begin producing mature milk sometime between two and ten days after birth. Ten days is on the long side and usually happens if mother and baby have been separated or if there has been some kind of problem.

Julie was still producing colostrum nine days after her baby's birth. This is a good indication that something is not right. In Julie's case, her son was not latching on correctly, so there was not enough stimulation to turn on the milk production machine. Remember, demand is what produces the supply. Low demand = low supply.

## Your New Vocabulary

In the beginning, I found all of the terms used to describe breastfeeding humorous. You know, "nursing," "lactating," "engorged." I had no experience with dairy farming, so like a kindergartner learning potty humor for the first time, I found my newly discovered lingo hilarious until I found out what it really meant. When we got home from the hospital less than 24 hours after my first delivery (I had an especially generous insurance policy), my milk hadn't come in. I was not conscious of the need to make sure my daughter was breastfeeding frequently these first few days. That is probably what led to my engorged condition.

Jill Dieteker, a labor and delivery nurse turned lactation consultant, says she tells women to start looking for their milk to come in two to five days after delivery. She says she can tell if their milk is coming in by feeling their breasts (she says, no, it's not a big turn-on for her). If the tissue is swollen, lumpy, or hard, it means the milk will be visiting in large quantities very soon.

## Tackling the Two Most Common Problems: Engorgement and Nipple Pain

Remember Lamaze and all that breathing you were supposed to do when you were in labor but were in too much pain to play along as your husband played track coach and led your breathing with a stop watch? Your breathing skills can eventually come in handy. If you become engorged, and your breasts are as big as Wyoming, you will need to remember your breathing techniques so that your screaming doesn't wake the neighbors.

Most women will feel breast *fullness*, which is very different from breast *engorgement*. If, when your milk is coming in and your breasts start feeling full, you do not keep breastfeeding often (very often), your fullness can turn into engorgement, which is unpleasant and can be very painful. Fullness is a temporary condition. Engorgement is also temporary, but if you don't find a way to get your milk flowing, it can lead to bigger problems such as breast infections.

The treatment for engorgement is breastfeeding—before you get engorged. Why do you get engorged? I know you're remembering that the baby's demand is what produces the supply. You're reasoning that can't you just decrease the supply by decreasing the baby's demand? No. But good thinking. It's your baby's job to bring your milk in. Without him (or a pump), your body will never stop producing colostrum. Stored behind the colostrum is the beginnings of mature milk. You want to turn that faucet on and keep it on until the milk is flowing without getting backed up.

If you keep your baby constantly slurping during those first few days, you'll get milk to start pushing through. So, the more frequently you breastfeed, the less likely you are to have painfully engorged breasts. Minimize your chances of developing two hard, hot lumps on your chest by keeping your baby close by and attached to your breasts as much as possible.

## Treating Engorgement

### It's Only Temporary

If you get engorged, first off, remember that it is a temporary condition and usually lasts twelve to twenty-four hours. Engorgement is a build-up of fluids as your milk converts from colostrum through a transition phase and finally to mature milk. I remember sitting in a new gliding chair with my newborn daughter suckling at my breast when she was just seventy-two hours old. Sounds so perfect, doesn't it? (Like watching *Baywatch* from your comfortably dry couch. It looks so sexy to see people making out on a white sandy beach. Of course, if you've ever kissed someone on a beach, the overriding sensation is of sand creeping up your crotch.)

But breastfeeding never lived up to my naive images until much later. At three days postpartum, my breasts were so engorged, they felt like someone had implanted gallon-size Clorox bottles into each one. When I tried to get my baby latched-on, she slid off. Theresa, who had always been flat-chested, was the only woman I interviewed who was thrilled to be engorged. "I was a 'B' for the first time in my life. I said to my husband, 'Look! Look! I have breasts!' I was so disappointed when the swelling went away." So was Theresa's husband. "He looked like he was about to cry and said, 'You mean, they're not going to stay that way?'"

### What to Do If You Find Yourself Engorged

Kristine's milk came charging in at 11:00 at night. "Everything was closed, so I told my mother, 'Find me a breast pump, and don't come home until you have one!'" This is one way to solve engorgement, though not the best method. Experts will tell you not to let yourself get to the Clorox bottle stage. But if you somehow find yourself already there, you'll know because you'll be in pain, your baby will not be able to latch on, and he will also be screaming. You scream, I scream, we all scream for breastmilk. The more swollen your breasts get, the less skilled you and your baby are likely to be.

I panicked because I envisioned my breasts making milk to the point where the breast tissue exploded. Just like your contact lens won't float around your eye, find an escape hatch, and meander into your brain, your breasts can't explode.

If you do decide to use a pump, you need to use one that provides intermittent minimum pressure. That means, not a steady, rhythmic harsh suck. Kristine's mother finally came home with a battery-powered one at 3:00 a.m. after a clerk at an all-night drugstore blew the dust off it and sold it to her. It worked for Kristine, but experts caution against using pumps when you're engorged. Your breasts are already traumatized by the swelling. You need to wait a few weeks so you don't damage your tender tissue further with a vigorous pumping session. If you use a pump, don't use it for more than a few minutes at a time. The other reason is that your baby needs the practice, and your milk will eject faster for the baby than for a pump.

## Better Ways to Ease Engorgement

Have your husband hold your baby and comfort him in another room. Calmly massage your breast tissue and follow the directions for hand expression (see Chapter 11) until your breasts start to leak.

### Take a Warm Shower

Hot showers (or warm compresses) are helpful immediately before you're going to breastfeed. In the shower, slowly and gently massage your breasts. The warm water will soften your breasts and may even cause the milk to start to drip so that you can express some milk in the shower. Your baby and your partner may be hysterical by the time you're out of the shower, but don't join them. Stay calm. Then get your baby on as soon as you've dried off.

### Get Your Baby Interested Again

If your baby is apoplectic and won't go near your breast, position him for breastfeeding and press a little drop of breastmilk out of your breast and let the drop roll from your breast onto his mouth. Remind him why he started screaming in the first place. Then start tickling his mouth with your breast to stimulate his rooting reflex.

## Take Advantage of a Wide-open Mouth—Whatever the Reason for It

I ultimately took off the kid gloves, and when my daughter took a breath and then opened her mouth to howl again, I saw that wide chasm and literally shoved her mouth onto my breast. Experts say to take advantage of crying and yawning. Once babies figure out what's in their mouths, they won't mind that you've done the bait-and-switch trick. They don't get to cry or yawn, they get to eat. As the milk flows out of the ducts, your breast will begin to deflate, and feel a lot less painful. Before the baby is full, make sure you move him onto your other engorged breast so that he can fix that side, too.

## Congratulations—You've Finally Become a Human Refrigerator

Once you've fed your baby, friends might tell you to continue to use heat. Yes, it probably does feel good, but no, it is not helping the swelling. You wouldn't put an ankle you'd just sprained in hot water, however nice it felt. You'd find ice as fast as you could. What you need instead of a hot shower after a feeding is ice. The general rule for relieving engorgement is: when you're not breastfeeding, keep your breasts on ice.

### Buy Frozen Peas

Instead of trying to balance a bag of ice cubes on your chest, buy bags of frozen peas. (Make sure you mark the breast-peas so that you don't eat them.) Bags of peas are light but very cold and will conform to the shape of your breast. You can use them, then refreeze them (but remember not to eat them because thawing and refreezing encourages the growth of bacteria).

### Ice Flowers

Another trick is from a Martha Stewart wanna-be. Fill three plastic baggies with ice, then double-bag each. Put a wire twist tie around each bag. Arrange the bags into a flower shape and attach them to each other with a fourth twist-tie. Voilà! You have a pliable, reusable ice-flower centerpiece to arrange on your breast "table." You'll only need to remove it when you have company.

### Cabbage Leaves Work, Too

If you've heard that cold cabbage leaves work, the person who told you this is not out of her mind. There is a natural astringent in green cabbage leaves that seems to help to relieve swelling. You can chill the leaves in the refrigerator or freeze them, roll them with a rolling pin, and apply them directly to your breasts or put them between your bra and your skin. April did this and walked around with cabbage leaves on each breast for a day. "I forgot how long I'd been wearing them, and I started smelling this weird smell in our bedroom. I got my husband, and kept saying, 'Do you smell *that*?' Then, I moved into the laundry room, and I smelled it there, too! I said, 'There! Do you smell that?' We were smelling it in every room of the house, until finally, I looked down and realized I had cooked the cabbage on my breasts!" Another reason not to overdo the cabbage treatment is because the leaves can reduce your milk supply.

### Don't Bind Your Breasts

I happen to have big feet (and small breasts: somebody up there thinks he has a very good sense of humor). When I was a budding gymnast in the seventh grade, I remember a petite blond girl who looked like Cathy Rigby. She decided it was her duty to tell me my feet were huge. I was already incredibly self-conscious, since I was 4'7"—and had size 8 feet. "You should bind them," the Cathy Rigby look alike said, turning up her pert little nose at me and doing a perfect flip-flop, landing, of course, on her tiny feet. I went home and bound my feet with an Ace bandage. But it was so painful, I decided to ask my mother if this would really make my feet stop growing. To her credit, my mother suppressed what likely would have been a long and hearty laugh and broke the news to me: no, it would not. It would only cause me more pain than my eventual size 9½ feet would cause me.

Do not bind your breasts if you're engorged (or if you want to wean). If anyone tells you to do this, practice your "I'm pretending to listen but I'm ignoring everything you're saying" skills. You can get yourself in big trouble. Binding will put pressure on your swollen breasts. It's like putting a kink in a garden hose. You'll put pressure on your milk ducts and can even kill off your milk-producing cells. You will likely also give yourself a whopping breast infection. Valentina, a recent immigrant from a farming village, says women in her country still bind their breasts. She showed me how by tightly wrapping circles of ripped sheet around her breasts. Ouch!!!

## Yoo Hoo! Milk Delivery!

Your milk goes through a rapid change from colostrum through the transition phase and finally to mature milk. That's what you'll be making for as long as you breastfeed, though it will constantly adjust itself to supply your growing baby with what he needs at each stage of his development.

## "It Looks Kinda Thin"

Did you know that your breastmilk, as loaded with fat as it is, looks watery and often has a bluish tinge to it? It looks like skim milk. Given its calories, you'd think it'd be the consistency of buttermilk. But just because it looks thin doesn't mean there's something wrong with it. Rachel's doctor told her she was breastfeeding too much and her milk had turned to "skim." If anyone tells you this, particularly if it's a medical professional, report them to the Myths and Morons Agency. (I wish there was such a thing.) This is what experts refer to as, "Horsesh—."

Samantha was worried that there wasn't enough fat in her milk, so she pumped some into a bottle. Then she put her milk in the refrigerator, intending to bring it to a lab for testing to make sure it had enough fat. When she went to get it, she noticed that a layer of white creamy fat had risen to the top. She stopped worrying.

## Foremilk and Hindmilk

Your breastmilk has two stages: foremilk, the thinner milk to quench your baby's thirst and hydrate him, and hindmilk, the thicker milk full of protein and fat. Babies need to stay at one breast long enough to drink all of the foremilk before they get to the hindmilk. The hindmilk is rich in nutrients and fat. It's the stuff that makes them grow.

There's a restaurant chain called Fatburger, and every time I drive by I crane my neck to see the size of the bottoms of the people eating inside. We've gone nuts in this country over fat, but babies, especially new babies, need fat. For once, fat is good. The fat in human hindmilk is what promotes brain development. If you're taking your baby off your breast too quickly, or if his latch isn't great and he comes off soon after going on, he'll never get to the hindmilk.

## Time at Your Breast

The average amount of time babies stay at each breast is between ten and twenty minutes. The normal range is five to thirty minutes on each breast. Your baby can stay on longer, but don't try to get him to finish in less than five to seven minutes.

But there are mothers like April. Her milk supply was so plentiful and ejected so easily that daughter Rachel was usually done at each breast after five or six minutes of breastfeeding. April knew Rachel was done because Rachel came off by herself. April was worried that Rachel wasn't staying on each breast long enough to get hindmilk, though the baby was growing and looked healthy. A worried April told her pediatrician that Rachel wasn't getting enough milk. The doctor looked at Rachel's chubby cheeks and her weight, which put her in the 90th percentile of babies her age, and said, "Well, she's either getting milk or she's sneaking off at night and eating Häagen Dazs."

My first daughter was two weeks overdue and a robust eight pounds, so she was a fast learner. I let her stay attached to each breast for as long as she wanted, which turned out to be fifteen minutes each. A nurse told me I should have kept her on for eight minutes each to avoid sore nipples.

There is a lot of controversy over timing your baby's feedings. Some doctors and nurses still like to specify exact amounts of time to put your baby on your breast. Don't tell this to your doctor or nurse if you're afraid of offending him or her (though you'd be doing other patients a favor), but that's old information. Studies have shown that if you're putting your baby on for regimented amounts of time to avoid sore nipples, you are simply prolonging the amount of time it'll take to develop sore nipples. Even if you're doing it right, you may be a little sore anyway, whether that happens at the second feeding or the fifth.

Also, the more the baby sucks, the more stimulation your breasts will get and the more milk they'll know they have to produce. Your baby will be growing rapidly throughout the first year, and there will be times when your baby will suck more. That's to clue your body to speed up production. "I'm bigger now. Make more." If you let the baby take the lead and let him tell you when he's ready to come off, you'll likely have fewer problems. That means, sometimes he won't make it through both breasts. He may want to suck for a long time. He might want to go back and forth between breasts.

Soon, you'll figure out what your baby's breastfeeding personality is. Some babies are rapid, get-down-to-business slurpers. Others are leisurely stop-and-smell-the-flowers nursers. I have some very bad news for you if you're a control freak. You have no control over how your baby wants to eat, just as you'll eventually have little control over the clothes he wants to wear and the friends he wants to have. Oh, well....Is your appreciation for what your mother put up with growing by the day?

## Getting Enough to Eat and Dehydration

Many mothers worry about whether their baby is getting enough to eat. The best way to know if your baby is getting enough is to count his wet and dirty diapers. "What goes in must come out," most lactation consultants will tell you. Remember that breastmilk is 88 percent water and 12 percent solids. If your baby is urinating enough, he's getting enough to drink. If he's pooping enough, he's getting enough to eat.

Your baby should be soaking six to eight cloth diapers per day or four to six disposable diapers. Waste a diaper so you know what a "soaked" newborn diaper feels like. Pour one-fourth cup of water into one of your baby's diapers. That's what a wet diaper should feel like. It's heavy, isn't it? As for the poopy ones, some infants have a bowel movement with every feeding. Most have three to four a day. But make sure that during the first month he's having at least one bowel movement daily. One counting trick is to put two empty trash bags near your changing station. Put wet diapers for one day in one bag, and the same day's poopy diapers in the other bag. That way, you'll know exactly how many wet and how many poopy diapers he's made during a specific time period. You'll also know if you need to call a doctor.

The first few days, your baby should be making yellow, green, brown, or black bowel movements. They can look watery but they shouldn't smell bad, and you shouldn't see blood or mucus. Look for at least one in a twenty-four-hour period and probably more like three to four.

If you need more reassurance that your baby is getting enough to eat, look at him. Does he look healthy? Is he gaining weight? Can you hear him swallowing? All good signs. If your child has good skin tone, is alert, doesn't sleep for long periods of time, sucks at your breast, and makes small swallowing sounds (sucks, swallows, takes a break, then repeats all of that), he's probably getting enough. You will also be able to see the baby's ears wiggle (an indication that the jaw is drawing milk from the breast) and that your baby is growing (although not necessarily as fast as growth charts indicate he should since they're based on the weight of bottle-fed babies, who tend to take in too much at every feeding). You will worry, but your baby is probably flourishing.

Diarrhea is uncommon in breastfed babies. But if your baby is having a run of poopy diapers (twelve or more a day) that seem watery and smell, get him to a doctor—and keep breastfeeding him to get fluids back into his body.

Watch for the following signs that your baby isn't getting enough milk: sleeping all the time, eating all the time, skin that doesn't pop back up if you press on it, dry mouth, or not enough wet or dirty diapers. Your baby should also have good skin *turgor*, meaning he looks plump, round, and well-hydrated because his cells are full of water. If your baby is alert, has good skin tone, seems content, and is gaining weight, he's fine. (Check Chapter 9 for more information on dehydration.) If you do call or see a doctor, *always* ask him or her *how long* the problem should take to resolve itself, so you're not waiting days for the baby to get better if it's supposed to be hours.

## The Biggest Complaint: Sore Nipples

Sore nipples are the biggest complaint about breastfeeding, and the number one reason new mothers give up breastfeeding in the early days and weeks. I'm here to tell you I know how awful sore nipples can be firsthand, but know this: the pain can be relieved until you've figured out the underlying cause. If you're tempted to bottle feed, let me put it to you this way: it would be like standing in a long movie line for a film you've been dying to see. You get your ticket, popcorn, and all the junk you never eat, and you're sitting in your seat, when suddenly, you decide you're sick of waiting and walk out before the film begins. You've missed the best part of the experience, and all you will remember is the tedious, difficult part. This is what happens if you abandon breastfeeding in the early weeks—you'll never get to the good part.

## "Is It Possible to Breastfeed Initially Without Any Negative Sensation?"

I hope you'll be able to avoid describing breastfeeding the way one popular sitcom actress described it to me: "It feels like your tits are on a grill." Initially, breastfeeding may be sort of uncomfortable. But it's not supposed to be teeth-grindingly painful and have you wishing for an epidural. "Don't think that breastfeeding should hurt," says Dr. Jane Heinig, a nutrition research scientist and expert in breastfeeding. "Many women suffer through blisters, cracked nipples, terrible pain, etc., believing that such things are part of the breastfeeding process. Maybe we get numbed by childbirth!"

## "What Does a Sore Nipple Look Like?"

If your nipples look and feel like chapped lips, have blisters, open sores, cuts, are scabbing or bright red, you probably have a problem with your baby's positioning, his latch-on, or his suck. Remember how much a paper cut hurts even though it can be just a little tiny cut? That's because there are a lot of nerve endings in your fingertips. The same is true of your nipples. Your nipple is supposed to be one of the most sensitive areas of your body. And incidently, if you do happen to bleed while you're breastfeeding, the blood is not harmful to the baby.

## "Could You Define Pain?"

Before you assume you have a problem, figure out how you define *pain*. If it lasts for the first twenty seconds of sucking, or the first ten sucks or so, you're having normal pain. If it stings as your baby gets the nipple to fully extend in his mouth, that's normal, too. If your nipples are more sensitive, that's normal, too. If it's so painful that you are breaking through skin as you bite your knuckle, you need help.

## Don't Grin and Bear It

I have a reasonably high threshold for pain (except when somebody's mean to me on a day that I have P.M.S.). That was part of my problem, and it's the problem of a lot of women who believe they should just put up with pain so they don't sound like complainers. By day two, I had blood blisters (I wish I was kidding). Here's the good news (for you, not for me): I was doing it wrong. You don't have to endure pain to breastfeed. Pain is an evolutionary protection. It's a signal that something isn't right. Breastfeeding is supposed to feel good or at the very least neutral. If it doesn't feel that way, something is not right.

"I thought you were supposed to have problems," Rachel says. Rachel had developed a whole host of problems, including sore nipples that began with a bad latch-on. "I just assumed I would have problems, so I didn't know to get help." By all means, get help.

## "But I Was Fine at the Hospital!"

Many problems can take a few days to develop. Jill, the registered nurse who visits women a few days after they're released from the hospital, says most of the women she sees complain about some pain. But slight irritation is vastly different from blood blisters.

## How to Fix Sore Nipples If You Couldn't Prevent Them

### Check for Positioning Problems

Before you put your baby on your breast, look at his body. Is his chest pressing against your chest? Is his face turned to face your breast? Don't let him lie on his back and stretch your nipple into a faucet shape.

### Check for Latch-on Problems

If he seems to be doing everything correctly but it still feels like someone's using your breasts as a pincushion, you may want to take him off and start again. He won't be happy, but he'll be so anxious to get back to your breast that eventually he'll do darn near anything, including opening his mouth wide enough to take in your head. Remember that he needs to take enough of the areola tissue in his mouth along with the nipple. If your nipple is still hurting, slide his lower lip down and check out where his tongue is. If it's visible and is resting on his lower lip, he's doing it right. If you can't see it, it means he could be sucking on his tongue or on your nipple.

### Don't Soap Up

Be careful when you shower or bathe to use only water on your nipples. No soap. No fancy talcum powder. And try to use the open-air-drip-dry method to dry your breasts after feedings and showers. Your breasts don't need to be disinfected or sterilized for the baby. Nature has already thought of this, and your breasts secrete oils that cleanse and lubricate the breast tissue.

### Breast Shells

No, you will not look like Xena, the Princess Warrior, with your breast shells on. Breast shells serve two purposes: 1) to help you evert inverted nipples—see drawing in Chapter 9, and 2) to protect sore nipples from chaffing against clothing while you heal. They cost about $20 for a pair and look like little frisbees. Once they're in place in your bra, your nipple is protected. I used them with my second baby Julia, who as you'll remember was nicknamed "the washboard" because of what happened to my nipples after a good scrubbing in her mouth. The shells were comfortable and couldn't be detected under loose clothing.

### Do your Pilot-Co-pilot Thing. Position? Check. Latch on? Check. Pain? Check.

Once you're sure the position and latch-on are correct, there are things you can do to make your nipples feel a little better until they heal. Moisten your nursing pads with water before you take them off to keep them from sticking. While ice between feedings and warm compresses right before feedings offer the greatest relief, some women swear by lanolin, and new research seems to back them up.

### Try Pure Lanolin and Go From Feeling Like a Cow to Feeling Like a Sheep

My second child, Julia, tested my own resolve to breastfeed because my nipples were so sore, even the thought of her tiny mouth opening for her next meal made me perspire with the anticipation of pain. I was so desperate for pain relief, I would've applied motor oil if it'd been recommended (it wasn't, so don't try it).

Breastfeeding consultants didn't traditionally treat sore nipples with anything, other than to tell women to be vigilant about how the baby latches on and to keep the sore area dry. But thankfully, new research has changed that thinking. I was given a tube of Lansinoh for Breastfeeding Mothers™, which is modified lanolin endorsed by La Leche League International. It seems to spur healing by keeping the wound moist and lessening pain by blocking the nerve endings. Other kinds of creams, ointments and lanolin can actually be harmful because they may contain high levels of pesticides, free lanolin alcohols, and detergent residues. I don't know about you, but I didn't drink coffee while I was pregnant, so I wasn't about to feed my babies high levels of pesticides. Suzan says she patted a little on when she was in pain. "Usually, the cracks cleared up the next day. I thought it worked great." You don't even have to wipe it off before feedings. Apparently, babies consider it a welcome condiment. (If your baby notices, gently wipe it off before a feeding.)

### Breastmilk: The Sure Cure

Believe it or not, breastmilk helps bleeding, cracked nipples. What most experts recommend is rubbing a little breastmilk on your sore nipples. Express a little onto your clean fingers and gently rub it on. It also helps to let your breasts air-dry after every feeding. The more they're exposed to air, the quicker they'll dry and the better they'll feel. Breastfeeding experts used to advise women to "blow-dry" their nipples with a hair dryer. Bad idea. You nipples are skin—you wouldn't blow any other wound dry.

Another little tip: breastmilk cures pinkeye. No joke. A doctor visiting from England noticed a student in his lactation class with a baby. He pointed to his swollen, red eye, and said ever so politely, "Might I trouble you for a little breastmilk?"

#### Ask For Help

If nothing is working to correct your sore nipples or, as in my case, your blood blisters, have a lactation consultant assess the baby's sucking style and the position you're nursing in. There could be something going on in the baby's mouth that you can't see. It could be that he's got an oddly shaped palate or he's curling his tongue in his mouth. There are other positions to feed him in, where gravity can help—for example, having him lie on your chest. Talk to a lactation consultant for help.

#### Keep a Sense of Humor

While you're working on this, try to find a way to laugh. I was in so much pain, I walked around with the flaps of my nursing bra in the down position. One time, I answered a knock at the door without remembering to put the flaps up. The UPS man got a thrill (and showed up for days after that with packages addressed to my neighbors. "Whoops, sorry, wrong address"). I was too tired to be embarrassed. So I laughed (even though I did not find it *that* funny at the time). Cheryl did the same thing at a fast-food drive-thru window. Baby Gabriel was having a fit, so she calmed him down while she waited in a long line of cars. "I'd forgotten to put 'Mrs. Happy' back in her harness. I think I made everybody's day at the drive-thru. When your baby is that upset, you don't give a hoot who sees what, but I bet they still talk about it," Cheryl says.

### Things Nobody Tells You about the First Few Days

#### Did You Know the Milk Doesn't Come Out of Just One Hole?

The milk actually comes out of the tiny holes distributed on your nipple. There are between ten and twenty of them. You'll see them squirting milk out of various holes if you pump or hand express.

### Did You Know That If You're Fair-skinned, or Have Very Pink Areolas or Are a Redhead, You Might Have a Slightly Tougher Time because Any or All of Those Things Make Your Skin More Sensitive?

There seems to be a direct relationship between certain physical characteristics and skin sensitivity. How do I know this? I'm fair-skinned, have very pink areolas and red hair, and have very sensitive skin. Experts disagree, but I don't think those experts are fair-haired, have pink areolas, or have red hair.

### Did You Know That You May Have to Walk Around with Your Breasts Exposed?

This means that the first week is not a good time to have houseguests, like your father-in-law, for example, who might be startled at the sight of your naked chest.

### Did You Know You Might Squirt?

Sometimes your milk will come out so fast, your baby will pull off of your breast. I squirted my daughter in the face a number of times when my milk came out so quickly, she couldn't swallow fast enough to keep up with it. If your baby is gulping and gasping, grab a towel and press it against your breast to slow the flow and mop the excess. Then try again. If you have a fast milk-ejection reflex, it may work to put your baby on when he's sleepy. If he's ravenous, he'll pull so hard, the milk will eject even faster. If he's tired, it should come out more slowly. If this is really a problem, you might want to get into the habit of pumping or hand expressing some of the excess before you put your baby on your breast. We'll get to both of these techniques later.

### Did You Know You'll Leak?

I hope you have a small supply of nursing pads. Don't get pads with plastic backs, because plastic prevents air from moving around and encourages the growth of bacteria. Also, your nipples could get sore because they'll never dry. Change the pads as soon as they seem wet. Don't try to save money by leaving them in for long periods of time. You'll only spend that savings trying to cure your sore nipples or a breast infection.

It's a good idea to carry around two cloth diapers: one for the baby, one for your breasts. Sometimes, when the milk starts to eject from one breast, the other breast will think it's her turn and start to eject, too. This is normal. Your breasts are still amateurs at this. Eventually, most women find that each breast will be able to wait in line. If you do start to leak, press the diaper against your breast. A little pressure will usually stop the flow and mop up the excess.

### Did You Know That the Poop of Breastfed Babies Doesn't Smell?

You will not change an offensive-smelling diaper until your baby starts on solids or you feed him formula. The poop of breastfed babies doesn't smell because breastmilk has less bacteria in it, so when it goes through the baby's system, it doesn't turn into that rank stuff that carries the distinctive eau-de-poop smell. Even one bottle of formula will change the balance in the baby's gastrointestinal tract and lead to smelly diapers.

## Common Questions and the Mistakes That Lead to Problems

### 1. Question: "How Often Should He Eat?" Mistake: "Everybody Says Every Three to Four Hours"

Feeding your baby every three to four hours is a thing of the past. Nurses or doctors may tell you to feed your new baby every three to four hours, and in fact, a lot of people still think this is how to feed a breastfed baby. This is bad advice. It is also wrong. It is based on directions for bottle feeding. After the first few days of life, newborn breastfeeding babies need to eat every two hours—sometimes even more frequently. On about day five, you'll have a rough idea of the next six weeks because your baby will probably have developed a breastfeeding pattern. Listen to him. He can tell you when he's hungry. Remember to watch for early signs, hand sucking, activity to avoid the late sign of crying. It's harder to get a crying baby latched on.

"My doctor told me to feed Ben every three to four hours," Rachel says. "It took me a week of listening to him scream before I finally thought, 'Ben knows when he's hungry! To hell with that advice.'" Once Ben was being fed more frequently, he stopped screaming and his weight gain, which had been faltering, picked up.

It's not abnormal to have a ravenous newborn who wants to nurse every one to two hours. You should also expect periods of marathon nursing that are of longer duration than normal. Feeding in general, not breastfeeding in particular, can be a full-time job in the beginning, but it will not be a life-long occupation. Keep that in mind if you decide that breastfeeding might take too much time. Feeding a baby formula often takes almost as much time or more because of round-the-clock bottle duty.

Don't try to put your baby on a feeding schedule. Think about it. You have a well-regulated, adult system. And yet, you don't eat the same portions at precisely the same times every day. Some days you eat less. Some days you *wish* you had eaten less. You eat, if your eating thermostat works, when you're hungry. So do babies. In order to keep up with their growing demands, you need to breastfeed very frequently, particularly at the beginning. We'd all probably be healthier if we ate smaller, more frequent meals and didn't go to bed full of potatoes and pork chops. Babies have this figured out better than we do.

2. QUESTION: "HOW DO I KNOW IF I'M MAKING ENOUGH MILK?"
MISTAKE: FEELING INSECURE AND ANXIOUS

Only about one-quarter of the milk your baby gets at each feeding is actually stored in the ducts. Even though you feel like a cow, you aren't one. Milk isn't being stored in your body. Even if your breasts feel excruciatingly full, most of the milk will be manufactured as the baby starts to suck.

3. QUESTION: "HOW DO I KNOW IF THE BABY IS GETTING ENOUGH MILK?"
MISTAKE: GETTING OBSESSED AND SWITCHING TO FORMULA OR SUPPLEMENTING

We have a real interest in measurable quantities in our culture. How much time? How much money? How many calories? Precisely, exactly, to the second, penny, ounce. According to Canadian doctor, Jack Newman, "The reason many women do not seem to succeed at breastfeeding has nothing to do with their ability to produce milk. Most have been undermined by the health system which mistrusts breastfeeding because it is so difficult for us to measure. We would much rather feed the babies by bottle, which measures, by the clock, which imposes limits, and using doctors' advice, which controls." The best way to make sure your baby gets enough to eat is to pick up on his cues. You may just have fed him, and he may still be signaling that he wants more. Your best guide is your baby. Put him on, let him drink to the point where he's sated, then let him initiate coming off.

### HOW TO TELL IF HE'S HUNGRY

You need to pay attention to the cues newborns give. When they start rooting, it means they're hungry. If they're sucking on their hands, they're probably hungry. It's best to try to get your baby on your breast before he goes ballistic. He'll be less frustrated waiting for your milk to be ejected if he's just beginning to feel hunger and isn't yet ravenous.

If your baby seems hungry or inconsolable unless he's at your breast, even if you just fed him, he may be hungry again. Breastmilk really is "made to be gentle" (I'm stealing that line from a formula commercial). It's digested rapidly and easily, within an hour to an hour and a half. Digesting formula is a much more complicated process for a new baby. There's a bunch of stuff in it that his immature system wasn't meant to digest. (That's why babies have more gas, smellier poops, more burping, and more spitting up with artificial baby milk.)

Just be aware and notice subtle changes in your baby. This is good practice for when he's a teenager and suddenly barricades himself in his room.

### "Can He Eat Too Much?"

Mothers often ask if it's possible to overfeed a breastfed baby. It's not. If your baby eats too much, he'll let the excess go in the form of spit-up. The next question mothers ask is whether spitting up is a problem. Rachelle, mother of two, has a good response: "Spit-up isn't a baby problem. It's a laundry problem." (Projectile vomiting is another story. If he's throwing up and it's hitting the wall on the other side of the room, get him to a doctor. It can be an indication of a serious problem.)

## 4. Question: "How Do I Know When He Needs to be Burped?" Mistake: "I Try to Burp Him After Every Sip"

I watched a new mother in a hospital bed telling the lactation consultant the baby was crying all the time because he couldn't burp. The lactation consultant asked the mother to show her what she was doing. The woman put the baby to her breast and started counting as he sucked. "1-2-3-4-5-6-7-8-9-10!" At ten sucks, she triumphantly pulled the baby off her breast while he struggled to stay attached and said, "Now burp!" The baby screamed. "Burp!!" More screaming. "See?" the woman said. "If only he'd burp!!" No, if only he could eat in peace. Someone in this woman's family had told her to let the baby suck ten times, then burp him. Then suck ten times, then burp him. The baby was crying because his mother kept yanking him away from the dinner table.

Not all babies need to be burped after every meal. But that's not to say they won't ever need to be burped. Listen carefully to your crying baby; he's trying very hard to let you know what he needs.

If your baby is contentedly finishing one breast, then pulling off and signaling he wants the other, he's not telling you he wants to be burped. If he comes off of your breast and seems fussy or in pain, try burping him. Sometimes, it's trial and error. This can be upsetting, particularly if you have an audience. Sasha's mother-in-law was suspicious of breastmilk because she'd formula-fed her children, and was ever-vigilant for a chance to feed her grandson Oliver artificial milk. At one feeding, Oliver popped off of Sasha's breast, looked plaintively at his grandmother, and howled. The mother-in-law said, "See? He doesn't like the taste of your milk. That's why he's crying." For a second, Sasha was upset. Maybe Oliver really didn't like her milk (actually, the foods you eat do flavor your breastmilk, but babies like the variety). But Sasha needed to silence her mother-in-law and her screaming son, so she tried burping Oliver. He let out a loud "errrp," and went happily back to breastfeeding.

### Effective Burping Technique

Most people try to burp a baby by holding him upright and giving him a gentle little tap on his back. Hmm, geee. Why's he still crying? Because no gas came out. The biggest favor you can do for your gassy little kid is to put pressure on his belly. If you put pressure on his gut, you should be able to dislodge the gas that's making him cry. If you just pat his back, he'll probably cry harder because he's feeling pressure in the wrong place, and he may or may not burp.

If he's crying after a feeding and you think he needs to burp, sit him on your lap and drape him over your arm the way a maître d' holds a towel. Your arm will be pressed against his abdomen and he should burp. You can also sit him in your lap, put your hand around the front of his neck (gently), press the heel of your hand into his stomach, and pat his back with your other hand. If you want to lie him across your legs, you can, but make sure his belly isn't hanging between your legs because then his stomach will be the only part of his body not getting pressure.

You can put him over your shoulder, but you need to put him pretty far over your shoulder. If you put your thumb under his armpit, you can get him all the way up so that his chest and belly are getting pressure from your shoulder. I know, I know. You're thinking, "How could this be comfortable?" But remember, your baby was upside down in utero for months. He likes being upside down! You only stop liking being upside down when you're out of grade school.

Of course, your baby may spit up wherever you've got him, so burp at your own risk—and with towel in hand.

### 5. Question: "How Long Do I Have to Breastfeed My Baby?"
### Mistake: "My Friends Say Just A Few Weeks to Pass Along Immunities"

We discussed all of the bare minimum numbers earlier. Yes, the baby will get a lot of benefits in the first few weeks. Yes, this is a very important time to breastfeed. But you are constantly passing along your immunities, so the benefits don't diminish if you continue to breastfeed. Your baby's brain is growing all through his early childhood. He is being exposed to illnesses, his fat cells are being laid down, and his immune system is maturing. Breastmilk contributes to helping him fight illnesses and stay lean and healthy. Breastfeed for as long as you can. That's how long it will take for your baby to receive the maximum benefits.

### 6. Question: "Can I Give Him a Bottle Yet or Supplement with Formula?"
### Mistake: Giving Him a Bottle or Supplementing with Formula

You may be wondering why experts go nuts about using bottles. The reason they want you to wait three to six weeks before you give your baby a bottle is to avoid "nipple confusion." I have been told that some lactation consultants advise women to alternate nipple and bottle earlier than this, but DON'T DO IT.

If you introduce a bottle too soon, your baby could fall in love with a rubber nipple. Breastfeeding takes work and jaw action—two things a bottle doesn't demand. Until infants have learned how to coax milk from your breast, the milk from a bottle that just drips down their throat takes much less work (the difference between watching someone work out and doing some exercise yourself). Sucking from a bottle and compressing the sinuses of the breast are distinctly different activities. It's pretty unlikely that you'd try to learn to play tennis and racquetball at the same time. They look a little bit alike, but they require completely different and often contradictory skills. It's the same with breastfeeding and bottle feeding. This is also the reason why breastfed babies have straighter teeth and better craniofacial development. They worked at it.

Some babies won't get confused. You'll hear stories from mothers who gave their babies bottles within the first three weeks and the babies easily went back and forth. But some babies do get confused. Yours might be one of them.

### 7. Question: "Can I Give Him a Pacifier?"
### Mistake: Giving Him a Pacifier

My husband and I were ignorant about pacifiers and did not tell the nurse in the baby nursery not to give my daughter one. I was no ace at even holding an infant, so figuring out how to get her latched-on was like skipping addition and subtraction and beginning with geometry. But right after birth, she latched on right away. After she'd been to the nursery for a bath, the nurse brought her back with a pacifier in her mouth. This time, she couldn't latch on. A friend who'd just been through it all arrived at the hospital to give me pointers. She noticed the pacifier and advised us against it. I still wasn't convinced, because babies like pacifiers, right? Why else would companies sell them and all of your shower gifts come with one attached? But I began noticing that if my daughter had been sucking on a pacifier before nursing, she had trouble using her reflexive sucking action to get milk. Finally, we just stopped giving her a pacifier. Six weeks later, when she was an expert nurser, we stuck one in her mouth when she was crying. She spit it out. We pushed it in. She spit it out. We got the message.

One more thing: studies show that the use of pacifiers cuts down on milk production. Significantly. That's because when he uses a pacifier, the baby spends too much time with rubber in his mouth (which doesn't make milk) and not enough time with your breast (which does).

### Is the Pacifier For You or For the Baby?

A lot of people who routinely give their babies and children pacifiers lose the ability to figure out what's really wrong. Hungry? Here's a pacifier. Tired? Pacifier. Want to be held? Pacifier. Turned over? Pacifier. Changed? Pacifier. Think about it. You and I have similar emotions when we're hungry, tired, need a change of position or a restroom. Only as adults, we're expected to know how to control ourselves—and some of us even succeed at this. But what if the person closest to you shoved rubber in your mouth each time you tried to tell him or her that you were having a problem? You and your offspring will survive—for at least the first few weeks—without a pacifier.

However, that said, let me quickly contradict myself. Miriam, Lucas's mother, says Lucas seemed to want to suck twenty-four hours a day. When Miriam says this, I believe her. Some women think half an hour attached to the breast is all day, but in Miriam's case, it probably was close to twenty-three and a half hours. "Finally, I called the pediatrician. He said, 'Obviously, he has a great need to be sucking a lot, so have you thought of trying a pacifier?'" When Lucas was about three weeks old, Miriam gave him a pacifier. Lucas was full-term, normal, and never had any trouble attaching himself to the breast. Three weeks is about the bare minimum to wait before getting into the routine of using a pacifier. For Lucas, the pacifier seemed to make no difference in his sucking ability at the breast. Be watchful. If you notice no difference—no fussiness, no slowdown in weight gain, no slowdown in appetite—the pacifier is probably okay.

### 8. Question: "How Do I Get Anything Done?" Mistake: Trying to Get Anything Done

Marian liked to make long lists of things to do. One day, she fell in a tired heap on her bed but jumped up and started running water as soon as she heard her husband taking the baby out of his bassinet.

"What are you doing?" he said. "I'm going to give the baby a bath," Marian said. When her husband asked her why she felt the need to get out of bed when she was tired to bathe a perfectly clean baby who was perfectly happy being held by Dad, Marian responded, "Because it's on the *list*!"

There is an old poem by an unknown author that's kinda schmaltzy but makes the point:

> Cleaning and scrubbing can wait 'til tomorrow.
> For babies grow up, we've learned to our sorrow.
> So quiet down cobwebs, dust go to sleep.
> I'm rocking my baby and babies don't keep.

Oh come on, it's cute. Here's the updated version:

> Chill. The cleaning can wait. The baby can't.

This goes for doing shopping, too. Even though *you* have to buy groceries and maybe even like to shop, your baby may not. Sure, you can put him in his stroller and he'll sleep. But as soon as you're first in a long line at the post office, he'll wake up. And if he seems fussy and upset, even hours later, it's because he didn't feel like spending his day bargain shopping. You'll get tired, too, and you may find that it's difficult to find places where you can breastfeed comfortably.

Babies love to just hang out at home with you. Even when they're bigger, they'd take a day of you sitting on their floor reading to them over a day at Disneyland (unless you tell them that Disneyland is an option).

### 9. Question: "Will My Breasts Look Like My Grandmother's When I'm Done Breastfeeding?" Mistake: Looking at Your Grandmother's Breasts

Your breasts won't look any worse than they would have if you hadn't breastfed. Doctors will tell you that stretch marks have more to do with genetics, hormones, and weight gain than with breastfeeding. For some women, pregnancy does change the size, shape, and general elasticity of their breast tissue. This is the burden we bear. Depending on whom you ask, if you stick to a slow, steady weight gain during pregnancy and apply some kind of heavy-duty moisturizer, you can reduce the likelihood of getting stretch marks. But there is no guarantee that you won't get them. The good news is that even if you do get stretch marks, those angry purple lines will eventually fade to match the surrounding tissue. And look on the bright side: unless you're a nudist, who but your partner and baby are going to get a good look at your stretch marks anyway? (And if you *are* a nudist, I'm sure there are far worse things you've been treated to at your nudist hang-outs.)

It's kind of sad when your breasts go back to their old size. For me, it was a mixed blessing to go from a big C cup back to a B. I say mixed blessing because I'd always wanted big breasts, and I never thought there'd ever come a day when I'd wish for smaller breasts. But that day did come.

### 10. Question: "Will I Ever Have a Life?" Mistake: Thinking You Don't Have One Now

Sure, it's different, but it's a life all the same. Try to enjoy this little sliver of time. You'll get sick of hearing everyone tell you how fast it goes; but for once, all those nosy strangers are right.

Marian, the list-maker, is a policy analyst who had her son at age thirty-nine. She says slowing down and watching for her son's cues was hard for her. "My whole identity was tied up in my job. I kept making lists of fifty things to do every day, and I'd only get one thing done. Finally, I'm starting to figure out that *this is* the job—carrying him around and watching him sleep." So now she writes those two items on her list and crosses them off again and again.

You won't have to do this for long, but when you first have a baby, this new schedule takes some getting used to. You'll be sitting around a lot. Now here's the contradiction: you'll be sitting around with nothing but time on your hands and you won't be able to get anything done. No reorganizing your closets, trying out that new dessert recipe, sewing all the buttons back on your suits, writing all of those thank-you notes, and doing the laundry before grocery shopping. Forget it. If you need to, think of the time spent at your breastfeeding station as work. Clock in, clock out, heck, pay yourself if it makes you feel better. Just don't feel like you're being useless. Every minute you spend with your child is a minute well spent (unless you're being what my daughter now calls "Mean Mommy," when I'm being less patient with her. That happens to the best of us. I prefer the terms, "Had-a-bad-day Mommy," "Paid-the-bills-today Mommy," or "P.M.S. Mommy").

# Chapter 7:

# The First Six Weeks: I Think I Can, I Think I Can, I Think I Can

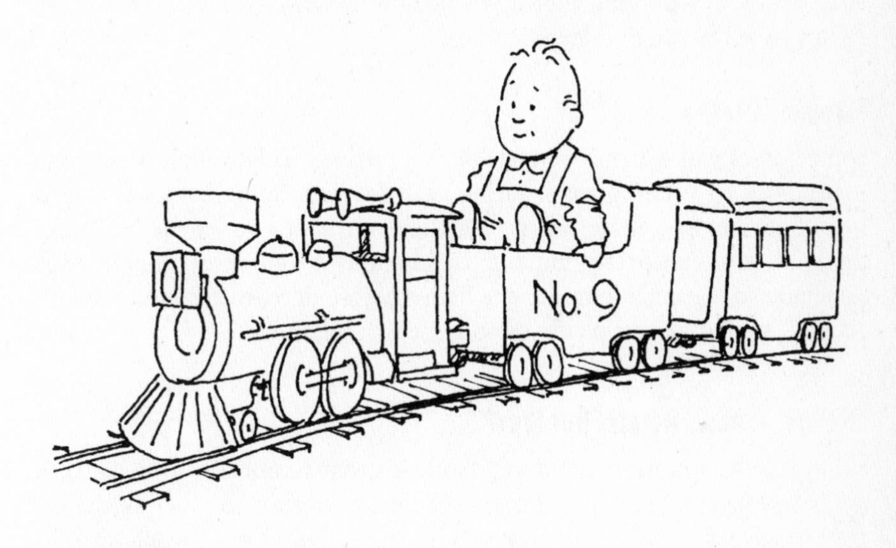


### In a Nutshell

What's his poop supposed to look like?
Seedy yellow mustard.

When does he regain his birthweight?
By about two weeks.

## "Give Me a Rough Idea of Feedings . . ."

Here is the information your poor breasts have been waiting for. When do they get to switch from overtime, swing-shift work to more normal hours? When your baby is a newborn until about six weeks, he'll be eating up to twelve times a day, usually every two hours. When he hits six weeks, he'll go to about ten feeds, every two and one-half hours. (Incidentally, when you're calculating this, figure from the beginning of one feeding to the beginning of another. For example, if he's eating every two hours and starts at 10:00 and finishes at 11:00, he'll be hungry again at 12:00. By three months, he'll be eating about eight times a day, every three hours, *or* he'll feed constantly during the day and sleep through the night. Don't expect him to sleep through the night yet or even by the time he is three months. This is no indication of whether or not you have a "good" or a "bad" baby. It's only an indication of how far away people should stay from you while you are sleep-deprived.

## Feeding Patterns

Some babies will use only one breast at a feeding. This will blow sky high that advice to rotate breasts during each feeding. Some babies will feed from both breasts. Some will go back and forth. If you let the baby take the lead, you can pretty much trust his body to guide his hunger. But remember not to take him off one breast before at least five minutes have elapsed, so that he gets plenty of nutrient-rich hindmilk.

## "Rotate, Rotate, Rotate. But Why?"

Some lactation consultants don't think it's that important to make sure the baby takes both breasts at every feeding, even though much of the literature suggests this is the only way to breastfeed. One consultant told me, "That's the big thing right now: doing each breast, one at a time." Instead, this consultant suggests that you feed your baby one breast at a time and let him give you the signal. That signal is very recognizable. It'll say either, "I'm done. Move me to Breast Number 2" or "I'm in blissland. When I look like a drunken sailor, it means I've had enough." If he only nurses at one breast, try to remember to offer him the other breast at the next feeding.

There is some preliminary research that keeping a baby on one breast per feeding is a good way to help some babies get over colic. Behind the cherubic face of my second daughter was an arsenal of enough baby gas to float the Hindenberg. Once my milk supply was established, I fed her one breast at a feeding. She stopped spitting up, wailing, and clearing the room after every feeding.

## "What's All This Sucking About?"

Babies nurse for comfort, in addition to food. Remember Freud's "oral fixation?" This is the period of life devoted to experiencing the world through the mouth. Even if they *have just eaten*, they may still want to latch on and suck.

It's likely that no one has told you that part of their early development is getting their sucking need met. If you don't always want to be the human pacifier, wait about six weeks until breastfeeding is well-established, and then try a pacifier. But don't let the pacifier become the all-purpose crying deactivator. Sucking is only one of your baby's needs. Plus, your baby is better off meeting his sucking needs at your breast to keep the milk supply up.

## Germ Warfare

Did you know you protect your baby from germs every time you breastfeed? There is an amazing thing that happens when your baby is at your breast. In addition to transferring your immunities, your body will make antibodies to combat whatever he's been exposed to.

Let's say your husband comes home with a runny nose and a cough. He kisses the baby's head and exposes the baby to what he has, a cold you and your baby haven't yet caught. When your baby breastfeeds, the germs your husband handed over will make their way into your breasts. Then your mammary glands will catch a whiff of the germs now beginning to find a new home in your baby. These germs get to the glands through the ducts as your baby breastfeeds. Your mammary glands will rapidly produce a *specific antibody* to the germs in your baby's mouth. The antibodies to your husband's cold then get passed right back into your baby to help him fight it off. I know you think I'm making this up, so I'll tell you that this is based on at least three studies.

You'll probably notice this happening a few times during the period your baby is breastfed. I remember it happening at least four times, though at the time, I didn't know what was going on. My husband and I would get sicker than dogs. We would worry that our daughter was going to get bronchitis or laryngitis or whatever other nasty illness we had. But she was fine. She breastfed during our illnesses and didn't get sick. This is why breastfeeding babies are safer out in public than bottle-fed babies.

This is not to say your baby will never be sick. Michelle complained that Jenna was congested. "And I'm breastfeeding! What's the deal?" Don't get mad at your breasts if your baby gets sick. But you should know that research shows that the duration and severity of any cold, congestion, virus, bacteria, ear infection, upper-respiratory disease, and so on is likely to be much less if the baby is breastfed. If one of your bottle feeding friends says, "I thought breastfed babies didn't get sick," tell her that even though they do, they're usually far less sick than babies who are fed artificial milk.

## "He Likes Me! He Really Likes Me!"

It's easy to get maudlin when you start talking about how you feel about your baby and how your baby obviously feels about you. It's the most magnificent feeling to be that important to someone, particularly when you are a breastfeeding mother. Research shows that women who breastfeed have a physically closer relationship with their child. Though mothers who bottle feed say they hold their infants just as much, studies have shown they don't. They couldn't possibly. A breastfeeding mother of a newborn is feeding him, on average, twelve times in a twenty-four-hour period. A bottle-feeding mother is doing it six times. A breastfeeding baby stays at the breast longer. It takes more time, it's more fun, and it's about more than just getting food. You have to get close to breastfeed, no way around that.

You may sometimes be envious of your friends who put their babies in an infant carrier, prop up a bottle, and then get some work done. Don't be. Your baby is getting *you*. Your breast, your focus, your attention, your love. Not a plastic object. The payoff for being a loving parent is not immediate; it is long term.

Jane said she loves it when her daughter holds her hand or "laces her fingers in mine while nursing. That's probably the most wonderful feeling of love and contentment I've ever experienced." Carolyn, who breastfed her second child but not her first, knew what was coming when I said I was going to ask her a hard question. "Do I feel closer to number two than I do to number one?" she said. "That's a hard one because they're five years apart. Did I feel closer sooner and bond more quickly to number two? Yes. I feel bad saying it, but yes, I definitely did."

## Better Eyesight

Breastfeeding offers more stimulation for the baby, too. Because it requires moving from side to side, even subtle things like shifting him from arm to arm is better for him. Since new babies can only focus eight to twelve inches away and your face is their favorite thing to look at, you're at just about the perfect distance and perfect angle for them to see you while they breastfeed. These two things may help account for the fact that breastfed babies wind up with better eyesight. Also, check out the way a baby is bottle fed. He's held away from his mother's body usually, there's no skin to skin contact, and his focal point is the ceiling or the bottle.

### Illness—Yours

You shouldn't stop breastfeeding your baby if you come down with a cold or the flu. You'll be giving your baby immunities through your breastmilk, because he's been exposed to what you have. Your breastmilk does not get contaminated if you're sick. Check with your doctor, but you should be able to breastfeed through most illnesses, depending on the drugs you've been prescribed.

### How to Get a Sleepy Baby Up for Mealtimes

There are all kinds of techniques to get your sleepy baby interested in eating. The first thing you should do is take off all the blankets and undress him. Cool air passing over him will usually wake him up (he'll be warm again soon when he's next to you). You can tickle his toes. You can pick him up and try to gently rouse him.

### Once You Start Using Bottles

Some experts believe you'll be more likely to confuse your baby if you use a nipple shaped like a cylinder. Those same experts say these nipples are the worst ones to use if you're using bottles at all because, contrary to the marketing hype, those rubber tips resemble pegs, not nipples. They're too short, and that little peg is what the baby will latch onto. Ultimately, you will be teaching the baby to suck on just your nipple. Nuk nipples or any orthodontic nipple (they say that on the packaging) are better for most babies if you're using bottles to feed your baby breastmilk when you're away. However, most people (I'm including my own bonehead self) don't use these nipples properly, so you could end up with the same problem the Playtex nipples cause. The baby needs to take about an inch and a half of the entire Nuk nipple into his mouth, not just the little nipple-shaped tip. They were designed to get the baby to mirror the action he's making when he breastfeeds, and the bulbous-looking rubber below the tip is supposed to be a stand-in for your areola. If you do plan to use bottles because you're going back to work, you may need to experiment with different nipples. Buy a couple and see if your baby has a preference.

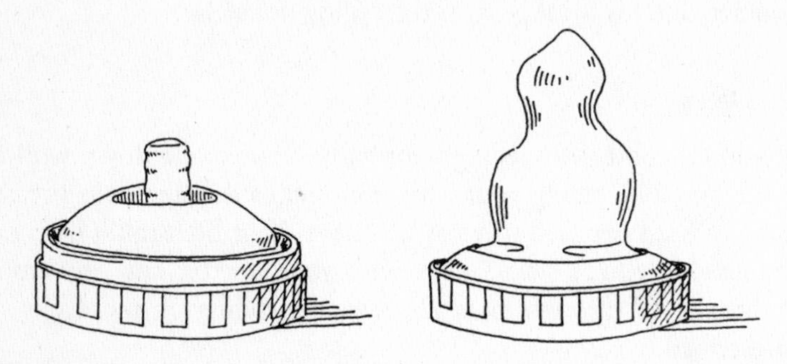

Plastic nipples: The Playtex nipple (left) is not a good choice for breastfed babies. The NUK or orthodontic nipple (right) is the best choice for feeding a breastfed baby pumped milk.

On average, breastfeeding is not considered well-established until three months. By that time, babies who've been exclusively breastfed will have little or no interest in any form of a rubber nipple (if there's a choice). Some babies won't take bottles at all, no matter at what age they're offered. Marilyn couldn't leave her daughter for more than an hour until she was six months old and eating solids. Marilyn didn't know she could have had whomever was taking care of Daisy use a feeding cup, an eyedropper, or a spoon. Terry, a radio newscaster, reported a similar experience. When she was on her eight-hour shift, her daughter simply went on a hunger strike. Her baby waited until Terry came home in order to be fed. Babies are very smart, and they like you. A lot. Some will reverse their habits so that they can be awake when you're home. That's what Terry's baby did. She figured out when her mother was gone, and that's when she slept. During the night, she wanted to be with her mother, so that's when she ate.

Don't avoid breastfeeding because you are afraid of getting stuck like this. Some babies simply can't switch easily back and forth from breast to bottle. Some don't want to. Would you? "Hmmm, warm, soft, cozy Mommy-skin, or hardened petroleum?" But most take it in stride, and if not, there are many other ways to feed a baby.

## "But I Have to Go Back to Work!"

If you want to breastfeed but your maternity leave is finite, you may want to think about introducing a bottle of pumped milk at about six weeks. That's about the bare minimum. By that time, your baby has figured this breastfeeding thing out and should be able to make the switch. Remind him what a bottle is by having someone else give him a bottle of pumped milk every couple of days. Ignore people who rush you on the bottle by scaring you with this advice: "If you wait too long, your baby won't know how to use a bottle!" Babies can simultaneously learn several different languages. They can certainly figure out a way that they're comfortable eating when you're away.

## What's Wrong?

Mothers often complain that their babies seem fussy at the breast, won't latch on, or cry unless they're given a bottle. *This is nipple confusion.* If you want to stop this vicious cycle and continue breastfeeding, lay off the bottle feeding. You may only have to wait another few weeks until your baby is more neurologically mature.

## Bottles Can Undermine Your Confidence

Claudia has had to work at breastfeeding because her nipples invert. She never was able to get her son to breastfeed, but she's having much more luck with her daughter, Canelle. That said, at Canelle's last weighing, the doctor was afraid she was not gaining weight quickly enough. He urged Claudia to give Canelle a bottle.

So Claudia did. "There was such a difference," Claudia says about the way two-week-old Canelle took the bottle. "Her eyes were open wide, she was just guzzling it down." Claudia started to wonder if this was a better way to feed Canelle, because clearly it seemed to her that's what Canelle preferred. This is exactly why lactation consultants get hysterical about bottles. Sandra Jansen, a nurse and lactation consultant who also owns Birth Plus, a pump rental station, says she gets calls like Claudia's all the time. "Mothers have a screaming baby. They're frustrated. They don't think the baby's getting enough to eat. Everyone else is saying, 'Give him a bottle.' And then, to make things worse, the mother tries this, and the baby glugs it down. No fussing. It doesn't matter how the nipple is placed in his mouth. He's instantly appeased."

When your child gets older, he'll likely prefer eating a bag of chips and watching cartoons to doing his homework. But you know that just because he appears to be working hard when he's doing his homework and he seems more content glued to the television it doesn't mean that he should be watching television, all the time. That's how you have to think of the early stages of breastfeeding.

A lactation consultant finally got Claudia to start feeding Canelle extra pumped milk with a syringe, by a method called *finger-feeding*, which is discussed in Chapter 9. It's a good way to avoid nipple confusion in young babies and to help babies get on the breast if they have a poor sucking ability. You'll have to have an expert show you how to do this. But there are other ways to feed a baby that take no special expertise.

## How to Feed a Baby with Something Other Than a Bottle

I know you are probably feeling skeptical because bottles are everywhere. Everybody uses a bottle. (Everybody also used to use formula.) Try to keep an open mind, because these other ways to feed are not harder to learn than drinking from a bottle. There are special feeding cups for very young babies. They're flexible and the sides can be squeezed together so that you can literally feed your baby drops at a time. In fact, any cup with a flexible rim will work. You can also use an eyedropper, which lets you squeeze the milk in. If your baby has a hard time at any age going back and forth from bottle to breast (you'll usually know this because his latch-on and suck will feel different or you may develop sore nipples), discard all those bottles and use a cup, spoon, or eyedropper until your baby is older.

These other ways to feed have a hidden advantage. You will insure that your caregiver is not propping up a bottle and leaving your baby alone in his bouncer while she talks on the phone. All these other ways of feeding require that your baby be held and attended to while he's eating.

## Crying Babies

If your baby has a fussy period in the late afternoon or around dinner time, he is normal. Some experienced baby handlers call it the "grandmother's hour." I prefer to call it the "How'd-you-like-to-hold-the-baby? hour." Babies can get really cranky and uptight right around the time you'd intended to eat dinner—and that goes for bottle-fed babies, too. Don't think if you switch to formula, as Sharon thought, the crying will stop. For Sharon, the crying intensified when she gave son Adam formula because artificial baby milk is much harder to digest. Sharon's son was much gassier and fussier on formula. When she switched back, Sharon says, "Adam went back to a little squawking instead of the screaming he did the two days I had him on formula."

"For two hours around dinner time, they'll hear the fork and start to cry," says Sandra Jansen. It doesn't seem to matter when you eat, either. Six o'clock one night, eight o'clock the next, your baby is still apoplectic during dinner time. "Who knows why—maybe because of the shift in your attention," Jansen says.

It's likely that your baby is tired and overstimulated. If you think about it, this is probably *your* least productive time of the day, too. Babies are usually at their gurgly best in the mornings. As the day wears on, so does a baby's ability to tolerate stress.

Some babies are soothed by rhythmic movement, like a baby swing. Most babies are also soothed by rhythmic "white noise." We had a broken kitchen fan that was so loud, if you screamed at the top of your lungs, you wouldn't be able to be heard over it. I kept meaning to get it fixed, but one day when I was cooking and my first daughter was screaming, I turned it on. Presto! Like magic, she quit crying. Now, in truth, I can't tell you what was more annoying to listen to: her "waahh" or the "argh-argh-ARGH-ARGH" sputtering sound of the fan, so I rotated. Crying, fan noise, crying, fan noise. It was also obviously a genetic trait. Daughter number two liked the fan more than a lullaby, too.

If you don't have a broken kitchen fan, try a vacuum cleaner as your source of white noise. Some babies will even get into those New Age sounds of the ocean. Just as long as it's repetitive.

## "What's Colic?"

"Waaahhhh!" That's crying. "WAAAAAHAHHHHHH!" That's colic. That's about the amount of help you'll get if you ask friends about the dreaded *colic*. Many doctors aren't much help, either. Most will tell you that they don't know what causes it and that it will go away. Here's one simple rule to determine whether your baby has colic or he's just crying: normal crying can last up to two hours. Colic-induced crying will go on for three to five hours or more at a stretch. The baby's cry will be higher-pitched and more irritating, and the baby will pull his legs up in seeming agony.

## THE ONE-BREAST SOLUTION FOR COLIC

Recent research advises mothers of colicky babies to offer just one breast at each feeding, instead of moving the baby back and forth. One study found that foremilk, which contains most of the lactose, could stimulate colic by putting too much lactose into the bowel. Hindmilk, the richer, fattier milk that comes out a few minutes after the foremilk, squirts out more slowly and has less lactose.

Also, emptying one breast at a feed will help keep your infant from swallowing air. Breastfed babies don't swallow nearly as much air as bottle-fed babies because of the air-tight seal their mouth makes around your breast. But your baby might be more sensitive and might be taking in air when he's being pried off one breast and then put back on another. Try it. What can it hurt?

## "IS IT SOMETHING I ATE?"

If your baby's colic fits seem sporadic, and you can remember what you ate, try to avoid gas-inducing foods. Use Beano (grocery stores and health food stores sell this) if you eat a lot of beans (and you should because they're a good source of complex carbohydrates and they're lowfat). Try avoiding cauliflower, broccoli, chocolate, and spicy foods for a week and see if it makes a difference—though a lot of experts will tell you that what you're eating probably has nothing to do with your baby's crying jags. If you're smoking at all, that could be what's causing the crying.

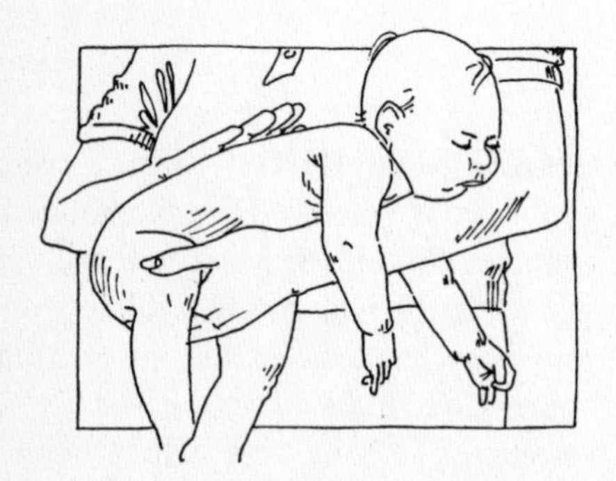

The colic hold: Crying, gassy babies or fussy babies often feel better if you try to gently sway them with the palm of your hand, putting pressure on their gut to get the gas moving.

## Daddy's Turn

This was often my solution. I gave the screaming baby to Dad. No, wait, that needs more explanation. A lot of men like to fix things, and you can tell your husband there is something called the "colic hold."

If he places the baby in the crook of his arm, the way he would carry a football, holding the baby's head in his hand and putting the baby's body and legs along his forearm and up to his elbow, he can gently rock the baby up and down his body. Often, the baby will stop crying. According to some pediatricians, it's because the cerebral fluid in the brain is being redistributed.

This almost always worked for my daughter. Since my husband's arms were bigger and stronger than mine, he didn't worry about dropping her in this position, and an added bonus: my husband was incredibly pleased with himself when she stopped crying and started cooing at him. He was even more excited than he was the day he fixed the kitchen fan (when my daughters were done with it). Letting your baby's father "fix" his baby will increase his confidence in his paternal skills and will make it easier for him to be supportive of breastfeeding, because he'll be bonding with the baby, too.

## "Sometimes, I'd Like to Be Doing Something Else"

I'd be remiss if I didn't tell you the truth: breastfeeding is *very* time-consuming. You will likely be spending one hour out of every two breastfeeding in the beginning. It means you won't have time to cook, shower, or go to the bathroom—at least for the first six weeks. Although this is a temporary condition, you're entitled to feel depressed, resentful, and overwhelmed. Somebody else is dictating the pace of your life and that's weird. It takes time to absorb this change. Do what you can to get help lightening the load. If there is any way you can scrounge together a little extra money, hire a cleaning service to come once a week or once every two weeks to do the heavy cleaning for awhile.

## Don't Quit Now

The worst part about quitting during the first three weeks is that you are just coming to the end of the hardest part. That means, you get the pain but not the goodies. Once you are through your first month of breastfeeding, the experience will radically change. You won't be in pain. You won't have to do it in only one position. You will actually enjoy it. Hard to believe? Cheryl, mother of Jared and Gabe, said, "Even though it hurt the first month, I knew this was *it*."

## "Can't Somebody Else Do This?"

Before I started breastfeeding I thought that I couldn't wait to let my husband take over the feeding "chore." By the third week, the most amazing thing had happened to me. I really didn't feel like sharing this warm, fuzzy ritual with my husband (okay, the truth is I still felt like sharing the 3:00 a.m. shift). And by that third week, my daughter was a full partner in the breastfeeding business. Cool, eh?

## Did You Know About Growth Spurts?

You may not understand what the heck's going on when all of a sudden, out of nowhere, your baby wants to breastfeed every time you want to sit down. The nonstop, marathon nurser. Why? Is he hungry? Are you not making enough milk? Should you supplement? All your friends are giving their babies some artificial baby milk. Maybe you should, too.

Babies grow, obviously. That's why that cute little outfit you meant to put on him before now will no longer cover his legs. He's growing, and he's growing fast! Check the calendar if your baby is suddenly wanting to breastfeed around the clock. He's probably going through a growth spurt. This can vary, but to give you an idea, expect growth spurts at two weeks, sometime between week three and week six, and three months. If you need to reassure yourself, circle the weeks around these rough estimates in red. That way, when all your baby wants to do is breastfeed, you'll remember why.

During a growth spurt, you should not supplement. Any time you supplement, you *decrease* your milk supply because your breast won't be stimulated to make that milk that's now being guzzled in the form of a supplement. Your body is making plenty of milk. (In fact, by now, your baby is probably taking in a quart or more in a twenty-four-hour period.) Typically, there is a three- to four-day lag period between your baby's request for more (or less) milk and your body's adjustment in supply. That's why the baby power-nurses for a few days ahead of time. He's giving you cues to get your milk supply up to meet his new needs.

These growth spurts are one of the reasons why lactation consultants advise working mothers to try to stay home for three months. If you're back at work during days when your infant would usually be building up your milk supply, supply can often dip below demand. Frequent pumping won't accomplish the same thing, but it will keep your milk supply up better than not pumping frequently. Babies are more efficient—and a lot more fun—than pumping, but pumping is definitely better than nothing.

### Dealing with a Perceived Six-week Milk Crisis

Dr. Jane Heinig, a researcher at the University of California at Davis, says that if there's one thing she'd like new mothers to know, it's that they shouldn't wean or supplement at six weeks just because they suddenly feel they aren't making enough milk. "This seems to be the number one time to wean because two new things are happening that moms don't expect: first, your body suddenly adjusts to making milk, and your breasts won't feel full anymore. Second, your baby is going through a growth spurt and will be at the breast sometimes constantly in order to build up the milk supply." Dr. Heinig says that mothers start worrying at about six weeks that they aren't producing enough milk because they can't really feel stored milk in their breasts anymore and because the baby seems so hungry (actually, what you were feeling before was swelling, not quarts of milk). This is normal. Expect this, and you won't have to worry that your child isn't getting enough to eat. Yes, he is hungrier. That's why he's eating all the time, but his increase in demand will cause the milk-producing cells to step up production.

### Did You Know Both Breasts Might Not Work the Same?

Don't be surprised if one breast works differently than the other—one may be easier for your baby to latch on to, may become less irritated, and may produce more milk. This is normal. My left breast always seemed to produce more milk and have a faster let-down response. When I pumped, I'd sometimes get 30 to 40 percent more out of my left breast, though I thought I was faithfully rotating. My left breast was also less sensitive than my right breast. All of this may have been because my daughter seemed to prefer my left breast. Even though I thought I was letting her breastfeed for the same amount of time on both sides, she probably spent more time on the left breast. Eventually, this became a problem. You want your baby stimulating milk production on both sides. If you heavily favor one breast, you'll end up looking very lopsided in clothes. If your baby doesn't take both breasts at every feed, try to remember to rotate them next time. To remember, some women will put a safety pin on the bra strap of the last breast used. This seemed like too much trouble to me since I barely had the energy to snap the flaps closed on my bra. Rebecca says she transfers a ring from hand to hand to remember. With my second baby, I sometimes helped myself to my older daughter's stickers and moved them from hand to hand, but she eventually caught me and limited me to little ones, which didn't stick.

## Did You Know You'll Lose Weight If You Breastfeed?

Yes, read that sentence again. It says, "you'll lose weight." Your body stores a lot of extra weight, particularly in those swinging, pendulous breasts. Studies show that if you breastfeed past three months, by the end of your baby's first year of life, usually with no extra dieting, you'll be back to your prepregnancy weight. Those same studies show that mothers who use artificial baby milk or wean before three months, on average, keep an extra four to five pounds. This can start to add up if you plan to have more than one child.

## Dealing with Depression

Your body won't hit equilibrium for a while. You may occasionally feel depressed. If you suspect it's chronic, get some medical help. If it hits you in waves, little things that may seem to take a lot of effort to do are the things that will make you feel better right now. Make an effort to wear something that makes you feel pretty, and put on a little mascara. My husband came home one day, took a look at me and said, "You look like you slept under an overpass." I didn't even look *that* good. But remember, you're pulling yourself together not to get compliments from your partner, but so that you'll feel better about yourself. If you look decent, you'll feel decent. If you look like you slept under an overpass, you might feel like a bag lady.

Exercise is another thing you will not feel like doing, because you are out of shape. But the only way to get in shape is to start doing something. The time will pass, anyway. You have no control over that, so you might as well lose the weight rather than keep it.

## Dealing with Other Worries: Is Breastfeeding Sexual?

Sandra Jansen, a registered nurse and lactation educator who educates groups of breastfeeding women and couples, says one of the most frequent questions she gets goes something like this: "Women will call me, and say in a whisper, 'I really like breastfeeding.' And I'll say, 'Umm-hmmm,' and they'll say, 'No, you don't quite understand. I really like it.'" A big fear of many women is that there's something wrong with them if they enjoy breastfeeding. Many also worry about being stimulated in a sexual way. "It's normal if you are," Sandra tells worried mothers. "Your breasts aren't that specific about what feels good. You don't have to feel ashamed. It's totally normal."

Chele Marmet has a different take. "It is definitely not sexual," she says. Even though oxytocin is the same hormone that gets released during sex, your breasts are being used for a very different purpose. But depending on you, this could be a very sensual area of your body.

Here is one of those things that nobody will tell you because it is embarrassing. Some women have actually come to orgasm while they're breastfeeding. You don't have to worry that your body will behave like Meg Ryan's in *When Harry Met Sally* in that famous scene when she fakes an orgasm in a crowded deli. I never had an orgasm while breastfeeding. Most women don't. Some women, in a calm, quiet, private, dark atmosphere—like perhaps lying down, half-asleep might. Don't panic if this does happen. Your brain has just secreted a hormone that is telling your body to feel good. This does not make you a child molester, and it doesn't make breastfeeding immoral. You just need to know this is a possibility, so that if it happens, you won't turn yourself inside out wondering what you did wrong. But it's not that likely, so try not to worry about it or let it stand in the way of a comfortable breastfeeding relationship with your baby.

## Dealing with Leaking in Public

You may have to keep nursing pads around for about a month. Some women don't need them at all. Some don't need them after the first few weeks. But if you continue to leak, keep a pair in every bag you use. (Just what you need. More junk to carry in your purse.) The one day you forget to put them in will be the day you're wearing a dark green silk blouse to a business meeting with ten men. No, I didn't do this, but I know someone who did. Mary, an accountant, was discussing changes in tax law with a roomful of executives. The other woman in the room kept motioning with her head. Mary failed to pick up the signal. She did notice that all the men were squirming uncomfortably and not laughing at any of her jokes. In the office restroom during a break, she saw the reason: she had two dinner-plate-sized wet spots on her chest. Susan, a police sergeant, had another solution: "My bullet-proof vest helped with the engorgement, and it's waterproof." God forbid you have a let-down response while asking your boss for a raise, or, in Susan's case, in the middle of reading a suspect his Miranda rights.

Within a few months, sometimes even a few weeks, your body gets the hang of it and stops deciding to squirt milk every time it feels like it or because it's had some kind of stimulus. Merilyn reported that she leaked every time she heard anything that resembled the sound of a crying baby. For her, that meant a squeaking door, someone sneezing, high-pitched phony laughter.

There are some handy tricks you can use if you feel yourself starting to leak, and you've forgotten to bring along pads. Cross your arms tightly across your chest. Pressure alone should stop the milk-ejection reflex. Or, if it's not going to be too conspicuous, it works better to put direct pressure on your nipples. I know, you're howling at the idea of Mary continuing to lecture the male executives while squeezing her nipples. I'm just offering suggestions. Don't take them if you think they'll get you arrested.

## Weight Charts: Did You Know They're Based on Bottle-fed Babies?

Before you compare your baby's weight to the weight on the chart at the doctor's office, you need to know something. Those charts were put together years ago by formula manufacturers and are based on the weight of bottle-fed babies. This is important to know because bottle-fed babies tend to gain weight at a much faster rate. Researchers now say this is because bottle-fed babies are getting fed too much. Pediatrician Robert Hamilton says this is an especially hard concept for the fathers of breastfed babies to understand. "There's no question that growth charts can interfere with breastfeeding," he says. "Fathers in particular just want to know what 'percentile' their kid is in. They don't listen to me when I tell them not to focus on the percentiles."

Dr. Heinig has done pioneering studies called the DARLING studies (Davis Area Research on Lactation, Infant Nutrition, and Growth). "We've been able to show that breastfed babies are normal weight and artificially fed babies are overweight," Dr. Heinig says.

In general, breastfed babies grow rapidly their first two to three months. Then, they tend to grow more slowly. Bottle-fed babies are "significantly heavier than breastfed infants at each month between seven and eighteen months among boys and between six and eighteen months among girls." There was no significant difference in length (height) between the bottle-fed and the breastfed group. Breastfed babies are leaner during the period of life when a lifetime supply of fat cells are laid down (at about eighteen months). This certainly helps to explain why breastfed babies may tend to be leaner during their lifetimes.

## Breastfeeding in Public

Since too many people don't know the extraordinary benefits of breastfeeding, you may still feel like you're on your own once you leave your house with the baby. Many states have begun passing laws to protect your right to breastfeed anyplace you're legally allowed to be. Some states don't have these laws. But in the past five years or so, women have stopped getting arrested or thrown out of places for breastfeeding in public. Notice I said *in public*, not *publicly*. Contrary to some legislators' arguments that laws allowing breastfeeding in public places will encourage women to take their tops off at restaurants, in shopping malls, and in places of business around the country, most women I know didn't have babies or breastfeed because they secretly wanted to be exhibitionists. The last thing, and I mean the last thing, that I wanted anyone other than my husband and baby looking at was one of my breasts. Don't hyperventilate at the thought of breastfeeding outside of your locked bedroom. You can breastfeed discreetly. So discreetly that you can have a conversation with someone, up close and personal, who likely won't know that you're doing "it."

## Remember How You Used to Feel

I have a confession to make. Before I had a baby, I think I was one of those people who was uncomfortable about breastfeeding. I conveniently can't quite remember, but I have some vague recollection of looking the other way when I saw suspicious movement under the large T-shirt of a new mother about to breastfeed on a park bench. It wasn't as bad as being seven and imagining my parents having sex, but it made me, and I know it makes others, squirm a little.

Be prepared for this. In some ways, and depending on the part of the country you live in, you are still a pioneer. You are not a small minority, though. And think of all of those early joggers running past tables of fat smokers.

## Dealing with Your First Time

Eventually, even the most private, modest woman—the kind who won't go into a communal dressing room—will want to start resuming a life outside the walls of home. Before you've actually done it, taking your baby out of your breastfeeding sanctuary is a lot like those dreams you have in fourth grade in which you're swinging on the jungle gym, realizing too late that you've forgotten to wear underpants. Here's the shocker: no one ever gets a look at your breasts but your baby. You don't have to expose anything to give your baby breakfast, lunch, and dinner in public. And necessity is the mother of relaxed standards. There's no way in hell you'll listen to that baby scream if the solution is mounted on your chest. Even in Los Angeles, where bare midriffs, necklines that plunge to the navel, and exposed thighs are the norm, I was still occasionally subjected to strange looks and was asked at least a hundred times, "Are you *still* breastfeeding?" when my first baby was still so young, she couldn't turn over by herself.

I was having lunch at a sidewalk diner right off of the famous Venice Beach boardwalk, where Deadheads mingle with runners, cyclists, and roller skaters in various states of undress, when my daughter Olivia was a few weeks old. It looked to me like a place where you could try out any fashion, as long as your outfit covered the same parts a Las Vegas showgirl is required to keep under wraps. In the middle of lunch, my baby woke from her nap and started crying. The sound of an infant wailing to be fed is about a million times more offensive than the mysterious occasional slurping sound from under a blanket. My friend and I had just been served lunch, and there was really no place to go. So I decided to feed her.

I'm a reasonably modest person, and this was also my first time "outing" myself, so I was careful to make sure no part of my chest was visible. Still, I found myself embarrassed and uncomfortable as people stared at me and then looked away with downcast eyes and made those little tsk-tsk expressions. I felt like a thirteen-year-old caught making out in public. When a woman skated by wearing a string bikini top with a thong bottom, no one stopped talking or stared. (Well, maybe the men stared. But with stupid smiles, not disapproving scowls.) And my friend (my ex-friend) said, "Can't you give her something else?" Like what? A cheeseburger? Chili fries? A chocolate shake maybe?

Sally was a shy and modest woman, who would only breastfeed in front of her husband. When her second daughter was born thirteen months after the first, she had to get over her modesty and breastfeed wherever she happened to be. She figured this out one day at the park when they'd been there less than five minutes. Sixteen-month-old Miranda had no intention of getting off the slide and coming to the car so that Mommy could breastfeed three-month-old baby Sarah. "I kept saying, 'Please Miranda,' while Sarah screamed at the top of her lungs. Finally, both children were crying: Miranda because she didn't want to leave five minutes after she'd arrived, and Sarah because she wanted to eat—five minutes after her last meal." Sally let Miranda play and sat down on a park bench. "It wasn't nearly as bad as I'd thought it would be. I laugh at myself now. It seems weird that I was so worried about doing it outside of my house." Jennifer says that when she and her husband went "out" to dinner in the beginning, "We ate in the car. Then I got braver, and I thought, 'Oh the hell with it. No one can see anything anyway, so what difference does it make if they know what I'm doing?'" Most of the time, if you're discreet, no one will know what you're doing.

## Most People Are Nice

Looking back, I realize I was overly sensitive to what I perceived as critical looks. Most people, though they may feel slight embarrassment at first, are tolerant. Marybeth tells a story of breastfeeding her newborn in a shoe store. She went to the back of the store and sat in an aisle full of dusty platform shoes. No one bothered her. Then a woman walked by her. And turned around and walked by her again. And again. Finally, Marybeth said, "Would you like me to leave?" And the embarrassed woman said, "Oh, no, no. I'm pregnant, and I was just wondering if I could ask you about breastfeeding."

## Dealing with a Baby Who Likes to Eat

As you've probably discovered by now, infants who've just spent three hours sucking before you bundle them up and charge to the car can decide within the first thirty seconds of your outing that they're hungry again. It is still always best to breastfeed your baby right before you go out, even if you have an infrequent feeder, because if he has something in his tummy, hopefully he won't begin wailing the second you get stuck in traffic on the freeway.

Jane, like many mothers of round-the-clock feeders, often had to climb over the back seat and breastfeed Alyx Anne, who had to stay strapped in her carseat (her husband was at the wheel). Jane had to be a contortionist to get her breast near enough to Alyx Anne. "I was just terrified my husband would have to jam on the brakes while I was caught in her mouth." It is much safer and more comfortable to pull the car over to the side of the road, stop, and then breastfeed.

Once, when I was a guest on a radio talk show, a woman called in to tell me that she thought women should "plan" better, so they wouldn't have to breastfeed in public. This woman did not have children. There is no such thing as a scheduled breakfast, lunch, and dinner break with babies. They are like cars with a broken gas gauge. They're puttering along when suddenly they seize up and stop. Sometimes you'll get no warning that they've run out of gas. They need to eat and they need to eat now.

## Dress for Success

The easiest way to deal with the inevitability of having to breastfeed on the spot—let's say, when you're already trying to be inconspicuous in the "ten-items-or-less" line while you're trying to slide through eleven—is to dress for the task. That means, no matter how much you like the tight ankle-length slip dress that zips up the back, this is probably not the best outfit to wear. Even if you decide you won't be breastfeeding in public because you're going to a wedding or some other place where you won't be comfortable breastfeeding in front of people, still dress so you can breastfeed in a pinch. Feeding a child in a restroom or some other private place will be unbearably uncomfortable if you're stuck sitting on a toilet seat in your bra and panties.

I'm intimately acquainted with how this feels because I learned my lesson the hard way. I wore a tight dress that buttoned down the back to a friend's spring wedding. (Oh that dress was sooo cute—for the short periods of time I was actually wearing it!) I sat in a restroom getting goosebumps, with my new dress around my ankles and my baby slurping leisurely, while the reception went on without us.

## "But I Don't Want to Breastfeed in Public"

If you're too modest to breastfeed in public, there is always the restroom. If there is no other choice, and you don't feel comfortable on a park bench, in the furniture section of the department store, or at a back table at a restaurant, you may have to use a restroom. But if you're in a mall, take a few minutes to scope it out, or ask a mother if she knows of a restroom that has a lounge area. I checked out all the malls near my house, and I can still give anyone a rundown of all the mall bathrooms, including which ones have the nicest wallpaper, the most comfortable chairs, the best changing area; which are the most frequently scrubbed with cleansing powder; and which are the most likely to get a raised eyebrow if you're breastfeeding there.

At the same time, if you just can't face ever, ever having to breastfeed in public and you don't want to do it in a restroom, there are still plenty of options. Susan, the Los Angeles police sergeant, was always afraid she'd run into an officer she knew, someone she'd arrested, or, worst of all, a subordinate officer whom she supervised. When she was off duty and out in public with baby Ada, she'd bypass the women's restrooms and mall benches and breastfeed in her car. I would suggest that if you plan to do this, spend some money and get your car windows tinted. Some states only allow you to tint the back windshield and passenger door windows. But that's okay. You can't safely or comfortably drive and breastfeed anyway.

Some women pump their milk and carry a bottle of pumped breastmilk when they go out with the baby. If this makes you more comfortable, try it. It does have a downside, though, so be forewarned. Your body will still be making milk during that bottle feeding, so while your baby has a bottle, your breasts may get engorged. If your baby is six weeks or younger, you're likely to start leaking as soon as your baby starts drinking. And your baby may not take a bottle from you, so you may end up having to breastfeed, anyway. But find out what works for you. If this is the only way you're comfortable, then pumped milk in a bottle is still better than formula. But try not to do it so often that it cuts down on your milk supply.

## Tips for Discreet Breastfeeding

When my daughters were really young and nursing every five seconds, I would put them in a front baby carrier and wear a nursing shirt. They could ride around in the carrier, and I could shop at a leisurely pace. When they got hungry, I'd just maneuver them into place to nurse, and everyone smiled and cooed at us. They thought the baby was sleeping. "How cute!"

Some women use a piece of cloth knotted at the top, then slipped like a sling over one shoulder. The baby can ride along with you, and you can breastfeed even while walking. Others get two dozen baby carriers at their baby showers, so they have plenty of choices when it comes to how to get around with a newborn.

## How to Soothe Relatives, Friends, and Other Well-Wishers

Everybody and his brother has an opinion about breastfeeding and most feel compelled to express it. I don't suggest you say any of the following rejoinders out loud, but if you need some relief, you can smile and nod sweetly while someone delivers his opinion—and think these responses in your head.

**Your mother:** "You'll turn him into a sissy!"
**You:** "Actually, we're hoping he has a fine career in fashion design."

---

**Your mother:** "I didn't breastfeed and you turned out okay."
**You:** "Mom, you were a great mother, and I have no regrets (except I would've loved the extra I.Q. points). But now we know a lot more about breastmilk, so I'd feel guilty if I didn't do it."

---

**Your mother-in-law:** "Don't you think he'll remember that he sucked his mother's breast?"
**You:** "We've already set aside his therapy fund."
**You:** "Wouldn't that be great? His wife will be so appreciative."
**You:** "Maybe he'll be nicer to me when he's a teenager."
**You:** "He'll remember all the bad things I ever did to him so isn't it nice that he can remember one of the good things?"

---

**Your single friends:** "Are you still doing that?"
**You:** (innocently): "Feeding her? Yes. Can't I get arrested for child endangerment if I don't?"
**You:** "Yes, but only until she's old enough to cut her own meat."
**You:** "Yes, and I'm doing it just to bug you."
**You:** "Yes, but I know I'll have to wean her so she can attend a college out of state."
**You:** "Yes, we ran out of formula."

---

**Your husband's single friends:** "Are you still doing that?"
**You:** "Yes, but only because it's such a thrill for me."
**You:** "Yes, we want to make sure he lives at home until his pension kicks in."

**You:** "Yes. And your point is . . .??"
**You:** "Doing what?"

## How to be Nice to People You Won't be Able to Kiss Off

The hardest people to dissuade are the people you'll have to see again. Those people may even be your mother and/or your mother-in-law. They can't help but have an opinion. Laura counsels new breastfeeding mothers and hears the same story over and over. "These new mothers feel like they're being criticized. Their mothers are not only *not* supportive, some of them are downright subversive." Theresa, a Mexican American who married a man from Thailand, said that her husband's family associated breastfeeding with being poor. When her first baby was born, each time she fed him, her mother-in-law would make comments like, "Your breasts are too small. You won't make enough milk."

But what mothers and mothers-in-law are saying between the lines is not, "I was a much better mother," but, surprisingly, "Reassure me that I was a good enough mother.'" Try and hear that what sounds like critical nagging might be the sound of a mother who's insecure. Mothers worry until their dying day about the things they did wrong (as perfect as you are, you will worry, too). Even though you're a grown-up, your mother may still feel guilty that she did not breastfeed you. She may be feeling bad about this, and now she's discouraging you. As nutty as it seems, she may really want to believe that breastfeeding isn't that big a deal, and that you would still have had allergies—and wouldn't have been a Rhodes scholar—even if she had breastfed you. The best way to disarm her or your mother-in-law is to say, "You were a wonderful mother, and I'm so thankful that you raised [fill in "me" or your husband's name]. We'll probably do some things differently but I want you to know I think you are a terrific mother!" Okay, so lie a little. It'll be easier to get along with her and to preserve that all-important grandparent/grandchild relationship if you say something kind instead of what you want to say.

# Chapter 8

# Getting Some Sleep (Some What?)

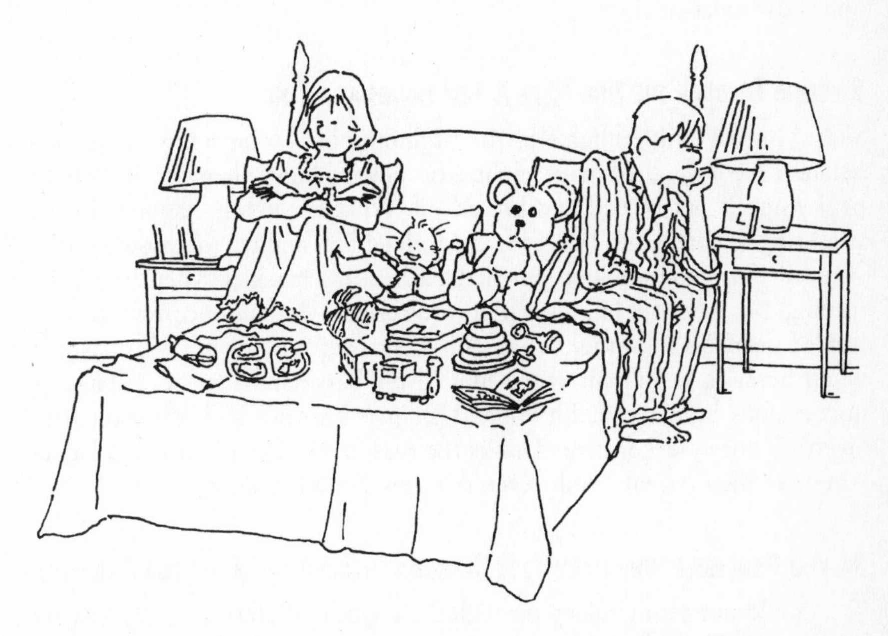

Dr. James McKenna, a professor of anthropology and a leading researcher in the sleep patterns of infants, says, "We need to determine if unrealistic parental expectations, rather than infant pathology, play a role in creating parent-infant sleep struggles." Dr. McKenna goes on to say that this struggle is "one of the most ubiquitous pediatric problems in the country. It may well be that it is not in the biological best interest of all infants to sleep through the night in a solitary environment, as early in life as we may wish, even though it is more convenient if they did so."

Dr. Jay Gordon puts it a bit more succinctly. "If your goal in life is to get your sleep, you made a mistake about nine months ago."

If sleep is a sore topic around your house, consider yourself part of the majority. Infants don't sleep the way we do, and we shouldn't expect them to, any more than we should expect them to walk and talk when they're born.

When people complain about being new parents, they are mostly complaining because they're exhausted. There is a good reason why prisoners of war are tortured with sleep-deprivation. And now you know what kind of prisoner you'd be. "Name, rank and serial number? Sure, and I'll also tell you the time and place of the secret invasion—as soon as you show me a cot."

### Sleeping Through the Night . . . A Few Hours at a Time

Since you have little choice in the beginning but to be following an on-demand feeding schedule at night, you never know when you'll have to haul yourself out of bed and breastfeed. What frequently happens is that you bring the baby into bed with you to feed him and try to get some sleep yourself, fully intending to put him back in his bassinet when he's done feeding. But when he falls asleep on your breast, you fall unconscious from lack of sleep. Your partner, whose job it is to get Junior out of his bassinet when he cries and then return him to his bassinet when he doesn't, is unconscious beside you. Eh voilà. That nice bassinet with the expensive layette is purely decorative. That is the reason why many breastfed babies end up in their parents' bed—even if it's just for a few hours.

### Do You Remember When You Took Sleeping Through the Night for Granted?

You should not plan to sleep through the night until your baby is about six months old. We lucked out with Julia, the second baby, who came into the world able to read our lips: "Go to sleeeeeep." She did, sleeping through the night at the age of about three months. But don't be envious. On the nights Julia enjoyed a full night's sleep, we still did not since her big sister Olivia suddenly developed sleep problems. Many parents have to wait until their children turn three—years, that is. Some babies will sleep for long periods before six months. But most need the extra food. They are waking up not to bug you but because they are hungry and need to be fed.

If your friend brags that her baby sleeps through the night, have her define what she means. Mary told me her son "slept through the night," but what he was doing was sleeping a four-hour stretch from 2:00 a.m. to 6:00 a.m.—and it only felt like it was a full night.

## "Can't You Teach Them to Sleep?"

Some women think that weaning their baby off the breast is the way to sleep at night. It isn't. (You'll still have to feed them and formula feeding is even harder at night.) Rebecca wanted to know how she could "teach" ten-week-old Justin how to sleep through the night. "My friends kept asking, 'Is he sleeping through the night yet?' And every time I said, 'No,' they gave me that look like, 'Well, guess he won't be going to Harvard.'"

Some research done in the early 1990s and published in *Pediatrics*, the journal of the American Academy of Pediatrics, seems to indicate that, yes, maybe you can influence a baby's sleep patterns. But when researchers talked about "sleeping through the night," they were referring to a five-hour stretch between midnight and 5 a.m, which isn't exactly a full night's beauty rest for most people.

The researchers began with a "focused" feeding between 10 p.m. and midnight. That was the only regimented feeding the mother had to do. The idea was to put a well-fed infant to bed. Then parents were instructed to "gradually lengthen intervals between middle of the night feeds by carrying out alternative caretaking behaviors." They were not instructed to let the baby cry himself to sleep, but to try things other than feeding first when he woke up crying: reswaddling the infant, changing his diaper, or walking around with him. If none of that worked, then they were told to feed the baby. Parents also went out of their way to make a big deal out of the difference between night and day. The study showed a high rate of success getting young babies to sleep for a five-hour stretch. The babies didn't drink any less milk than those who were breastfed during the night. They just made up for it by breastfeeding more at the first feeding in the morning and throughout the day.

## Take Your Baby into Account

Even the researchers acknowledged that temperament played a key role in sleep. Infants who had a "low sensory threshold," that is, seemed more sensitive to anything affecting their environment, were the ones most likely to have night waking problems.

Don't get upset if your baby seems "difficult." Some of the most "difficult" babies grow up to be some of the brightest, most creative people. Yes, it is harder on your nerves if your baby isn't always giggling and smiling. But nobody's baby does this all the time.

And even among the 50 percent of parents who reported that their baby slept through the night, when the researchers recorded the baby sleeping, only 15 percent actually slept through the night. The rest woke up, then settled back to sleep without waking up their parents.

## "But Everybody Says He Should"

It's not a race. Not yet, anyway. Not until preschool. Yet sleep is the number one issue in this part of the world. We like our sleep and we want babies to fit into our sleep/wake patterns as soon as they come home. Unfortunately, it doesn't work that way. Remember when you settled down to sleep when you were pregnant and your baby decided, "Oh goody! Everything's quiet, must be Gymboree time!" Your movements during the day rocked your baby to sleep in your womb. You can't expect your new baby to appreciate the difference between night and day the way you do. Your baby will eventually figure it out, and you're not doing anything wrong if he's waking you up. But there is much more at work here than figuring out the difference between night and day.

"Grown-ups spend 80 percent of their sleep time in deep sleep, and 20 percent in shallow sleep," says pediatrician Jay Gordon. "Babies reverse that: 80 percent of their sleep time is shallow, 20 percent is deep. They're meant to eat, rest, eat, and grow."

## You Really Are Their Blankie

Babies come into this world with certain biological expectations. One of them is close proximity to you during sleep. Until relatively recently in human history, parents and infants slept together. In our culture, the goal is to get babies to be as independent as possible. This need to be free of babies, particularly at night, is in direct opposition to what babies seem to be needing from their parents, particularly at night. That's why the struggle to get your baby into his own bed can get so difficult. Just as researchers are learning there's more to breastmilk, they are also learning there is more to this sleep thing.

Getting your child to sleep, in your bed or in his crib, may become an obsession for you when even toothpicks won't keep your eyes open. You need to know that there is a range of options as to where your baby or child sleeps, and that even if you find yourself in a pattern, you can still change it.

## "Oh, But the Nursery Is So Cute!"

I spent months of my first pregnancy searching for just the right fabric for the perfect quilt and for girlish curtains and festive pillows (which babies aren't supposed to have, anyway). It was that stupid nesting hormone. I think my body overdosed on it. Finally, I had put together the perfect room—a room my daughter will probably want to change as soon as she starts to notice decor.

But when she came home from the hospital, even if she'd been old enough to notice, she didn't see enough of her room to pass judgment on the pink and green motif. She was so little for that big, imposing, cold, crisp white-and-pink-sheeted crib. I couldn't put her in that. So I put her in a tiny little bassinet next to our bed. That arrangement lasted one evening. By the end of the night, she was in our bed. We might as well have covered her perfect room in sheets because by the time she used that crib, there was a layer of dust on it nearly a year old.

## Sleeping Family Style

Many couples end up bringing the baby into bed with them. "It's simply the best survival mechanism for the first six months," Sandra Jansen, lactation consultant, tells parents at the childbirth preparation classes she teaches. Letting your baby sleep with you is called having a *family bed*.

I think all of us envision a family bed as a pile of people huddled together for warmth on a dirt floor. I think of the television show "The Waltons." Even though they had separate beds (it *was* big-budget network television), whenever I hear of the family bed, I think of John-Boy and all of his brothers and sisters in one bed sharing a tattered blanket with their toes hanging out.

I hadn't planned to have my daughter in our bed. I just had to learn how to sleep with her in my bed for a while, like a lot of parents. It was the only way we all could get some sleep. Sandra Jansen, who has two children, says she was against having her first baby sleep with her in bed until one night, she found herself nodding off in the rocking chair and woke up to find her baby somewhere between her knees and the floor. "I was so tired, my arms were just releasing her. I decided that it was dangerous to breastfeed at night anywhere but in bed."

Getting up, breastfeeding, settling the baby down, getting back in bed, falling asleep again, then having this cycle repeat itself three or four times a night would drive even a saint insane. If you are letting your child sleep in your bed, I'll let you in on a little secret: you are part of the majority, not the minority. Feel better?

## "If I Let Him In, Won't He Think He Can Stay?"

Many people will also tell you never, ever to bring a baby into bed with you because you'll never get him out. This is also not true. If you and your husband are both comfortable with the idea of temporarily sharing your bed, then there is nothing wrong with it. Any pattern *can* be changed.

## "Who's Making All That Noise?"

Babies are not quiet sleepers. They poop, burp, sigh, cough, and sputter like little old men all night long. If you find yourself continually being woken up, you might want to try earplugs, though make sure you can still hear your baby if he starts to cry.

## "Can I Hurt Him If He Sleeps with Us?"

I was so terrified I'd roll over and kill my daughter that I remained ever-vigilant, frozen in a position I thought I'd never break myself out of. Jansen tells new parents not to worry about rolling over and smothering their newborns. "When I had children, I had to remind myself that I hadn't fallen out of bed since I was six and sleeping at my friend's house," she says. However, co-sleeping is not a good idea if you have a waterbed (the baby could suffocate or roll around), if you are intoxicated by alcohol or drugs, or if either you or your partner is grossly overweight.

## "What If I Don't Like the Idea of Sharing My Bed?"

Some babies sleep very peacefully with their parents. I did not have that experience. My first daughter liked to sleep with my breast in her mouth. As soon as her mouth sensed she'd lost contact with the breast, she'd start to scream. That meant that if she slept with us, I had to stay glued to her, and this was uncomfortable for me. Laura says that John thought bedtime in Mommy and Daddy's bed was playtime, even when he was very small. "As soon as we'd start to go to sleep, I'd hear him gurgling and playing with my hair, trying to get me to stay up and coo at him."

Michael says his son Jared slept between him and his wife Cheryl for two and a half years. "I wasn't angry so much as I was resentful." Though Michael had hunted for a California king-size bed, a good foot wider than a regular king-size bed, there was still no room for Daddy. "My son would sleep sideways. He was kicking and rolling, and his foot was in my ear, and I'd think, 'Geez, it's not even *Cheryl's* foot!'" With Jared between him and his wife, Michael was unable to get near Cheryl. And there was another, more immediate problem. Baby Jared wasn't in danger of rolling out of bed, but his father was. "Here we were in this huge bed, and Jared had most of it....I was left trying to sleep on about fourteen inches of bed."

When son Gabe came along three and a half years later, Michael and Cheryl had only recently reclaimed their bed. Jared had moved out of it but still slept on a blanket at the foot of their bed until the new baby came along. Michael and Cheryl decided they couldn't repeat this sleeping arrangement with a new baby. Michael says, "We let Gabe sleep in our bed until he was two months old, then I said, 'Sorry buddy, but this is where you sleep.'" Gabe fussed at being put in his crib, and Michael still got up an average of six times a night, this time to get Gabe out of his crib and bring him to Cheryl to breastfeed, then to put Gabe back in his own bed.

But even Michael, who now has the full seventy-two inches of bed all to himself and his wife's foot in his ear again instead of his infant son's, says he can't decide which method was better. "They were just different ways to eventually achieve the same thing," he says. "I definitely had a very close bond to Jared because he was with us at night."

## Some Ways Around a Family Bed

Some new parents decide to sleep in close proximity to their baby instead of with their baby. Roberta and Tom pushed their bed against one side of the baby's crib, then took the side of the crib off, so that the two beds became one sleeping arrangement. They slept in their double bed, but they were literally right next to their baby.

Jim worked during the day and his wife Rhonda stayed home with the baby. When he came home at 6:30, he took care of baby Alexandra while Rhonda slept until 11:00 p.m. Then he slept by himself in another room until 6:30 a.m., while Rhonda and Alexandra slept together in the master bedroom. At 6:30, he got up and took the baby again for two hours so his wife could get some sleep. If you are at home and your husband or partner is working, you will still be tired from "working" all day, too. You may be able to work out a similar arrangement so that you can get a little bit of sleep, too.

You can also rotate nights, the way Carrie and Robert did. She would wake up and breastfeed one night, and he would get up and give his daughter pumped milk the next. This was more trouble than it was worth for Carrie, though, because on the nights it wasn't her turn, her breasts would become engorged, and half the time, she'd wake up in pain and pump anyway.

### How to Breastfeed While Sleeping

When I was getting my daughter to go to sleep at night, I'd first put her on the outside edge of the bed to give her the first breast while I was still conscious. I sleep on the left side of the bed; ergo, she got my left breast first. Once she'd milked the left breast, I'd put her in the middle of the bed, between my husband and me, for the right breast. That way, I didn't have to worry about her rolling off the edge of the bed while we slept.

As she got bigger, and I got back in shape thanks to my aerobics classes, I was eventually flexible enough again to offer her my right and my left breast while lying on my right side so that she always stayed in the middle between us. Tricky, eh? Some women also like sleeping on their backs and propping the baby on their chest and stomach to nurse.

### "Don't Ever, Ever, No Matter What, Let Him Fall Asleep While Breastfeeding"

Many books recommend that you do not ever allow your child to fall asleep on your breast. This may be good advice, but it's very impractical advice. I'd bet money that most of the people who tell you this do not have breasts. Breastfeeding a baby who is dropping off to sleep is something that you will probably not be able to prevent. It just happens. Babies sleep a lot, and sometimes they sleep at your breast. It's a nice experience for you and for your baby to nurse until the eyelids droop, the mouth loses its grip, and the baby relaxes into a deep, blissful sleep. The books are right about one thing, however. Once your arm begins to fall asleep and you ever so carefully ease yourself up, being careful not to move your frozen arms, and tiptoe to the crib to gently lower your baby into it (while still attached to your breast) you have a problem. The problem is, you do not fit into your child's crib. Once you are no longer serving as the human pacifier, guess who wakes up?

One cautionary note: There is something called "baby bottle mouth" or "nursing caries" that you do not ever want to have to experience firsthand. It is a devastating type of tooth decay. Since your baby probably started sprouting teeth at about six months, here's what you need to know about what dentists' officially call, "Baby Bottle Tooth Decay" or BBTD. To have a problem, your baby needs four things: teeth, bacteria, food for the bacteria, and time to develop. Food for the bacteria is any *fermentable carbohydrate*. That includes breastmilk. Time to develop means night after night of milk or juice hanging around new teeth. The bacteria is a specific type that you and the rest of the family may also have in your mouths.

Usually, BBTD is found in bottle-fed babies who are put to bed with a bottle. As the baby sleeps, that last bit of milk or juice he sucked but never got around to swallowing because he fell asleep, pools around his teeth and can begin decomposing those cute little pearly whites. BBTD is less likely in breastfed babies because the nipple where the milk comes out is usually back in their throat away from their teeth. But dentists report they do occasionally see BBTD in breastfed babies who feed all night long. Watch for chalky white spots or lines on teeth. Get a baby toothbrush or little plastic finger cap brush sold at most grocery stores. Use it on your baby's teeth as soon as the teeth are visible. Fluoride in your diet should reduce the possibility of BBTD. Check to see if the water you drink is fluoridated. Check with a dentist, doctor or lactation consultant if you're concerned about your nighttime feedings.

## Sleep Rituals

As children get older, the way they put themselves to sleep evolves out of the way that you teach them to do it. If they associate falling asleep with having your breast in their mouths, eventually this will be the only way they can get to sleep, and then you may have to teach them another way.

Laurie has a two-and-a-half-year-old son named Jack. She and her husband have developed an elaborate ritual to put Jack to sleep: "You have to sit at the very edge of the bed, not in the middle or on the side, put your finger in his mouth so that he can suck on it, jiggle him on your lap, and sing 'Walk Like A Man!'—oh, and the vacuum cleaner has to be on. And then, I breastfeed until he goes to sleep." Any pattern children have learned can be changed. It is not engraved in stone, or Jack's future wife would have to repeat this ritual for him every night.

### Develop a Ritual You Can Live With

I tried to develop a bedtime ritual for my first daughter. When she was a little baby, I read her a book, then said "Goodnight" to each of her toys in the same order. But this never caught on. When my husband put her to bed, he read a book, kissed her little pink blanket, pulled it up around her chin, and sang three songs. She liked his ritual better.

## How to Tell When Your Baby's Getting Tired

To tell when your baby's tired you'll need to watch for signs of sleepiness. Usually, your alert, sweet baby will begin to fuss. If it isn't food he's fussing about, it is probably sleep. Then he'll move to the next stage of sleepiness: he'll spit out pacifiers, cry when you try to breastfeed him, rub his eyes, squirm and be generally inconsolable.

Get going with your sleep ritual sooner rather than later. (You'll eventually need to develop a naptime ritual as well. The naptime ritual can just be a shorter bedtime ritual.) Try to start your bedtime ritual before your baby or toddler gets past the point when he's rubbing his eyes and whining a little. In our house, when my first daughter was tired, we got "noodle girl." She turned into a wet piece of spaghetti and wouldn't sit in her chair, get in her carseat, or help in the changing process. At my friend Suzan's house, they call Francesca "2-x-4 girl" because when *she's* tired, she stiffens into a plywood child. If you miss your opportunity to settle your baby down for the night (because you're taking a phone call, you got home late from work, or you forgot the time), you'll find that it may take much, much longer to get your now anxious, unhappy, and crying baby to sleep because he's so wound up from fatigue.

## Practical Tips for Bedtime

Don't take phone calls after a certain time, even if they're work calls. Turn on your answering machine so you won't be tempted to interrupt bedtime by picking up the phone. (You can even change the message, so people know you're home and will be available to return calls after the baby's in bed.) If there's a television show you want to watch and it starts in three minutes, forget it. Either tape it, or watch the show that follows it. Allow enough time to complete the sleep ritual, and don't be impatient. Know that it'll take at least fifteen minutes (more if bathtime is included) to get your child to bed (yes, this will be for the rest of your life, or until your child decides he wants his own apartment).

Aside from breastfeeding, reading a story is probably the most common ritual, even for young babies (though young babies are more interested in eating books than in reading them). Read slowly. Speak in your nice, soft, warm storytime voice. Make slow transitions, that is, don't slap the book closed, say "Good night!" and walk out of the room. Let the baby know that the story is over, it's time to go to sleep, and Mommy and Daddy will be leaving the room now. Tell the baby where you're going to be: "Daddy and I are going to be right next door in our room."

Stick to a predictable routine from the beginning so that, for example, your baby comes to expect one story and three songs. Babies don't need variety—they like sameness. The predictable routine settles them down and prepares them for sleep.

## Breastfeeding, the Ultimate Sedative

Most mothers don't deliberately set out to use breastfeeding as a sedative. It just seems to happen. There's no quicker way to soothe a baby and get him drowsy than to breastfeed.

Helen had a writing class every Monday night, but Lily wouldn't go to sleep if Helen's husband Eric tried to put her to bed. That's because Eric doesn't have breasts and Lily liked to fall asleep at her mother's breast. This was fine with Helen, except for Monday nights. Finally, Helen started pumping a bottle of milk and leaving it with Eric so that Lily could fall asleep. This is a solution that ultimately will cause problems, however. As babies get older, they don't need food at night, but if they learn to associate falling asleep with eating, they won't be able to put themselves back to sleep when they wake at night. Also remember that any kind of liquid (other than water) left to pool around budding teeth may lead to decay. If you can help it, don't get into this routine. Give your baby (when he's six months or older) his final feeding of the day when he's still awake.

## Working Parents

If you work, your job is harder because you'll need to be semi-coherent during the day. Of course, it depends on the kind of work you do. Maybe you work in a profession where it's a benefit to be semi-coherent, like the job I once had licking stamps.

Many parents who work outside the home take shifts so that each one gets a good night's sleep every other night. One night one parent takes care of the baby, the next night the other parent does. Since you're breastfeeding, this may not work. But even if every few days your husband can give your baby pumped milk, you might be able to keep severe sleep deprivation at bay. Sleep research on subjects who were up for several days at a time (to the point of keeling over) recovered from their ordeal with just one good night of sleep. One full night can make up for three nights without. Even if you still feel tired in the morning, your body is nearly back to its normal state.

### Babies Will Take the Graveyard Shift

Some babies will actually reverse their feeding schedule once they figure out your new hours. My first daughter did this, so nighttime for her was time to make up for all the feedings she hadn't had during the day. She was a nighttime marathon nurser. There wasn't a whole lot I could do to change this, and frankly I couldn't blame her. I didn't like it that she had to be the one to shift her life around to accommodate mine, but I marveled at how clever babies are and the lengths to which they'll go to maximize their time with Mommy.

### "Easy for You to Say . . ."

Do not despair about this sleep thing. You will find a solution. You may have to tackle the problems individually. For example, if your baby is old enough to make it through the night without food but still wakes up to eat, you'll have to solve the eating part first. If your baby is sleeping in your bed with you, you can deal with that part second. And if your baby needs your help to put himself to sleep, you'll have to tackle that part last. But it will all work out.

It doesn't help all that much, especially when you're so tired you could cry, to hear that this is a temporary condition. But it is. I know you don't feel better, and you're still weeping. Work on slowly changing whatever it is about sleep that's got you down. You will not be able to just say, "Okay, tonight it's all going to be different." Make it different one part at a time.

# Chapter 9

# Problems: From Small Ones to Big Ones

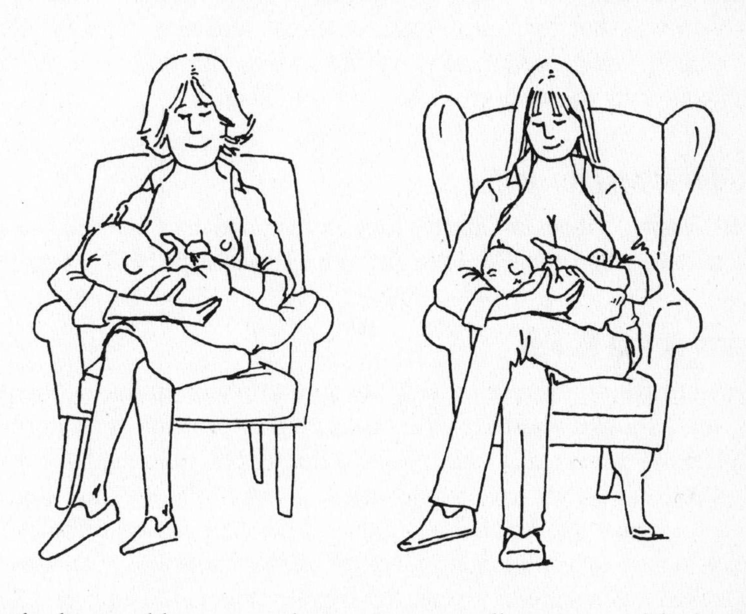

Breastfeeding problems range from minor to really serious to life-threatening. Once you've tried simple solutions, move on to the more complex. If you're sure that you're in the right position and the baby is correctly latched-on and you're still having problems, you may need intervention from a good lactation consultant. Many problems can be fixed, often simply by one phone call to a professional. If you aren't producing enough milk, there are a myriad of reasons why this may be happening. It is not necessarily because you have insufficient mammary tissue, though in rare cases, that happens. Your baby may not be stimulating your breasts to produce enough milk because of a problem he's having. He might have a receding chin (a problem that can be remedied with a different position, which a lactation expert can show you), or he might have a very poor suck (either because of anatomy or because he got confused by various nipples along the way). He might have a short frenulum, which makes his tongue bunch up and prevents him from sucking properly. Your baby might have severe allergies. He might have a neural tube defect. He might have something else that doctors are missing.

First, you need a doctor to determine whether there is something physically wrong with the baby. Once the baby is given a clean bill of health, it's time to have a consultation with a certified lactation consultant. Either one may advise you to buy a precise scale to carefully monitor your baby's growth, but these scales are expensive and may actually increase your anxiety. Most pediatricians will let you stop by so that a nurse can weigh your baby on the doctor's scale (free of charge).

## Still Having Sore Nipples?

Reread Chapter 5 about latching the baby on and positioning him and you. Also, check the sections on nipple soreness and pain relief in Chapter 6. Then read this.

## Inverted or Flat Nipples

Inverted or flat nipples are actually not an uncommon problem. You probably won't know if you have either because they probably look normal to you. The word *inverted* makes you envision nipples pointing back toward your spine. But if they have a tendency to invert or flatten, they'll only do this in the baby's mouth. Before Leah had her first baby she thought her nipples looked totally normal. What she didn't know was that when her son sucked on her areola tissue, her nipples inverted. Think of a bottle with the nipple pushed in. That's what Leah's nipple did in the baby's mouth, so her breast didn't get formed into a teat. Samantha, another new mother, knew her nipples were flat because unless it was cold out, her nipples were even with her breast. She just didn't know that flat nipples also make breastfeeding more difficult.

To see if you have flat or inverted nipples, you can do a simple test.

Stand in front of a mirror. Cup your hand under your breast and at the areola tissue press your breast together with your fingers. If the nipple pops out, it is normal. If it flattens so that it's level with the surrounding tissue or turns inward, that means it will flatten or invert in your baby's mouth. Guess what? You have flat or inverted nipples.

## What To Do if You Have Inverted or Flat Nipples

Someone might tell you to stretch, roll, massage or pull the nipple. This is outdated advice. You won't be able to do it enough to make a difference and you could damage your breast tissue.

Check with your doctor and find out if you are a candidate for breast shells. They look like small, round plastic saucers with holes. They go directly on your breasts and your nipples go through the holes. The shells will gently press the tissue around the nipples and hopefully get the nipples to evert by putting pressure on the base. Women who know about this condition before birth can wear shells beginning in the second trimester. (The exception is women who've had a previous miscarriage, because shells could cause contractions.) If you've already had your baby, you can still wear shells in between feedings. You'll have to be extra vigilant when you latch your baby on. But once the baby is latched-on properly, your nipples will gradually evert. Some lactation consultants don't believe shells will make a difference, but Cheryl told me she read about shells in the first edition of STWTF!, spent the 20 dollars on shells and by wearing them around in her last month of pregnancy, got her nipples to evert. You can't see the shells under clothes, though if you bump into someone, they might be surprised to feel hard plastic where your breasts should be.

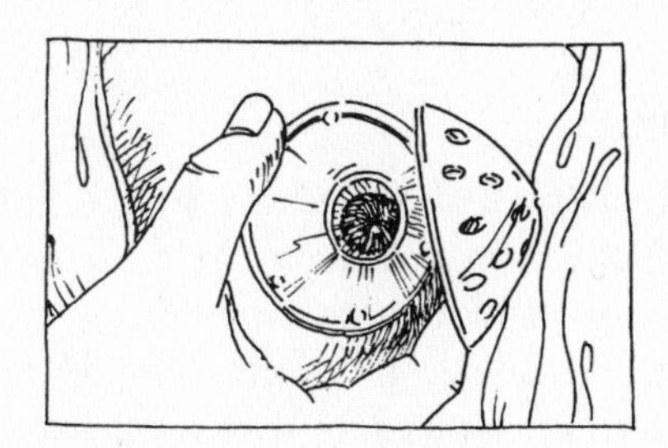

Breast shells: Make sure to buy *shells*, not *shields*. The nipple is gently coaxed into everting through the hole, while the protective top keeps fabrics from putting pressure on your nipple (this can also be used in between feedings to protect sore nipples until they've healed).

Make sure what you are buying are called shells, not shields. This is an important difference. Mothers with sore nipples used to be routinely handed breast shields. The idea was that you could simply cover your breasts with rubber and the pain would go away. But since the shields were essentially rubber nipples attached to your breast, for many babies, they caused nipple confusion and didn't relieve sore nipples. But some lactation consultants recently reported in the *Journal of Human Lactation* that they use them sparingly, and sometimes find they will help a mother over an early hump. Jena used shields for twenty-four hours with her baby Paris, who wouldn't latch on. After just one day, Jena removed the shield and got

Paris on. Before using shields, get help in the form of a good lactation consultant, who can rule out everything else before resorting to shields.

### Short Nipples

You probably won't know you have short nipples until your baby is on your breast and has trouble getting latched-on. If this is happening and you've done everything right, you might need to get him farther up on your breast or to get expert help.

### Extra-Large Nipples

Nurses refer to really large nipples as *champagne corks*. They do this out of the earshot of patients, of course. Most of the time, large nipples won't be a problem. The exception is a premature baby or a baby with a very small mouth. Dawn had premature twins and the largest nipples the hospital staff had ever seen. Her twins were never able to latch on, but Dawn diligently pumped breastmilk and gave it by bottle for six months. Don't assume, though, that because you have large nipples, you'll have to pump or give your baby formula. Most babies will eventually be able to get on after they've grown a little.

### Soreness Caused by a Short Frenulum

Another woman, the mother of triplets, had incredibly sore nipples. (Incidentally, she had breastfeeding down to a science. She'd breastfeed two at a time, giving each his own breast, and then give the third baby the leftovers from both breasts. At the next feeding, the triplets would rotate, and the baby that got the leftovers at the last feeding would get his own breast, and so on. She had to write it down and number the children with a marking pen to keep it all straight.) A lactation consultant went to see this mother and discovered that two of the three triplets had normal sucks but the third triplet had a short frenulum, the piece of skin that holds the tongue down from the underside. A short frenulum results in a tongue that is tacked down too tightly and doesn't stick out far enough. That means that when the baby sucks, he can't get his tongue to the right spot and he grabs the nipple with his tongue, causing friction and soreness. Usually, this anatomical problem is quickly discovered because the milk supply drops or never becomes sufficient (since there is not enough stimulation of the areola tissue). But in this rare case, the other two babies were keeping up the milk supply. A doctor can clip the frenulum to loosen the tongue and allow it to stick out further. A drop or two of blood comes out and then the baby can immediately go back to his favorite pursuit, breastfeeding. Some doctors say this isn't necessary, but if you're having problems due to this, you might consider it.

## Soreness Caused by a Bad Suck

If you and your baby are doing everything right in terms of latch-on and positioning, and you still have sore nipples, you'll want to consider some more possible causes. Look at your nipple after you've gotten it free from your baby's mouth. It should not be discolored, creased, creviced or misshapen in any way. If it doesn't even resemble the nipple that went in there, it's an indication that there is a problem with the baby's suck. You will not be able to tell by looking or feeling with your finger if your baby has what experts call a *poor suck*. You'll need to call in a lactation consultant who deals with such difficult problems. A different position can often fix a baby's suck.

## Some General Rules about L.C.'s

In general, a lactation consultant will check position, then latch-on, then anatomy (yours and baby's), then pathology (medical problem). The consultant will look at the baby breastfeeding, will listen to the sounds the baby makes, and will probably put a finger in the baby's mouth to figure out how he is sucking.

If the lactation consultant only puts a finger in up to the first knuckle, take yourself to another consultant. Rachel complained that three doctors had done this to assess her son's suck. They all concurred. His suck was normal. But they were only putting a tiny piece of their finger in—in essence, they were mimicking a nipple, not a breast. The baby could suck on a nipple. That was the problem, doctor. Finally a lactation consultant put a finger all the way in the baby's mouth to the point where the soft palate meets the hard palate. That means about two-thirds of an adult finger. Eh voilà! There was a problem with his suck!

Because problems with suck range from very simple to very complex, you'll usually need an expert to evaluate your baby's suck. If you have a really complicated suck problem, your lactation consultant can refer you to a physical therapist, occupational therapist, or speech and language pathologist.

## Soreness Caused by Breaking the Suction

Are you sure you're breaking the suction before you take your baby off your breast? A tug of war in which the breast is slowly pulled out of his mouth causes a lot of friction on your nipple as he hangs on for dear life. Before you move your baby off your breast, slide your clean little finger between the edge of his mouth and your breast to break his suction-cup hold on you. Then you can ease him off your breast with your finger on your breast to keep him from reattaching. It also helps to tell him ahead of time that you're taking him off. As he gets older, he may let go himself after he hears your cue.

## Soreness Caused by Thrush, Eczema, or Allergies

You and your baby could share a problem that is causing sore nipples: thrush (a yeast infection), eczema, or allergies.

### Thrush

Look at your baby's mouth. Does it have a white coating? Is your baby gassy and cranky? Does he have a bright red rash, red dots, or a peeling rash on his behind? If you or your baby have just taken antibiotics, you or he may have developed a yeast infection. Check with your pediatrician. There are some over-the-counter remedies for his mouth and bottom and your nipples. If you or your baby have a thrush infection, you'll have to go back to sterilizing everything until it's gone. That means all toys, bottles, pacifiers, and breast pump parts. You should also change your breast pads more frequently.

### Eczema

If you have a history of eczema, you're more likely to have developed eczema on your nipple or areola. Is your nipple area burning, itching, flaking, oozing, scabbing, or crusting? If you've answered "yes" to any of the above, see a dermatologist pronto.

### Allergies

If you or your partner have food sensitivities or allergies, your baby might have them, too. On the other hand, even if you have an iron stomach and can digest anything, your baby may be intolerant of foods that you love. Allergies affect muscles, and because the tongue is a muscle, he might have trouble using his tongue to strip milk from your breasts.

If the baby is allergic to something you're eating and he's getting it through your breastmilk, you will have to eliminate foods one at a time for about a week each to narrow down the culprit. The Lactation Institute tells mothers to first monitor their milk—not their breastmilk, but the cow's milk they're drinking. Some babies have an extreme intolerance to milk protein in cow's milk. You may have to stop drinking milk and eating dairy products until your baby is older.

It could also be the cauliflower, cabbage, or beans that you're eating, because the baby isn't digesting the cellulose they contain. Wheat is often the culprit because it's a food we tend to overdo. Eggs could also be the cause and so could corn (corn syrup is a frequently used sweetener in prepared foods). If that doesn't do it, try eliminating fish, beef, or peanuts.

If you've eliminated the possible food culprits one at a time, and nothing seems to make a difference, you might want to see an allergist—not your baby, you. You'll be treating your baby by getting treatment yourself.

## Receding Chins

Some babies have receding chins, although this may be hard to tell by looking at them. If you have sore nipples and your baby seems to have a tiny or receding chin, he will need an alternate breastfeeding position. A lactation consultant can advise you about this.

## Problems That Can Happen to You: Plugged Milk Ducts

Debbie noticed that she was getting little white spots in her nipple. "I'd be in severe pain. I couldn't sleep on that side." Debbie had a filled milk duct, a duct that was clogged with dried or congealed milk. Debbie says her doctor told her not to push on the white bumps because it could cause bruising. But she says, one day, she was complaining to her husband and he said, "Why don't you dig around a little?" She took her husband's advice. She pushed on the most painful filled milk duct until it streamed milk so profusely, she "had to grab a diaper."

A plugged milk duct is a tender spot on your breast that may feel like a bruise. If you just push on the tip of the white spot, you will not unplug the duct. In the dairy industry, microsurgery is used to open clogged ducts. But most doctors don't know about this or do it for women. What you can do, as soon as possible, is gently massage and work the entire breast to get dried milk out. The sooner you do this, the less painful and serious the filled duct will be.

How did your duct get plugged? You may have been wearing a bra with an underwire or a bra that was too constrictive, your baby may have a sucking problem, you may have put too much pressure on your breast in one area for another reason (like sleeping on your stomach), you may not be breastfeeding enough, you may have given too many bottles, your baby may have spent too much time on a pacifier, or there may have been a radical change in baby's nursing pattern (such as sleeping through the night and not waking up for usual feeds).

If you catch a plugged milk duct early, you can do what Debbie did. Some lactation consultants will tell you to treat it like the flu: go to bed and breastfeed as much as possible. If you can work out the dried milk that is plugging the duct, either by yourself or with the help of a consultant, you should be okay. While breastfeeding, gently massage the area, use heat before breastfeeding, and keep emptying your breasts by frequent feeding.

## Mastitis or Breast Infection

Sometimes, a plugged duct that doesn't get unplugged leads to a breast infection, or *mastitis*. If you feel a hard, hot spot, like a pie-shaped slice of your breast, that is red and swollen, you probably have a breast infection.

Doctors used to tell mothers to wean when they got a breast infection. This is bad advice. Continue breastfeeding, especially on the breast that has the infection. You do not have to pump. Your milk is still good and will not hurt your baby. (You can continue to breastfeed even when you are sick with a cold, the flu, or a viral infection, with a few exceptions, such as being H.I.V.-positive.)

Keep the baby breastfeeding on the side that hurts as well as the side that doesn't (so that you don't get infections on both sides). That is the fastest way to get a breast infection to go away. Lie down and put your feet up. But not before you've taken a bottle of water with you. Keep drinking fluids (diet soda and coffee don't count as "fluids." Drink water and juice instead). You want your breast to keep draining. You don't necessarily want to jump to antibiotics immediately, but let your doctor make the call. We tend to overuse antibiotics. If you overuse them long-term, your body may stop reacting to their germ-fighting action.

If all of this isn't helping in the first half-day or so, call your doctor. He or she may decide put you on an antibiotic. Make sure you remind him or her that you're breastfeeding (even though it's obvious because you're calling about a breast infection). But you want to make sure he/she will prescribe an antibiotic that is safe during lactation.

### If You Keep Getting Breast Infections

Take the potato chips out of your diet. The Lactation Institute recommends getting rid of as many high-fat foods as you can, particularly those with saturated fats. They also advise women with repeated infections to avoid or reduce their intake of dairy foods (milk, cheese, yogurt).

Although it's possible to get a breast infection past the first few weeks, it's more likely early on. Even so, be aware that while you're breastfeeding, it *can* happen. I went away on business overnight when my first daughter was seven months old. The next day, my right breast got so big, it actually strained at the buttons of my suit. I had no idea what was happening, but my breast was hot and swollen and hurt to touch. The infection was gone in twenty-four hours after I went home, breastfed nonstop and took antibiotics (remember if you're prescribed antibiotics to finish the dose, even if you feel fine).

I've interviewed other working mothers who never had a problem until they too went away overnight. Pumping when you have mastitis is a possible solution, but it isn't nearly as effective as your baby. You need fast relief! You need your baby!

## Breast Abscess

A breast abscess is rare and much more serious than an infection. It feels like "a gel-filled tennis ball" according to Chele Marmet and Ellen Shell of the Lactation Institute. If you have an abscess, you will probably need a doctor to make an incision and drain it. As long as the abscess isn't near where your baby's mouth will be, you can continue breastfeeding, although it will probably hurt (until it drains, there won't be a time when it doesn't hurt.) If it's near the baby's mouth or hurts too much, you can use a piston-action pump on the breast that's healing to keep your milk supply up.

It's important that you find a doctor who has drained a breast abscess before. Check in the Appendix for organizations in your area that are familiar with breastfeeding problems. These support groups, including your local La Leche League, can probably recommend a doctor who can treat an abscess.

## Cesarean Births

Although C-sections aren't necessarily dangerous, they can be daunting to the women who have them. In my postnatal exercise class, a woman who'd had a C-section said she didn't breastfeed because "the C-section was bad enough." Here's a news flash: breastfeeding is not an enema. It'll probably make you feel better, not worse, especially if you're upset about having missed a vaginal delivery.

Lee, who had to have a C-section after thirty hours of labor, said, "I was so disappointed that I didn't get to push my daughter out that nothing would've kept me from breastfeeding her. It really did help me to keep my sanity when I was recovering from what in my groggy state I thought of as 'unnecessary surgery.'"

## Breast Enlargements

In most cases, women who've had breast enlargement surgery can breastfeed. Unless the silicone implants have been poorly put in or your milk ducts were severed in the process, you will likely make the same amount of milk you would have made without the implants.

Even though there recently was a huge settlement for women who complained of immune and other problems with silicone implants, there is still no hard data to prove this claim. However, that said, some preliminary studies seem to indicate that silicone in implants is not a harmless substance. But remember your baby, if you made him yourself, has already been exposed to the silicone in your body when he was gestating. All of the research is frustratingly premature. There simply is no way to know whether the silicone is harmful during gestation or breastfeeding. But to reassure you, many doctors believe that given the fact that an estimated one million American women have implants, you'd expect to see many more ill children. Those babies who do seem to be suffering from gastrointestinal illnesses may simply have a predisposition to this illness. Check the Appendix for more information and help lines.

Dr. Gordon, considered one of the leading experts in this country on breastfeeding, says the decision must be up to the mother, but he believes, "The known benefits of breastfeeding outweigh the theoretical danger of implants." Women in his practice who want a guarantee won't get one, though. "Can I guarantee there's no danger? No, I can't tell you for sure." Think carefully about all of the benefits of breastfeeding. Then, make your own decision. "I don't believe they're benign," one pediatrician says he tells expectant mothers.

Saline implants usually come in a silicone cover. That means you have the same decision to make as your friends who chose silicone implants. Lauren had saline implants. She had no trouble breastfeeding her son and was not concerned about an as yet undiscovered risk. "There are so many more things he could get into trouble over if he doesn't have breastmilk."

As for the mechanics of breastfeeding with implants, most women don't have any trouble. Their nipples may be slightly less sensitive because of the surgery. "The only thing I really couldn't get the hang of was hand expressing. I don't know if that was because of the implants or because I'm uncoordinated," says Lauren. "It just felt weird pushing against the implant."

## Breast Reduction Surgery

Carolyn had breast reduction surgery more than ten years ago, before surgeons had really perfected the art of keeping breasts functioning to breastfeed at a later date. Your milk ducts and all of the necessary biological equipment in your breasts is kind of like a tree with branches. If during surgery, the tree gets robbed of all of its branches and roots, you will probably not be able to breastfeed. Carolyn had one breast that produced a very small amount of milk. Because she had really wanted to breastfeed but could not, she still decided to always undress her baby and open her blouse so at least there was skin to skin contact. She was never able to increase the amount of milk that the one breast made, but she was able to do her best to create a breastfeeding relationship with her sons.

## Serious Problems: Dehydration

Getting breastfeeding going is a struggle. Lactation experts, doctors, and friends might tell you that if you're having a problem you simply need to keep trying. In most cases, this is true. But there are cases of babies who've become seriously dehydrated because they were not getting enough milk.

### Red Flags

Babies who are dehydrated will do one of two things: they'll either sleep a lot to conserve energy and will hardly eat, or they'll want to nurse around the clock. As you read earlier, we like to call babies who sleep all the time "good babies." While I'm not saying you don't have a good baby, you could very well have a dehydrated baby if your baby sleeps a lot. There are some warning signs to look for in your baby:

1. Your newborn should be nursing at least eight times a day, preferably closer to twelve after the first three days, with no more than one four- to five-hour stretch of sleep between feedings (this includes nighttime).
2. Your baby should wet at least six to eight cloth diapers or four to six disposable diapers a day. Try the experiment suggested earlier. Pour one-quarter of a cup of water into a diaper; this is how heavy a wet diaper should feel.
3. Look for at least one bowel movement a day, though three to four is more normal.
4. Dark-colored urine or urine that has a strong odor (of uric acid) can be a sign of dehydration. If there are uric acid crystals in his diaper, you may have a major problem and need to get the baby to the doctor.
5. Listen to the sounds your baby makes as he nurses. You should be able to hear and see him swallowing. Your breasts should also feel less full after a feeding.
6. Your baby will lose 10 percent of his body weight after birth but should be back at his birth weight within two weeks. If he isn't, have your doctor evaluate him for dehydration.
7. If your baby seems lethargic, sleeps and never cries, it is not a good sign.
8. If you put your finger in your baby's mouth and it feels dry, or if other mucous membranes appear dry, he may be dehydrated.
9. If your baby has poor skin turgor, or skin that isn't plump and springy; if his cute chipmunk cheeks are gone; if his skin folds around his neck, arms or legs; or if he's beginning to look like a little old man, he may be dehydrated.
10. If you press your finger against his skin anywhere on his body, the area should not stay depressed. It should pop right back up.
11. If there is an indentation in the fontanelle (soft spot) on top of his head, he may be dehydrated.

Any or all of these are danger signs. Don't take no for an answer from your pediatrician or a lactation consultant if he or she puts you off. One woman was frantic when she called her doctor's office because her baby had clear signs of dehydration. The office told her, "Just keep breastfeeding. We'll see you in two weeks for a check-up." But the mother knew something was wrong and finally barged in on her pediatrician without an appointment. The doctor took one look at the baby and rushed him to a hospital. The baby was severely dehydrated and narrowly avoided brain damage.

Chele Marmet has seen firsthand how quickly little babies can get sick. "Babies can go sour very quickly," she says. "If your baby hasn't urinated in twelve hours, it's serious." That means, get your baby to an emergency room. Don't fight doctors and nurses who may want to hydrate your baby with formula. If he's dehydrated, the first thing you'll need to do is hydrate the baby or you're going to have a very sick baby. The first rule is always to feed the baby.

### If You Think Something Is Wrong, Trust Yourself

It is up to you to take care of your baby and look for the warning signs. Dehydration left unchecked in an infant can cause brain damage, loss of a limb, and even death. It is among the most serious things that can happen. But remember, it is *rare*. Don't think you need to give your baby artificial baby milk to avoid dehydration. You just need to pay attention and know the warning signs.

## Failure to Thrive

Failure to thrive is not a disease. It is a blanket term for a baby who's not gaining sufficient weight and whose growth is faltering. There are many reasons why a baby may be failing to thrive. Listen to your doctor. But know this: a baby that is failing to thrive isn't necessarily a baby who needs to be fed with formula. If your doctor tells you your baby isn't gaining weight sufficiently, the first thing you need to do is feed the baby more often. If at this point, you have a very sick child and you aren't producing sufficient quantities of milk, your baby could be fed either pumped breastmilk, donated breastmilk, or formula.

### Curing Supply Problems

If the baby is failing to thrive you need to figure out why. You may need to help your baby improve his breastfeeding ability, or you may need your baby's help to build up your supply of milk.

Some lactation consultants will recommend taking the baby to bed with you for forty-eight hours if your milk supply is low. Monica had a baby who was diagnosed as failing to thrive. She had to take her baby in for frequent weighings, and her doctor told her to supplement with formula, but this seemed to exacerbate the problem (remember: demand produces supply). Finally, she won her doctor's permission to follow a lactation consultant's advice for forty-eight hours, during which Monica took Sam to bed with her and let him have free rein over her breasts. In just two days, he gained *one pound.* The doctor was elated. He'd never seen a formerly ill baby gain weight so quickly. "What did you do?" he wanted to know, so he could tell other patients. When Monica told him, his response was, "I'll be damned. It works!" He had never before tried this solution.

This may not work in all cases, and if your baby has been diagnosed as failing to thrive, you will need support from both a doctor and a lactation consultant. On the other hand, such a diagnosis does not doom a baby to a diet of formula. In most cases, once you fix the underlying problem, which could be caused by many things, you'll be able to breastfeed. A baby who is failing to thrive will do better on a diet of breastmilk, once he's getting enough, than he will on formula. Lois at The Lactation Institute says many milk shortages happen because, "Mom is doing too much." So slow down. Make sure you're eating and drinking enough good stuff. Some lactation consultants recommend brewer's yeast. That's why you've heard beer increases your milk, but usually only imported or expensive beer has brewer's yeast in it, plus along with that yeast, if you drink beer, you'll also be feeding your infant alcohol (See Chapter 11). You can buy brewer's yeast at health food stores, but lactation consultants say it often causes gas in both the babies and the mommies, so start with a small amount. You can also drink a combination of Fenugreek tea and milk thistle tea, another home remedy. You can try fennel, annis, or oats. All of these things are known to increase milk supply, plus unless you're eating bales full of any of them, they can't hurt you.

### Suck Training or Finger Feeding

A lot of babies who are failing to thrive aren't getting enough milk because something is wrong with their suck. They may be nipple confused, they may have been born with a poor suck, or they may just need extra help getting it right. Jennifer had some unusual complications. Isabella was born with Down Syndrome. The delivery was rough and Isabella had to be put on a respirator. She was extremely jaundiced and was separated from her mother and given bottles. Isabella ended up nipple confused. In addition, Jennifer didn't realize she had inverted nipples, a problem that can make it difficult for even a normal, healthy newborn to latch on. And

Jennifer was unable to get breastmilk using a manual pump that had been a shower gift. If you're just getting a milk supply going, even in the best of circumstances, a manual pump will be difficult to use. Given what Jennifer had going on, it's not surprising that after nine days of intermittent pumping, her breasts were still full of colostrum. And so, Isabella was fed bottles filled with formula.

At the Lactation Institute, Jennifer was immediately hooked up to one of the industrial-strength electric pumps that lactation consultants use for emergencies like Jennifer's. "Oh my gosh," Jennifer kept saying. "I can't believe how much easier this is!"

Because Isabella was nipple confused, when Jennifer put Isabella on her breast, Isabella did not take in enough tissue. She was using the same motion she used to get milk from a bottle. But of course, this doesn't work on a breast. Isabella had to relearn how to suck. Lactation consultants call it *suck training* or *finger feeding*. Until Isabella was a confident sucker, Jennifer would have to give her breastmilk some other way.

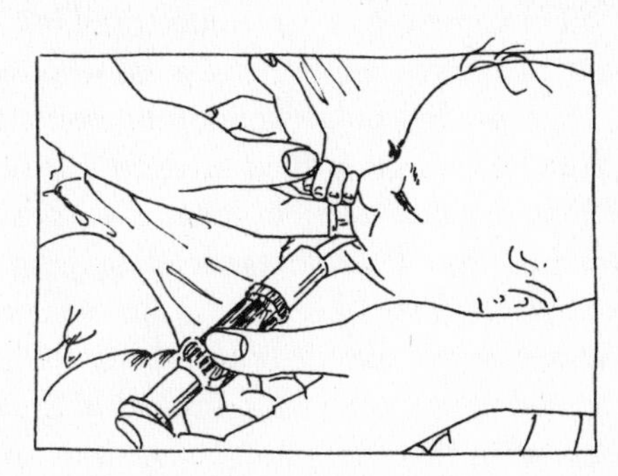

Finger feeding with periodontal syringe: This is a good method to use to teach a baby who's having problems with their suck. But get some hands-on advice from an expert before trying this one yourself.

Within a few minutes, Chele Marmet had shown Jennifer how to position her finger way up in Isabella's mouth, as far back as a nipple would go. Babies like to suck, so, of course, Isabella started sucking Jennifer's finger. As a reward for the proper sucking behavior, Chele showed Jennifer how to position a periodontic syringe on the side of Isabella's mouth and give her a little squirt of pumped breastmilk every time Isabella sucked. The syringe looks like a very large hypodermic without the needle at the end. Instead of a needle, it has a curved plastic tip that is sharp. The sharp tip of the syringe is pressed against your finger so that your baby's mouth is protected. The syringe fits into the corner of your baby's mouth. You want to get the baby to learn how to suck milk from your breasts. The syringe is to feed your baby, but in a way that rewards him for sucking. After he's sucked your finger, you give him a little squirt of either pumped breastmilk if you have a milk supply or formula if you don't. Suck, squirt, suck, squirt, and so it goes until, ideally, your breasts are making the milk and your baby is sucking it from them.

Jennifer says, "We had to do this for a week. Each time I finger fed her, I'd also try to see if I could get her on my breast. After about a week, I don't know what happened. Just all of a sudden, she latched right on to my breast and that was the end of finger feeding."

You will need help to learn this. It isn't hard, but it is time-consuming. Don't despair that you'll never get the baby to the breast and wonder what's the point of filling and refilling syringes, keeping your hands scrupulously clean and your fingernails short. In most cases you will succeed. And even if you don't, your baby has had the advantage of being fed breastmilk. Experts have found this is a very effective way to get a nipple confused baby or a baby with a poor suck onto his mother's breast. "I am so happy that we stuck with it," says Jennifer. "I thought it was hell at the time, but looking back it was worth it."

When the first edition of STWTF! came out, I remember thinking "I am *soooo* glad I never had to do this." That was before Baby Julia, who was right on time and robust at birth. She needed only twenty-four hours to turn my nipples into a sight that caused even Lois at the Lactation Institute to sigh over when she saw them. "Boy, it didn't take her long, did it?" she said sympathetically. Lois first watched how I was breastfeeding Julia. I passed that part of the exam. Then, she scrubbed her hands, put a rubber finger cap on, and let Julia suck on her finger. She determined that Julia's palate was more pronounced and arched than most babies. Instead of drawing my nipple back so that the nipple wasn't coming into contact with anything, Julia pulled my nipple to the roof of her mouth and then tried to get milk by ramming my skin against her palate. That's why it hurt.

Lois told me I needed to let my nipples heal, and Julia needed a lesson in sucking. When Lois brought out the syringes, I cried. No, please not the dreaded finger feeding. Fortunately for me, my husband likes to fix things. When we go to other peoples' houses, if they mention so much as a squeaking drawer, my husband Steve, instead of eating dip and making polite conversation, is on his hands and knees, eyeing the offending drawer runner. Teaching Julia to suck by feeding her with my finger was too much for me. But Steve loved the idea. Surprisingly, Lois told me fathers usually did the finger feeding because it gave them something to do other than hand tissues to their sobbing wives. (Bring your husband along when you go to see the lactation consultant just in case you end up having to finger feed.)

Steve got to trade places, and Julia was like that little bird in the children's story, *Are You My Mother?* She turned her head and rooted for Steve's finger, not my breasts. I think if I'd had to be the one to feed her by syringe, I would quickly have said, "the heck with it," and put her back too soon on my sore breasts. Steve called the finger he used to suck train her, "the magic milk finger." I felt a little left out as I took on diaper duty, pumped milk for Mr. Mom and his magic finger, and waited for my nipples to heal. But less than two days later, we had her back on my breasts. The suck training worked! I had no more pain, and Julia had had an early bonding session with her dad.

Suck training and finger feeding, when done correctly, is very effective. What you want is to get your baby onto your breast as quickly as you can, and not create other problems by starting bad habits, which some other methods (like bottle feeding until you heal) can cause. Find a consultant who knows how to do this if you're about to give up.

## Supplemental Nutrition Systems/Feeding Tube Devices

Supplemental nutrition systems (SNS) are usually sold by lactation consultants. They are used for adoptive mothers or mothers who need to supplement for some reason. Manya, who'd successfully nursed her first two, had problems with number three. A lactation consultant eventually fitted her with this odd contraption: two tiny tubes taped to her nipples and breasts snaking their way into a flat bottle of breastmilk (or formula) worn around her neck. Kind of like a necklace. That way, Manya's son Benjamin could keep breastfeeding. He was stimulating the milk ducts to produce milk, and getting fed with both the breastmilk that he was drawing out and some formula from the SNS tube until supply met demand.

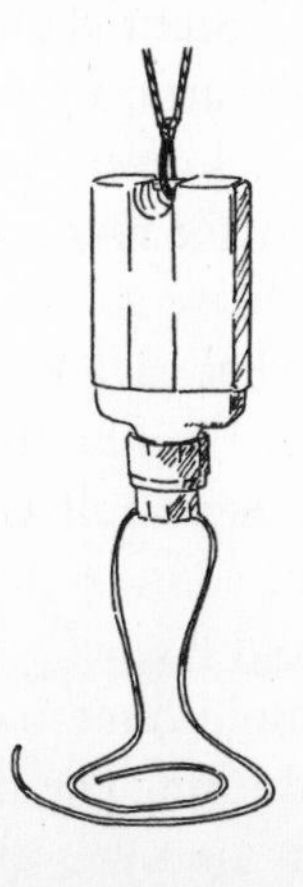

Supplemental Nursing System: Made by Medela, this is one of many feeding tube devices available for adoptive mothers, mothers with insufficient breast tissue, or other selected problems.

### "Congratulations! You've Pushed the Button Labeled 'Controversial.'"

There is currently a controversy over whether feeding tube devices help or hurt your attempts to build up your milk supply. Consultants at the Lactation Institute don't use them much. Instead, they use a periodontal syringe and the finger feeding and suck-training methods. These consultants say they've found that feeding babies formula through a tube usually doesn't help the mother produce enough of her own milk because the baby is not being rewarded for correct sucking as much as he would be if he were fed with a syringe. The flow of milk or formula from a tube is too fast and too much like a bottle, they say, so the same thing can happen that happens with a bottle: the baby takes in mostly formula from the tubes and a decrease in demand for breastmilk will lead to a decrease in the supply. That leads to more supplements, not a bigger milk supply. Plus, as inconvenient as you might think finger feeding is, wearing your Supplemental Nutrition System necklace might be a close second.

But I also interviewed lactation consultants and mothers who swore by these devices. They are especially useful if you are an adoptive mother or a mother who for some other reason is unable to lactate. You can have the benefits of a breastfeeding relationship and bond with your infant, even if you don't have breastmilk.

## The Wrong Help Can Be a Problem, Too

Be forewarned. Rachel's saga is just shy of unbelievable. She had help from three different doctors. None of them helped her to breastfeed. You may come across pediatricians, as Rachel did, who are good doctors but appear to know as much about breastfeeding as Howard Stern knows about tact.

Rachel took her son Ben to see the first pediatrician when Ben was a few weeks old because he was screaming through every feeding and did not seem to be getting enough milk. The first doctor told her to give Ben a bottle. The doctor diagnosed Ben as failing to thrive and attributed this to Rachel's inability to make enough milk. So Rachel gave Ben a bottle after every breastfeeding session because that is what the first doctor—and the second doctor—told her to do. But soon Ben was completely weaned, and Rachel, who hadn't been pumping, had no milk.

So she found a third doctor. This doctor told Rachel a few things that have no basis in medical literature. Rachel, who'd done some reading by now, asked about the possibility of nipple confusion. The doctor told her there was no such thing. "Sucking is an instinct, and you can't confuse an instinct," she said. Then the doctor went on to tell Rachel that Ben was nursing too much, causing Rachel's milk to turn into skim milk. The doctor was also against experts' advice to feed Ben on demand because she said if Rachel breastfed Ben too often, her milk would be thin and there wouldn't be enough fat in it. (If that had been true, Rachel would be the first nursing mother in history to skim fat from her milk inside her body.) And then more bad advice: the doctor told Rachel to put Ben on a rigid feeding schedule. "Three-week-old babies don't need to nurse more than every three to four hours." This is true only if you're putting your young baby on a starvation diet. Ben ended up hungry for an hour and a half to two hours between every feeding. Remember, formula is much harder to digest and takes longer to go through a baby's delicate system. That's why formula-fed babies don't eat as often and can overeat at every meal. Breastmilk easily rides through a baby's system. They can be hungry as frequently as every one to two hours in the first few weeks.

What Rachel later learned after this increasingly bizarre medical round-up is that she needed a lactation consultant. She found a consultant and with help eventually got Ben back on her breast. By now, she was a bit peeved at the lousy advice she'd gotten. In fact, when Rachel tried to ask the third doctor about her watery milk theory and her dismissal of nipple confusion, pointing out other experts' advice in print, the doctor told her that people who wrote "those" books were "earth-mother fanatic types." (Not me. I still wear uncomfortable shoes—as long as they're stylish.)

Some pediatricians are like Rachel's: they know next to nothing about breastfeeding and can actually do more harm than good. "We're taught to trust doctors," Rachel says in retrospect. If it had come from someone other than an M.D., Rachel might at least have questioned it. Instead, it came from doctors who were each described to Rachel as "an excellent doctor with a sterling reputation." Just not a reputation in breastfeeding. That doesn't mean that not one doctor could have helped Rachel. The right doctor, one knowledgeable about breastfeeding, could have helped her.

## Preemies

Babies born prematurely are the ones least likely to be breastfed—and the ones who need it the most. "They're the hardest to get going because a lot of them are too small to suck," says Corky Harvey. However, preemies who are fed breastmilk—by breast or spoon or tube—are likely to leave their isolettes (incubators) sooner than those fed formula. That was true for Erica's baby, who was home much quicker than the doctors had predicted. "I thought, 'He's starting out with a disadvantage. This is the least I can do for him.'"

### If Your Baby Is Premature

If your baby is premature, do not despair. Dr. Gordon, who's seen many premature infants, says, "All bets are off for severely ill, very early preemies." That means, you will have to first take care of all of the baby's medical needs. "Once they have the suck-swallow-gag reflexes, you can take them off of the [feeding] tube and put them directly on the breast," Dr. Gordon says.

You will probably still be able to breastfeed. You just have to be very vocal about your desire to do so. Many nurses are glad to help you because they know your baby is much better off with whatever breastmilk you can produce by pumping, even if it's half a teaspoon. I've watched nurses carefully transferring what appears to be an infinitesimal amount of breastmilk into an eyedropper and feeding a tiny infant.

Think of colostrum as medicine. You don't need a big bottle of antibiotics to get better. Premature babies don't need much breastmilk to get stronger and better. But you'll need to have a milk supply for them when they're ready to breastfeed. That's why you'll need to pump.

Very premature babies may need to be fed intravenously. But that shouldn't stop you from getting a milk supply going. First, get the name of a certified lactation consultant from the hospital. Have this person come to see you and the baby as soon as possible. You will probably need extra help when it comes time to get your baby on your breast.

### Start Without Them!

You will probably be able to rent a pump or borrow one from the hospital and start pumping to build up your milk supply. I realize you'd much prefer to have your baby on your breast, but if you pump as though it were your baby being fed, your body will kick in and treat the pump like your baby. You will have to pump as many times a day as a newborn would feed. That means twelve times a day or every two hours. You'll also have to get up at night and pump. (You'd be doing this anyway, if your baby hadn't been premature.)

When your baby leaves the isolette and is ready to learn how to suck, you will probably need your lactation consultant to help you. "The nurses were helpful," says Allison, the mother of premature twins. "But they just weren't educated about all of the special techniques you should use with a preemie."

Though there is a lot of equipment that various consultants use to get this process going, often your baby won't need anything but a little more time at the breast.

Some doctors and nurses won't be supportive because you'll be getting in the way of an easier routine for them. It means you may have to wear a beeper and get them to page you when your baby needs to be fed. It could mean you or they need to feed the baby breastmilk by eyedropper, instead of formula by bottle. But remember: that baby is yours, and it's up to you to enlist the help of a sympathetic pediatrician who supports breastfeeding or a lactation consultant.

## Twins

Because they share a confined space, twins frequently come early. Because they are often premature and there are two of them, they're a special challenge to breastfeed. (Is *that* why we come with two breasts?) Allison intended to breastfeed her twin boys, but they came very early and it took a while for her to pump up her milk supply. "They got preemie formula, which I wasn't real happy about, but I didn't have a whole lot of choice," she says. With help from a lactation consultant, she got her babies to take her breasts when they were about three months old. Many twins can go directly from a feeding tube to the breast. Some healthy twins breastfeed easily from birth.

## Jaundice

Jaundice is usually not a serious problem. Almost all babies will have slight physiologic jaundice, which is caused by an accumulation of bilirubin, a yellowish pigment, in the blood. The baby's immature liver and kidneys have to clear out these waste products, and sometimes the organs are a little overwhelmed or slow. That's why babies who are jaundiced have a yellow tint to their skin; kind of like one of those bad fake tans. Jaundice isn't a disease—it's a symptom. There is a lot of controversy over jaundice in the medical profession right now. Lactation experts say doctors and hospitals have always overtreated cases of jaundice. "Jaundice does not harm healthy, full-term babies," Dr. Gordon says, and research supports that statement. But there's a caveat to this. Bilirubin levels must be below 20 mg/dL in the first week of life and less than 25 mg/dL after that. Ask your doctor what your baby's bilirubin level is.

When hospitals see a jaundiced baby, in general, they'll treat him the same regardless of whether he's fine but needs to clear the bilirubin out of his system or he's jaundiced because he's sick.

Breastfeeding experts worry that routine separation of a mother and a healthy, full-term newborn to treat the infant under bilirubin lights in most cases does more harm than good. The baby has an immature liver and is born with an excess of red blood cells, which live only a short time. As the cells die, the liver must clear them out of the baby's body. If he was bruised during delivery, either through normal birth or because suction or forceps were used on his head, he'll have even more extra red blood cells to clear out. Colostrum is one of the great ways to flush them out of his system. But if he's been taken from you, he won't be getting breastmilk, and his problem won't be solved nearly so quickly. The hospital will probably expose the baby to bili-lights or phototherapy. In some other countries, there is a new technique in which the lights are wrapped around the baby's trunk so that the baby can stay with his mother.

Another kind of jaundice, late-onset jaundice or breastmilk jaundice, usually shows up five to seven days after birth. Some component or enzyme in the mother's milk causes the baby to be unable to process bilirubin. A lot of doctors will tell any mother who has a baby with any kind of jaundice to stop breastfeeding, even though the jaundice caused by breastmilk is extremely rare. If your doctor tells you to stop giving breastmilk, ask him if you can stop for just twelve hours. If by the end of twelve hours, your baby hasn't significantly improved, then breastmilk isn't the culprit, and in fact your breastmilk will help your baby get better faster.

Research backs up the notion of continuing to breastfeed even if your baby has to lie under bili-lights. In a study published by the American Academy of Pediatrics in their journal *Pediatrics*, researchers concluded that stopping breastfeeding "during phototherapy [treatment for jaundice] in most cases did not appear to be a useful adjunct to treatment." If the problem is simply "jaundice" and the hospital insists on keeping the baby under lights, you can still give pumped colostrum and, later, breastmilk to your baby.

## Cleft Palate, Down Syndrome, Neurological Problems

It's possible to breastfeed even very compromised babies, such as those with a cleft palate, Down Syndrome, or neurological problems. They may require a different latch-on or position, and you'll want to get guidance from the experts. Babies born with a cleft palate, even a small one, will have a difficult time breastfeeding because they will not be able to maintain a vacuum in their mouths. Remember that the vacuum or negative pressure is necessary in order to get milk.

Breastfeeding a baby with such a serious problem is a very big challenge. But breastfeeding will still probably make your life easier rather than harder. Babies with birth defects actually need nourishing breastmilk more than healthy babies do. They also need the comfort of your breast and the closeness of your body. In spite of all the trauma you and your family are enduring right now, breastfeeding can help you feel like you're doing something. You are helping your child in an important way.

If your baby is completely unable to learn how to breastfeed, you can still be a breastfeeding mother by pumping breastmilk and giving that to your baby in whatever way he is able to take it. If he is unable to go through the complicated choreography at the breast but is able to take a bottle, you might want to consider a Supplemental Nutritional System or feeding tube device. That way, you can have your baby breastfeeding from the system's feeding tube right at your breast.

## H.I.V., Tuberculosis, Hepatitis B, and Environmental Pollutants

If you are H.I.V.-positive, have active tuberculosis, or have hepatitis B, these conditions will prevent you from breastfeeding because these diseases are or may be present in breastmilk. But what if you've been exposed to some kind of environmental pollutant, either through your work, because of things you ate, or because of where you live? Unfortunately, your baby's already been exposed in the womb. But if you have some reason to be worried that you may be passing along serious toxins in your milk, such as high concentrations of PCB (polychlorinated biphenyl), you can have your milk tested. Milk banks usually are able to do this or you can contact your state health department to be referred to their lab.

## Epilepsy, Diabetes, or Thyroid Conditions

If you have epilepsy, diabetes, or a thyroid condition, you can breastfeed. You'll just have to be closely monitored by a doctor (so what else is new, right?). You'll need to make sure that whatever medication you take is safe for breastfeeding. For all three diseases, there are medications that are compatible with nursing. In the case of a thyroid problem, you should not nurse during any time when your doctor is using radioactive iodine to test for thyroid problems.

## Breastfeeding an Adopted Baby

Believe it or not, it is possible to get a milk supply going for an adopted baby. The Lactation Institute has helped dozens of adoptive mothers do this. But your goal going into this shouldn't necessarily be to get a full milk supply going. Skin-to-skin contact with your infant is just as important. "When I first put Eden to my breast," Nina, an adoptive mother, says, "I felt this incredible sense of love and acceptance." Nina felt she'd been accepted by Eden as her mother. Though Nina did it only for a few weeks, she's glad that she did. "It is a wonderful memory." You can still have a breastfeeding relationship with your baby, even if you do not have a full milk supply.

Some experts in the field hesitate to help a woman get a milk supply going before the baby arrives because they've seen so many mothers who are disappointed if the adoption falls through. But the disappointment over having a milk supply for a baby who doesn't appear pales in comparison to the disappointment over not getting that longed-for child.

Many lactation consultants tell adoptive mothers from the beginning that it will be the hardest thing they've ever done. So it is not surprising that some mothers give it up right there. But many don't. What mothers of adopted babies stressed to me during interviews is that the emotional relationship is much more important than their ability to make milk. Jane had one biological child when she adopted the baby of a young relative. She says she doesn't believe she made more than a few drops of milk initially, but she still decided to breastfeed her new daughter. "It seemed no different than having my own," she says. Though she initially was planning to breastfeed this second child because of the nutritional benefits, she says, "I could see the baby was getting some nourishment out of my breast, but the bonding turned out to be much more important than the nutrition."

Sara had two weeks' notice before baby David arrived. She wanted to breastfeed, and went out and found a lactation consultant and a pump. By the time David was home from the hospital, Sara was able to coax some milk from her breasts. Depending on how much success your body has making milk, your newborn can get some nutrition from your breasts, but you may have to supplement. That's okay. Nina, who quit breastfeeding Eden at three weeks, says she stopped because she thought the Supplemental Nutrition System was a "hassle." But many women don't mind the inconvenience and have better luck. Sara used the system for five months—and after that, she had a full milk supply!

### Inducing Lactation

Getting a milk supply going in a woman who hasn't been pregnant is hard. The body knows to produce milk because of all the signals it's getting from hormones while you're pregnant. Obviously, if you haven't been pregnant, your body won't know you're expecting a baby. But remember: even though hormones turn the machine on, it is the stimulation of the breast that makes the milk. And prolactin and oxytocin come from your pituitary gland—from your brain, not your breast.

Once you know you will be getting a baby, you need to get to a lactation consultant immediately. You will need to get a full-sized, professional pump (the consultant can recommend one that you can rent). Since your baby will be breastfeeding eight to twelve times in a twenty-four-hour period, that is how often you will have to pump. And those eight to twelve times have to include pumping at night, because your baby will be feeding at night.

At first, and perhaps for a long time, you will not see the fruits of your labor. Pumping isn't really a fun job even when milk is actually coming out, so be prepared for a not-especially-good time as you wait for your breasts to decide whether they feel like producing milk. You will just have to sit and listen to the racket your pump makes and pray that your breasts will catch on and start to make milk.

A biological mother is pregnant for nine months, so you can't expect to have a full milk supply within a few weeks. The lactation consultant assisting you will want to know your fertility history. If your hormones are normal, you will likely have some success. One adoptive mother I know had a full milk supply after she religiously pumped for only two weeks, but this is the exception, not the rule. Sara was able to breastfeed David the bulk of his feedings by the end of three months. Nina had almost no notice of Eden's arrival: she was told two weeks before Eden arrived. She began pumping like a fiend, and she managed to get a little milk going.

There is currently a debate over whether the milk begins with a colostrum phase, and if it does, exactly how much colostrum is produced. But keep in mind that you can't buy formula with colostrum, so whatever is coming out is better than anything you can buy. Even if you end up getting just part of your baby's meals out of your breasts, you have done great. If you get no milk at all out of your breasts, (and you use a supplemental device) you've still given the baby a huge gift. He gets the closeness, the eye stimulation, and the jaw and teeth alignment. Most importantly, the nurturing that comes out of a breastfeeding relationship is more important than the amount of milk that comes out.

# Part III

# Everything Else You Wanted to Know But Were Too Tired to Ask

# Chapter 10

# New Challenges: What's Next Now That You're Pros?

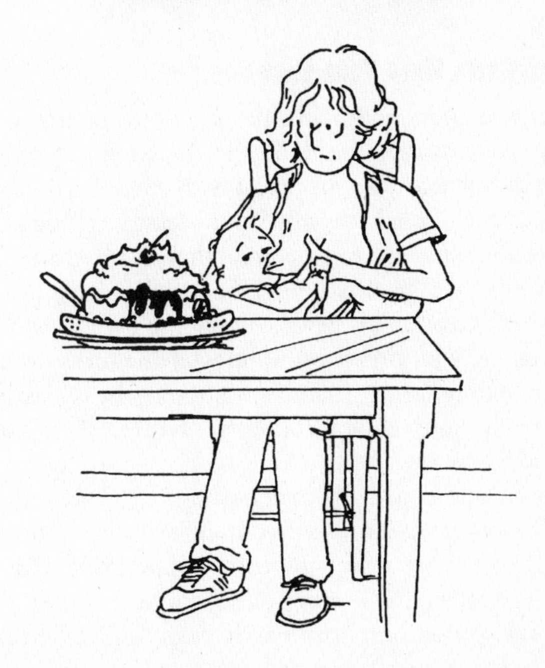

Helen calls her chest the "breastaurant." By the time Lili was three months old, Helen says, breastfeeding—oh, excuse me, eating at the breastaurant—became a piece of cake. "I was still walking around with pads, soaking them all the time and squirting Lili with milk. Except for that and the fact that my chest was a 42DDD—up from a respectable, prepregnant 36C—we were doing just fine."

At three to four months comes the first major transition for you as a mother. If you have to go back to work, you'll notice that just as your baby starts to be fun—that is, does more than sleep, poop, and eat—your maternity leave is up. Your baby is now probably smiling and laughing. I'll never forget the first time my daughter Olivia laughed. I was trying to get her to go down for a nap, but I was having no success. She must've been going through a growth spurt because she would not let go of my breast. I had to go to the bathroom. I put it off and put it off and put it off. I really just wanted some privacy. Finally, I couldn't stand it any longer so I took her into the bathroom with me, got her off my breast, and laid her gently on her back on the carpet. Then I sat down, closed my eyes, and let out a huge sigh of relief. I was startled to hear a little baby giggle. I looked down and saw her laughing at me.

## The Breast That Moves When Your Baby Does!

At about the age of four months, babies start paying attention to other people and like to turn their heads in the direction of any noise. Only problem is they also like to take the breast with them. If you have sore nipples about this time, this could be why. Your breast is a little like the bendable toy Gumby. It's supposed to be elastic, though it's not really meant to go wherever the baby's head is going. That will not stop a baby from experimenting with how far his new "Gumby the Breast" will actually go. If your baby is taking your breast with him while he turns his head to look around, you can tell him gently that this is not okay by taking him off your breast. If he's really hungry, he'll follow your rules. If he's just playing, he'll need to find a new toy.

It is important that your baby understand that breastfeeding is always a partnership. This is an easier task if your child is older, but even toward the middle of the first year, your baby will begin to understand where you will and won't breastfeed. You're the one who has to make the rules for yourself. How do you accomplish this? If dogs can understand that the sound of a leash means a walk and the sound of a can opener means dinner, babies, even very young babies, can understand simple commands. Talking to your baby from the beginning is important because he'll already know your voice (he's been listening inside for months), and he needs to hear the language he'll be speaking and learn ways to communicate with you. I've seen three-month-old babies who attempt to lift their behinds when their mothers say, "I'm changing your diaper now."

## A Quiet Place to Eat

Many babies are fidgety because they need some peace and quiet to settle into the business of breastfeeding. Karen noticed that Jake was so distracted by every sound in the room that she ended up having to find a quiet spot to breastfeed him. "If I didn't find a room with no distractions, and I mean none—no radio, television, phone, people, toys—heck, dust bunnies would catch his attention—he wouldn't eat."

## Hey! A Real Person Already!

Babies have distinct personalities, obviously, and, therefore, distinct breastfeeding preferences. Like Jake, who needed absolute silence to breastfeed, some babies don't want their mothers talking to anyone else while they eat. Some will become so attached to one breast that they won't willingly go to the other. Some don't want to be touched. Some need to be gently stroked. You may feel surprised that this early, your little pumpkin is already showing you just how "willful" he can be. It's hard to believe you are not in control when you are ten times your baby's size.

## "What a Cuuuuuute Baby!"

Since babies at around four months are more appealing than the sleeping body in the stroller, expect them to attract much more attention. They will want to interact with people as much as people will want to interact with them. Expect the unexpected. Your baby may decide to pop off of your breast to watch people go by—and leave your nipple hanging out to dry.

## The Next Big Challenge: Solids

Richard was feeding rice cereal to his eight-week-old. This is not a good idea for a lot of reasons. Anything other than breastmilk is foreign to the baby. Until he's about six months, his intestines lack the necessary digestive enzymes to break down foods other than breastmilk (this includes artificial baby milk for many infants, whose insides are too sensitive to digest it). This can trigger his immune system to fight the foreign food and stimulate allergies.

Another reason is that babies' stomachs are small. If you fill them with rice cereal, a tasty but not particularly healthy meal, you aren't filling them with breastmilk, a tasty and *incredibly healthy* meal. New AAP guidelines recommend that you wait to feed them solids (anything that isn't breastmilk) until they're six months old, because they have immature digestive tracts and aren't built to handle anything but breastmilk before that time. When you do start solids, pediatricians suggest that you start one food at a time so that you can monitor any allergic reaction your baby might have. All solids should definitely be delayed for six months if you have a family history of allergies or eczema.

Richard ignored his child's doctor and was giving rice cereal to his baby because he thought it would make her sleep longer, and "she seems to like it." Making decisions on what to do for your child based on whether they like it is not always the wisest way to run things. When my first daughter was eighteen months, she "liked" dog food. I know because I caught her helping herself to some from the dog's dish. By the way, when she was a two-year-old, a lollipop in her opinion, was a well-balanced meal.

### Is Breastmilk Enough?

Even though you may not have faith in your breastmilk, try to trust it. There is no need to rush your baby onto solids. In fact, the American Academy of Pediatrics reports there are no nutritional benefits to introducing solids before six months and there are some definite drawbacks to early introduction of solids. It's best to wait. If you're worried about him getting bored with the same thing, day after day, don't be. The taste of your milk is flavored by what you eat, and changes all the time.

### Why He Pushes Out Food

Your baby will push out foods because he has a protective mechanism called an *extrusion* reflex. To protect himself from gagging and choking when he's very little, anything that gets pushed in automatically gets pushed out—and that includes a spoonful of rice cereal.

### Baby Heartburn

You want to take your time starting solids because babies have immature gastrointestinal tracks. The wrong food can have nasty gastrointestinal consequences. Also, you can encourage the development of allergies to certain foods if you give them to a baby who's not equipped to digest them yet. The body reacts to food given before about five months as foreign and may produce antigens to it. This reaction explains why some babies cannot tolerate any kind of formula. To their sensitive systems, almost everything in formula is foreign. By the way, soy milk is equally far from breastmilk, and is *not* a better choice than other formulas.

## He Can't Get Fat on Breastmilk

While a baby can't overfeed on breastmilk, he can overeat solids. Like a goldfish who will keep eating as long as there's food, a baby isn't able to signal fullness quickly enough until he's more mature. You could conceivably keep shoveling it in long past the point where his tummy is full.

## You Mean It's Not a Contest?

Our mothers used to have contests to see whose baby could eat solids first. I've heard grandmothers bragging that their children were eating solids at two weeks. (These same children are now too big to fit into theater seats thanks to a lifetime of obesity.) *Our* generation is into talking, walking, and potty training contests. Trust your baby to let you know when he's ready to eat "real" food.

## How to Know When He's Ready for Solids

One of the first signs that your baby is ready for solids is that he'll be riveted by what you're putting in your mouth. Watching the first man walk on Mars couldn't compete with a baby's preoccupation with that fork poised to go into your mouth. Next? He'll start grabbing at your silverware and may even try to put food in his mouth.

But, since babies develop at different rates, your best guide that your baby is developmentally mature enough for solids is when he can get a pea-sized object to his face using his thumb and fingers, according to the guidelines at the Lactation Institute. When babies are little, they pick things up by first smashing them, then wrapping their palms around them. Once your baby demonstrates what separates him from the apes (by using his opposable thumb) he's ready for solid food.

Look to your pediatrician for guidance. Some babies will be ready for solids earlier than others. Don't rush. No one is scoring you, and just because your friend's baby is eating solid food doesn't mean he's smarter, a faster learner, or a better baby.

## One New Food at a Time

As a general rule, introduce one new food at a time, and no more than one new food a week. That way, if your baby reacts badly after a meal, you won't sit there scratching your head saying, "Was it the peas? Or maybe it was the pasta? Could it have been the yams? Bananas? Apples?"

## Rejecting Solids

Once your baby is underway with solids, sickness may cause him to reject them, even ones he really likes. While he's sick, there's nothing better that you can give him than your breast. You can provide his chicken soup. It's still milk, but it's a souped-up version. Because you'll probably have been exposed to the same thing he's got, you'll be passing along your immunities. You'll also be comforting him. Being sick when you're a baby is not fun. Just like you want to go to bed when you're sick, your baby will want to go to bed—and take your breast with him.

## New Breastfeeding Difficulties

Once your baby begins eating solid food, you may have to deal with some brand-new breastfeeding difficulties, completely unrelated to positioning and latching-on.

## The One-Breast Preference

Just when you thought you had all of your problems licked (sorry, bad pun), your baby may develop an obvious preference for one breast over the other. If so, you need to find a way to get him interested in the other one. It could be that you are unknowingly encouraging a preference. My right breast was more sensitive than my left so I favored the less sensitive left. "I have more confidence in the right breast," Kristine says. "Addison seems to prefer it." Addison probably prefers it because it makes more milk because she prefers it because it makes more milk . . .

To get your baby interested in the other breast, try feeding him when he's a little sleepy. He won't be as insistent that you do things his way. Offer him his least favorite breast first and don't take him off. Let him come off by himself. The less-stimulated breast will start making as much milk as the more-stimulated one after a few days of this extra stimulation.

## Nursing Strikes

Be forewarned. Some of your friends may tell you their baby weaned himself at three weeks. This baby was going on a nursing strike, not showing signs of readiness to wean. Babies don't self-wean before nine months—at the earliest. If your baby is younger than a year and is refusing to take your breast, it could be for several reasons.

### Look Mom! Teeth!

The most common cause of a nursing strike is that the baby got a new tooth and tried it out on Mommy. Mommy didn't like being bitten and probably screamed or jumped in surprise. Baby got the diaper scared off of him after hearing Mom's full-decibel range and is probably afraid of provoking that reaction again. You'll need to slowly woo your baby back to your breast by offering it gently, not forcing it. You can offer your breast while the baby is sleepy or asleep. He may forget that he's "mad" at you and take your breast.

### Stress

Stress can also cause a strike. If there's been a death in your family, your marriage is in trouble, or you are experiencing any other stressful event, your baby will know. He probably won't know what the exact event is, but he'll know that you're upset from the expression on your face and the tension in your body. You'll need to try to deal with your stress so that it doesn't affect your baby. Have you ever tried to have a meal when your boyfriend was breaking up with you? Did you eat much? (No, but you still ordered the lobster, took a bite, and made your soon-to-be-ex pay for it.)

Pretending to be calm when you're upset is easier said than done, but your baby will need you to reassure him. He has no idea what's going on, but he does know something terrible has happened to you. Severe stress can also cause your milk supply to dwindle.

Obviously, there are some stresses in life that cannot be avoided. Even so, if you're in the middle of a rough time, try to be extra vigilant when you are breastfeeding your baby. Even if you need to pack five hundred boxes to get ready to move, try to find a quiet place to sit down during breastfeeding sessions. Read a book or watch television to distract yourself while the baby eats.

### Pregnancy

Your baby may go on a nursing strike if you are pregnant. Some babies don't like the taste of their mother's milk during the second trimester of pregnancy. Yes, breastfeeding is a natural birth control method. No, it is not foolproof. You may not be menstruating, but that doesn't mean you're not ovulating.

### New scent?

Are you wearing a new, weird perfume? A new perfume or soap could confuse your baby right into a strike. You won't smell like yourself to your baby. Have you tried another kind of non-smelly soap? Or have you just finished exercising and you're wearing eau-de-gym? The taste of your milk changes after you've worked out due to the buildup of lactic acid, and some babies don't like the taste. I myself have never seen a baby refuse even a very sweaty breast.

### Garlic

Eat all the garlic you like because, contrary to popular belief, babies actually like the taste of garlic. It shouldn't cause a strike. In fact, when scientists fed garlic capsules to nursing mothers, babies latched on more readily and sucked more frequently. Apparently, they like garlic-flavored milk better than chocolate or strawberry milk.

## Teething

Teething is a long process. Some babies start drooling, fussing, and waking up at night for months before the teeth actually cut through their gums. Other babies only seem to be bothered when the teeth are rearing their little pearly white heads. Babies can start getting teeth as early as a few months, though my mother swears my sister had four—upper and lower—by the time she was six weeks. I think my mother's memory is a little foggy, though if you ask her about it, she'll still get all worked up about my sister's chewing on her breast. If you are worried about losing chunks of skin to your baby's teeth, here's reassurance. Your baby cannot bite you and breastfeed at the same time. He physically just can't. Remember how his tongue is draped over his lower gum? He's exerting pressure with his tongue, palate, and jaw, not his teeth. If he's biting you, it means he's retracted his tongue and is no longer getting milk. Time to take him off.

If you do get bit, don't scream at him (if you can help it—the first time is a surprise). If you make an unpleasant noise, he may think you're screaming because you don't want him breastfeeding, though the first time he bites you is likely to be the last time. Your reaction is usually enough of a deterrent.

The best remedy for teething pain is giving your baby something cold (that's safe) to chew, like one of those teething toys that you've put in the freezer. Check with your doctor about over-the-counter remedies. There are homeopathic teething tablets, which many mothers say work well. There's also a kind of gel that soothes flaming red gums.

## Habituating

Most babies eventually develop some little activity they like to do while they're nursing. Some babies will play with your bra strap. They'll fixate on one particular bra and have a cow if you're not wearing that bra.

Kitty's son Sam likes "twiddling," as she calls it. When Sam was about four months old, while he breastfed he began reaching for and twisting the other nipple. Many babies do this. The first time your baby starts running his little hands along your skin, you will think it is so cute. Many other mammals do this instinctively. There is a biological reason for this: they're actually priming the other breast for a quick milk-ejection reflex by massaging it with their free hand and giving your breast skin-to-skin contact. Left to find their own twiddling site, babies will habituate on a certain part of your anatomy, and often it'll be your free nipple. This is fine when their hands are an inch and a half across. But as those hands get bigger and small-muscle control gets more refined, twiddling can turn into an annoying and even painful habit.

Some babies also like to massage the breast they're feeding on. In the beginning, this massage is no big deal. But eventually, as your baby gets stronger and starts pressing harder, it can get very uncomfortable.

### What to Do If You've Got a Twiddler or a Squeezer

The first time you realize your baby is fixating on some part of your anatomy, particularly your free nipple, and the idea of that nipple being twisted, pulled, twiddled and stretched to within an inch of its life in the future isn't appealing, your best bet is to offer something else immediately. When your baby is older, gently move his offending hand to a spot you don't mind. Or you can give your baby something else to squeeze and poke while he's breastfeeding, like a special toy or a blanket.

I waited too long, and when I tried to get my daughter Olivia interested in twisting the ample flesh still left on my stomach, she wasn't having any.

She would begin twisting my stomach, then casually—with that, "whoo-de-doo, I'm not doing anything"—let her hand creep up until she had a firm grasp of my nipple. I would ask her not to pinch me because that's what it felt like to me. When she started talking, she'd always say, "I not pinching!" and drop her hand. But back it would go. Sam was just as indignant when Kitty would ask him to stop "twiddling." "I not twiddling!"

Twiddling or squeezing is a hard habit to control once it's well-established. Nothing, it seems, is quite as satisfying as flesh. So make sure whatever your baby decides to twiddle or squeeze is a part of you that you don't mind having kneaded.

Ellen had two little boys within a year of each other and was still nursing her first when her second came along. Both babies liked to push and prod a mole Ellen had between her breasts. As the newborn got bigger, the fight over the mole took on epic proportions, until finally, Henry Kissinger was called in to mediate . . . No, actually, Ellen told them the mole was off-limits to them both. Then they started twiddling each other until Ellen made them get in line and would only breastfeed one at a time.

## The Blankie that's Alive!

Your breast really is their blankie. Sometimes when you're out in public and in unfamiliar surroundings, you're likely to feel a little hand go down the front of your shirt, maneuvering to find a grip on some part of your breast. This is the place where your baby feels most secure. He doesn't realize that it looks a little funny to have your breasts groped in public—even by a baby. A couple of times when I was wearing a leotard, I feared that my first daughter would get me arrested when she stuck her arm in and the Lycra started to slip down my chest. I told her gently that it was not okay to take my shirt off when there were other people around.

Even very young babies will get the message when you start establishing some rules for breastfeeding in public. They may squawk the first time you move their hand or you insist on keeping your shirt down around your belly or up around your breasts when they're breastfeeding. But if you're consistent, eventually they'll get the message that "if you want to breastfeed in public, you need to do it my way or not at all."

## The Baby Competition

If you take your baby places where he's likely to see other babies, get ready for peer pressure. If one baby sees his friend getting some milk, he's going to want some, too. Gayle was at a "Mommy and Me" class at a mall and the "classroom" was in a storefront with a glass window. Gayle took the class with eight other breastfeeding mothers. One started nursing and then all babies followed suit. "It's this baby thing," Gayle says. "When you're around other mommies, you forget that other people might not see breasts the way you do. We were all breastfeeding in a circle, when a man walked by and peered in." He actually stumbled and fell over after realizing what all eighteen people (mothers and babies) were doing.

## Air Travel

Plane travel with a baby poses new challenges. Landing and taking off (and flying) can be difficult. When cabin pressure changes, the sensation of popping ears can last for fifteen minutes or more. Since little babies can't chew gum or swallow on cue to relieve the pressure, the best thing you can do for them is get them attached to your breast before the plane takes off. That said, you should also know that there is a push to change the rules for children under two, who can now fly free if they sit on a parent's lap. The change is for safety's sake. It would require the child to have a separate ticket and be strapped into a safety seat. Unless you're a contortionist, this could make breastfeeding rather difficult.

Right now, breastfeeding is still your best option to relieve pressure on your baby's ears, though it is obviously not as safe as strapping your baby in next to you. Keep in mind, the cabin pressure doesn't always change after the plane is aloft. Sometimes, the captain will begin to pressurize the cabin while he's taxiing, so begin feeding before take-offs and landings.

I flew across the country with my first daughter by myself twice—once when she was four months and then again when she was fifteen months. The first time, when she was tiny, I got myself into a position I thought I could hold, at least until the movie, and she latched on. She didn't cry when the cabin pressure changed, just sucked peacefully. I ate peanuts. She sucked quietly. I read the in-flight magazine with one hand, she sucked sleepily. I rented the headsets and watched a movie I'd already seen. She sucked. And finally snoozed. And groggily woke up and started sucking every time I tried to get some relief for my sleeping limbs. We kept this up for the five-and-a-half-hour flight. Nobody complained. I don't even think anyone looked, though what seemed like a plane full of weary business travelers thanked me for having such a good baby. I graciously said, "You're welcome," though I really owed the thanks not to my daughter's temperament, but to my breasts.

## Helping Out Your Seatmates

You can always purchase a pack of foam earplugs. You can buy a half dozen for a few dollars. If your baby goes nuts, you can offer those sitting nearby some free earplugs. Kellie did this on a flight from California to London when son Brett had a sudden crying attack. "When I held up the package and asked if anyone wanted a pair, everybody laughed. Then six hands flew up."

## "Where Should We Sit?"

If you're flying alone, there are advantages and disadvantages to any seat you choose. You'll have more privacy in the window seat, but you'll have to excuse yourself every time you need to get up and move around. In the aisle seat, you'll have more arm room and won't have to climb over anyone to get up, but will sacrifice privacy when you need to breastfeed on the side nearest the aisle. If you've done a lot of traveling, you may have noticed that frequent travelers invariably request the aisle seat.

Sometimes, if the plane isn't full, a nice ticketing or check-in agent might even give you a row or a couple of seats to yourself. It doesn't hurt to ask. Even though you may not like sitting in the back of the plane, it's usually less crowded.

If you and your partner are traveling with the baby, request an aisle and a window in the same row. This is a sneaky way to keep the row to yourself. No one requests a middle seat. And if the plane is full and someone does end up having to sit between you, you can ask to trade seats. He or she will probably happily move to either the window or the aisle.

Keep your infant carrier or carseat with you on the plane. At the check-in counter, ask for a large, clear plastic bag. (Most airlines have these. If yours doesn't, beg at other counters until somebody gives you one.) Also, bring along an extra address label. If there's an extra seat next to you, you can strap your baby in for take-off and landing. If you do strap your baby in, bring something along that he will suck, such as your finger, a pacifier, or a bottle. If the plane is full, you can put your carseat in the plastic bag you brought along, attach the address label, and hand it to the flight attendant before you board so it can be checked at the gate.

Before you strap the seat in, make sure you ask the flight attendant which seat to put it in. Some airlines want you to use the window seat so that nobody gets trapped next to the carseat. I've also had flight attendants request that I use the middle seat. Find out before you've labored to strap that seat in.

## Moving Right Along: Exercise

If you exercised before you had your baby, it's probably something you're thinking about doing again. Every woman I know who was in good shape before her baby was born is still in good shape. In fact, they all look pretty much the same as they looked before they were pregnant, though I haven't seen them without clothes. Don't despair if you've just had your baby. Or even if it's been six months or more. (I don't know what to tell you if it's been several years . . . though I suppose you can keep telling people, "I just had a baby." I did for almost two years.)

### You Can Look Like Yourself Again

"When I saw myself in mirrors, I didn't recognize myself," Kristine says. You *can* regain your prepregnancy shape. Wait until your doctor gives you the green light to exercise. For normal vaginal deliveries, it's about three weeks. C-sections take longer to heal, and most doctors will tell you to wait at least six weeks. A lot of aerobics studios, gyms, and health clubs have pre- and postnatal exercise classes. The one in my area allowed babies. This is actually ideal. Most of the newborns would sit placidly, sleeping or gazing around in those cumbersome carseats or better yet, on a mat covered with blankets, while their out-of-shape mothers griped and sweated through some badly needed exercise. It was comforting to have some camaraderie, and no one batted an eye when a mother stopped exercising to let a hungry baby latch on to her sweaty chest.

The class was also part support group. We traded anecdotes and advice. We whined about our fat thighs. We showed each other the sacks swinging from our upper arms. But ultimately, we encouraged each other. And every mother that I knew in that class eventually got rid of the excess baggage. In retrospect, I think the most important thing about it was to see other mothers breastfeeding. The first time I saw a nine-month-old breastfeeding, I remember feeling shocked. She looked so old! But it was a good thing to see other mothers doing what I would eventually be doing. I didn't feel like such a weirdo, and I saw babies in various stages nursing: from newborn to over eighteen months. The women who felt alienated were the ones using formula. If the class is full of bottle feeders, you might want to pass. No point in you being the one who's alienated.

### "I Have Big Breasts!"

I wanted to get in touch with the boy at the bus stop who'd called me "flatsy" all during junior high. "Get a load of these!" I'd have said, waving my new shape in his face. Getting used to very large breasts, particularly in the first few months of breastfeeding, means wearing a sports bra, maybe even two, when you exercise. (Buy them as big as they come so that you can get them on.) The woman who taught my postnatal classes encouraged us to hold our breasts with our hands if it was painful. We all laughed, then when the music started, ten pairs of hands immediately seized ten sets of breasts.

### Don't Blast the Baby

You'll need to make sure the instructor keeps the music low. I taught aerobics for five years during college and graduate school, and I am sure I lost about 20 percent of my hearing. If the instructor doesn't realize how loud the music is, make sure you tell him or her. You need to keep the music low so that you don't blast your baby's eardrums and so you can hear your baby if he starts crying. Some babies sleep all the way through. Some are wakeful and like to watch.

### Get to Class Early

If you can get to class fifteen minutes early, you can breastfeed your baby right before class begins. Also, it's more comfortable exercising with C-cups instead of D-cups, so any change of size you can manage before class will help.

### "Water! Water! Water!"

Stay well-hydrated. Drink water before you go, and always bring a water bottle with you. If you feel dizzy, spacey, or cold on a warm day or in a warm room or you feel nauseous during the work-out, obviously stop. Sometimes this isn't because you're so out of shape; it's because you are dehydrated. The next time you exercise, make sure you've had a lot of water in the hours leading up to your class. To test your hydration level, keep an eye on the color of your urine. It should be very pale yellow, almost without color. If your urine is very yellow, you're not drinking enough liquids. If you can smell your urine when you go to the bathroom, you are dehydrated. If you feel thirsty while you're working out, this is also a sign that you're dehydrated. By the time you feel thirsty, it's too late. Your body has needed water for a while and is giving you a late cue that it needs water. Drink!

### There's No Class for Me

If your gym or exercise studio isn't offering a postnatal class, find a few other women (most places require a minimum of three people) and approach the owners. See if they can begin a postnatal exercise class where women are encouraged to bring their babies. Insurance companies will accommodate these classes, so don't take "no, our insurance won't cover it" for the final answer. If you have enough of a demand, you'll usually find a supplier. If there aren't enough women in your area who want to get off their duffs after having a baby, see if you can get a combined pre- and postnatal class started.

### Don't Compete

If you don't have a prayer of finding or starting a pre/postnatal class in your area, find a place that offers a range of classes. Yes, you may hate organized classes, but it is a good way to get back in shape. You will have committed to the hour or so of class. There will be other people keeping you company, and if you have an ounce of competitive juice in you, you'll stay until the end. Take the easiest class on the schedule. Even if it's filled with women your mother's age, this is a good place to start. You can't help but be better than at least some of the people in class, and that will be better for your psyche—and your staying power—than getting your butt kicked your first time back. (If the only class that fits your schedule is high-level, don't be intimidated. Exercise at a level that's comfortable for you—regardless of what everyone else is doing. You might feel less obtrusive in the back of the room.)

### If You Can't Afford/Can't Find Classes or Child Care

If you can't find classes that offer child care or can't find or pay for someone to stay at home with your child while you go to a class, you can do something that doesn't involve leaving your infant. You can buy a step exerciser and some exercise tapes, find a class on television, or borrow somebody else's stuff, since a lot of people buy expensive equipment and then use it to hang their clothes on.

I know, I know. I hate exercising in front of a television set with a 115-pound model who has a washboard stomach (just wait 'til *she* has children). But just working up a little bit of a sweat will get you motivated. It'll also remind you that you are not recovering from being hit by a bus. Your body did not go through an organ transplant operation, even if you think it looks like it did. You simply put on a few pounds and had a baby. Okay, so you put on a lot of pounds and had a baby. Your body will eventually figure out that the baby's gone and it can let go of some of those sacks of calories it's been storing. When I was little and had a bad day, my mother would say, "Go to sleep. You'll feel better in the morning." I could've killed her. But the thing you're avoiding most is often the only thing that will make you feel better. If you can make yourself do just a little bit of exercise, you *will* feel better.

## Don't Diet

The only time in my life that I was fat was when I would regularly go on diets. I'd say, "Today, I'll eat celery sticks, fat-free cottage cheese—and an industrial-size bag of potato chips!" Even if you have dieted in the past, don't diet while you're breastfeeding. Dieting will cut down on the amount of milk that your body will make, and that is much more of a problem than the extra few pounds you may be carrying. You still need to think about somebody else's welfare.

You will lose all of that pregnancy weight, however. It'll come off reasonably easily if you go back to your old routines and eat normal amounts of food. I know it's easy to get paranoid and believe you are carrying around extra weight because your body is still storing fat to breastfeed. Except for the last few pounds, this isn't so. By six months postpartum, all of the women in my exercise class resembled very closely their old, prepregnant selves.

Remember that breastfeeding does help you lose weight. But you must breastfeed for longer than three months. Women who formula fed or weaned their babies before three months were still four to five pounds heavier than the breastfeeders, who were back to their prepregnancy weight. Lee, who exercised daily, decided to stop breastfeeding because she thought she was staying heavy since she was a breastmilk factory. She weaned her daughter at three months. But when she stopped breastfeeding, she also stopped losing weight.

# Chapter 11

# Pumping, and What's Safe for You to Eat and Drink

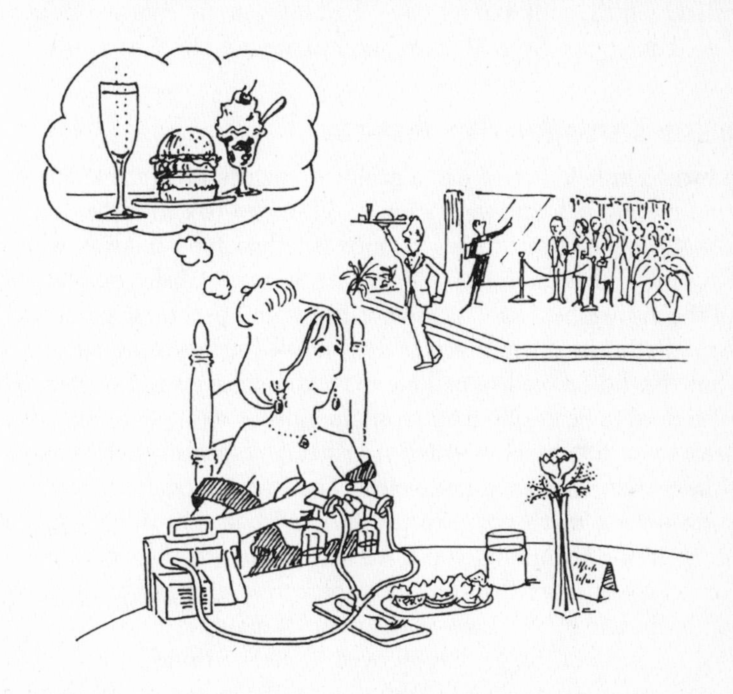

## PUMPING EVEN IF YOU DON'T PLAN TO GO BACK TO WORK

You may want to rent a breast pump even if you don't plan to go back to work. You will occasionally need an hour away so you can go do exciting things like go to the dry cleaners, return phone calls, or buy groceries (of course, you'll be so tired and so overwhelmed to be by yourself that you'll fritter away your golden hour trying to remember what you were supposed to do). You'll want to pump a feeding before you go out, so it'll be on hand if your baby needs it while you are away.

A lot of women want to pump or express milk so that their babies can still get the nutritional goodies even if they don't always have the breast. As silly as it seems, I was proud of the amount that I could express. I would occasionally count the number of bags I had stored in the freezer, calculating the number of ounces and the number of feedings that supply was good for. (I remember being really impressed with a mother of twins who told me she could express ten ounces—"like that," she said, snapping her fingers.) I was practically hysterical when my husband defrosted five extra ounces and left the milk out all day. I had tears in my eyes as I poured my liquid gold down the disposal (he refused to use it on his Cheerios).

## Cleanliness: Keeping Your Baby Germ-free

When I was a little kid and I had a problem, such as when the kid at the bus stop told me my red hair was "stupid," I'd try to talk to my mother, who was always doing fifteen things at once (she had four children who were close in age, and no help). She'd inevitably say, "Wash your hands and unload the dishwasher" or "Wash your hands and peel these potatoes." My mother didn't always help much when I needed help sorting out my problems, but she did succeed in making me a compulsive hand washer. This is what you need to be during the first six months or so of your baby's life.

Before you do anything, wash your hands, especially before pumping. Wash them well, with soap and water. Then you're ready to handle your child or anything that's going to touch your child. But don't panic about sterilizing. In the beginning, you'll sterilize the plastic diapers. Then you'll watch mothers of more than one child pick up a dropped pacifier, wipe it on their jeans, and push it back in their baby's mouth.

One of the cool things that allowed humans to survive is their ability to develop resistance to disease. You don't want to expose babies to every germ, but we've moved beyond old doctors' orders to keep new babies inside a plastic bubble until they're a few months old. Exposing babies to normal, everyday bacteria is a good thing. They'll slowly develop immunities and be better able to withstand bacteria and viruses.

## Sterilizing Your Equipment

The first time you use equipment, you should probably boil it, but I've seen nurses in hospitals open the packaging on breast pump attachments and just start using them. "We used to be hyperconscious about sterilizing everything," one lactation consultant told me. "Now we just use good hygiene."

When you do boil equipment, be religious about following the manufacturer's directions. Don't just dump all parts in a lobster pot and turn up the flame unless you want all of those parts to become one big part. Usually, the bottles and the heads (which look like a trumpet or funnel) need to be boiled because they'll be collecting the breastmilk. Some of the other parts should never get wet. Make sure you know which parts need to be boiled—and for how long—and which parts need to stay dry.

Once your instruments have been sterilized, you're ready for surgery, Doctor. (If you're pumping at work and the only place available is the bathroom, do not put the bottles or the pump directly on the floor. Lay some paper on the floor before you put down your pump.) One manufacturer must have gotten tired of getting melted pumps back, because the literature says, *"Don't Boil the Pump!"* No need to boil your hands before pumping, either . . .

## Types of Breast Pumps

Here's how to look at breast pumps: an old-fashioned cylinder pump is like walking. A battery-powered pump for $20 to $60 is like a bicycle. A good mini-electric pump ($150 or more) is a moped. The rental pumps (which retail for $600 to $1,000) are the Cadillacs. The Mercedeses of the pump world are the pumps you'll find in hospitals and at lactation centers.

Avoid the use of hand pumps shaped like old bicycle horns. These are known as "bulb" or "bicycle horn" pumps. They can hurt and do damage to your breast tissue. In addition, you won't get much milk and they are hard to clean.

### Battery-powered Pumps—The Bicycles

I have yet to meet a woman who was happy with one of those small, battery-powered pumps you will get as a shower gift or see in baby stores and drugstores. "My advice if you get one of these as a shower gift," says Sandra Jansen, R.N., "is return it and get something more useful like blankets." More than one lactation consultant said to me flat out, "Don't waste your money on those."

These inexpensive pumps have a reputation for either not creating enough suction (causing you to pump no milk) or creating too much suction (pinching your breasts and causing you to pump no milk). They also break down much more quickly than more expensive pumps.

*"I'm engorged, and I can't get up!"* That was the message Jane left on my machine on a weekend when we were out of town. Jane forgot her breast pump on her first romantic overnight trip with her husband. "We bought one of those cheap pumps at a drugstore, and I tried to use it in the car." It didn't work. Jane eventually bought three different pumps. None of them worked. Instead, she and her husband turned around and drove home. "Since it was a Sunday in a small town, I couldn't find a rental station that was open. Oh well, Alyx-Anne was sure happy to see us." Don't do what Jane did. If you're on the road, and you've forgotten your breast pump, you can still find one to rent. One manufacturer, Medela, has an 800 number, 1-800-TELL-YOU, that you can call for a referral to the nearest pump station, or breastfeeding specialist (you'll need to know what zip code you're in).

### Moderately Expensive Electric Pumps—The Mopeds

Some companies are now making pumps in the $150 range. For some women, these work great. Michelle has a very strong milk-ejection reflex and makes a lot of milk. She bought her pump for $150 through a catalog and is able to pump about four ounces of milk at a sitting. But before you invest in a pump, which even at $150 is still expensive, you might want to rent a pump for a day or try hand expressing. If your milk comes out in sufficient quantities using either method, you are probably a pretty easygoing producer and one of the less expensive pumps might work for you.

### Working Woman Pumps

There are also several new pumps on the market put out by companies like Medela and Natural Choice specifically for working women. They run from $100 to $180. They are designed to subtly whisper "I'm a briefcase," not trumpet "I'M A BREASTPUMP." They're lightweight and small, and touted to be almost as effective as the bigger breast pumps. (The downside to the Medela pump is that it has a finite life expectancy and was designed to be tossed after about a year's use.) Julianne rented Medela's Lactina (supposedly a bigger, stronger pump) for her first child, then bought Medela's "Pump and Style" portable pump for her second baby. She, like many women I interviewed, was very happy with the "Pump and Style" and noticed no real difference between the two. The "Pump and Style" she purchased was 150 dollars. She'd spent over three hundred dollars to rent the Lactina for a year.

### Piston-action Pumps—The Cadillacs and Mercedeses

The best pump is one with piston action (for those of us who aren't gearheads, that's one with a piston that gets moved back and forth by a motorized arm). It applies slow, steady, even pressure. Medela and Egnell both manufacture good piston-action electric pumps. If you rent one of these pumps, expect to spend about a dollar a day (still much cheaper than formula). Rented pumps are cheaper the longer you keep them, but you don't have to rent one for a year. Start with a month or two, then extend your rental time if you need to.

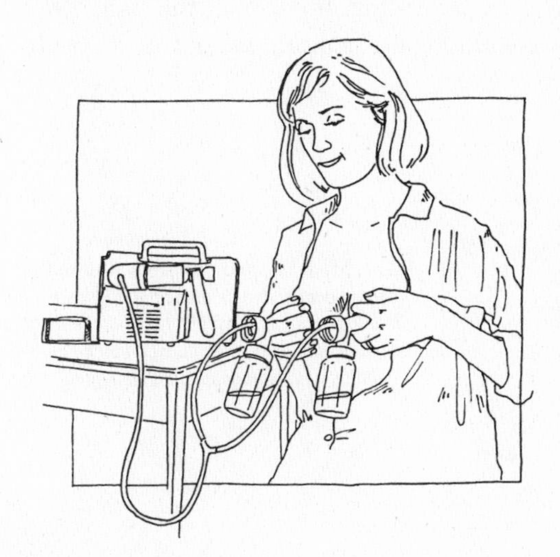

The Medela Lactina Dual Action Pump: This is one of the many pumps you can rent or purchase. This particular model is considered a "Cadillac."

### Detachable Hand Pumps

Some of the piston-action pumps come with a detachable unit that can also be bought separately and hand-operated. This is an option if you're carrying around other things and space is an issue to you. Some women have good luck with hand pumps. They are less expensive, but, generally, you will get what you pay for. They're inexpensive because the labor is supplied by you. You'll have to concentrate while you're hand pumping—no sneaking looks at the newspaper or the television—and you'll need both hands free as well as some arm strength. They're also slow (see? you knew there was a reason why they discovered electricity!). And unless your milk lets down at the drop of a hat, you may have trouble with these hand pumps.

Keep in mind, your baby is your most successful pump. Don't feel like a failure if you hook up to your machine and don't make much milk. "Every time I pumped, I got nothing, and I do mean nothing. A few drops here or there," says Janine. But son Derrick must've been getting milk, because he was steadily gaining weight. For some women, the hormone oxytocin isn't stimulated by pumping (and pumping takes longer if you're in a stressful environment). If oxytocin isn't produced, there is no milk-ejection reflex.

But just because you can't get milk when you pump doesn't mean your baby isn't getting milk when he's breastfeeding. Remember the signs? Wet and poopy diapers, swallowing sounds, and gaining weight at a steady pace, even if it's a little less than average.

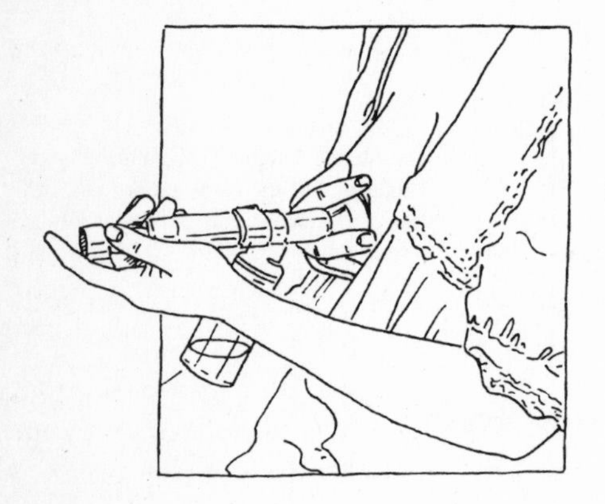

The Medela SpringExpress Manual Breastpump: This is one of the manual pumps you can buy for short-term or occasional use. It detaches from the Lactina, or can be purchased separately.

## Cycles

If you're comparing mechanical pumps and wondering which one to buy or rent, a good way to figure out how fast a pump is is to find out how many cycles per minute it does. This is kind of like figuring out how fast a computer is. The more cycles per minute, the quicker and more efficient the pump is. A baby sucks sixty to ninety times a minute, or sixty to ninety cycles. By contrast, a cheap, battery-powered pump runs six to twelve cycles a minute! For those of you who don't feel like doing math right now, that's about one-tenth as fast as your baby. No wonder you don't get much.

## How to Pump with an Electric Breast Pump

It takes a little practice to use an electric breast pump. Good pumps, like the ones rented through lactation consultants, are efficient and easy to use.

Hamida was in the hospital and began pumping for her premature daughter, Hena. Hamida said she'd been pumping for two hours straight and nothing had come out. When a consultant doing rounds at the hospital looked at the pump, she realized that the nurse had not told Hamida how to use it. Hamida's pump was set up for both breasts, but she was only holding it on one at a time. Have you ever tried to use a busted vacuum? You roll it over crumbs that even a manual sweeper would pick up and the vacuum just trots over them. The machine is called a *vacuum* because it's using suction and exerting negative pressure. That's what your pump is supposed to do. If there's a leak anywhere, there won't be pressure, and you won't make milk.

If you are pumping correctly, you should feel a little bit of suction and pressure on your breasts. There is a switch that controls this, so if it's hurting, look for that switch and turn the pressure down. If you're not feeling anything, turn the machine up (a little at a time).

It takes a few minutes for your milk to start to eject. If after three to five minutes, nothing is coming out of your breasts and you feel suction when you hold the pump against your cheek, you may simply be tense. (If milk comes out of your cheek, then you've got an interesting problem I'd like to hear about.) The more relaxed you are, the easier it is for your body to eject milk.

But if you're not feeling anything and hear the faint sound of wind, the seal may be broken, either where you're attaching the cups to your breasts or somewhere on the pump. It could even be a faulty pump. I went through two pump rentals before I realized I had faulty pumps, not faulty breasts.

## How to Get Milk If Your Pump Is Working But You're Not

If you've checked the seals, can feel a slight pulling on your breast (not painful, just a bit of a tug caused by the suction), and you're still not getting milk, it could be because you aren't relaxed. To stimulate your milk-ejection reflex, you have to think wonderful thoughts, but your body won't play this game until your mind is calm. It helps to think about your baby or look at a picture of your baby. The more tense you become about not stimulating your milk-ejection reflex, the more likely it is your milk won't come out. Don't give up after a minute or two at your pump. When I was at work, sometimes I would be attached for up to five minutes before I'd be rewarded with milk splashing around in the bottles.

## How to Save Time

If you're working (either outside or within the home), time is usually valuable to you. If you have limited windows of time in which to express milk, it's likely you'll want to plug in a pump or turn on a battery-powered one and get the whole thing over with quickly. Buy or rent a dual-action pump. If you use a single-action pump you'll have to double the amount of time you spend pumping, because you won't be able to do both breasts at the same time.

Attach clean bottles directly to the pump. With most pumps, if you put storage bags into the bottles and try to attach bottle and bag to the pump apparatus, you will break the airtight seal and the pump won't work.

You will maximize the amount of milk you produce if you do the massage-stroke-shake exercise (as explained in the hand expression section on page 220) after you've pumped each breast. Then pump once more. You'll soon get to know your body and have a good idea of how long it takes to empty your breasts—with an electric pump, anywhere from seven to twelve minutes for each breast. With a hand pump, it'll take more like twenty to thirty minutes for each breast.

## How to Store Pumped Milk

Freshly pumped breastmilk can last for up to ten hours without refrigeration, but you're probably safer if you stick closer to six. A new study has shown that milk stored at room temperature for ten hours has about the same bacterial level as milk refrigerated for the same length of time (as long as your hands, your bottles and your equipment are scrupulously clean). You're always safer if you refrigerate the milk after you've pumped it. When I wasn't home, I found it easiest to pour the two small bottles I'd pumped into one big bottle, then put that bottle in a refrigerator or on ice (any fast-food restaurant will give you ice).

## How Long Does It Keep?

In the refrigerator, breastmilk should last up to five days. If you have a freezer that keeps ice cream solid, it's cold enough. A freezer compartment inside a refrigerator will keep the milk for two weeks. If your freezer is separate, it'll keep the milk for three to four months. Put the milk in the coldest part of the freezer: on the bottom shelf, in the center, toward the back. At 0° F, plan on six months.

*Never* put defrosted milk back in the freezer and refreeze it. Also, never pour warm milk over frozen milk, because you'll thaw some of the frozen milk and encourage the growth of bacteria.

A simple formula for feeding is this: your baby will drink two and one-half ounces of milk per pound of his weight in a day. So if he weighs ten pounds, he'll probably drink twenty-five ounces a day (including nighttime feedings). Freeze milk in small quantities, though. It'll break your heart if you defrost twelve ounces and your child drinks two. If you freeze in two- to four-ounce quantities, you won't have to throw away milk. Helen's husband Eric opened the freezer one day and discovered that not only was there no ice cream, frozen pizza, or ice cubes in there, there was nothing except pumped milk. Every square inch of the freezer was taken up by the fruits of Helen's prodigious pumping. "I almost started crying because Eric said, 'Honey, can we throw some of this sh— out?' The freezer was Fort Knox to me. He wanted to throw out GOLD!"

After the Los Angeles earthquake, Sandra Jansen had to provide counseling services to women who'd lost power and had to throw away their spoiled breastmilk. Forget about their condemned houses—these women were devastated because they lost pumped milk! Try getting your insurance to compensate you for *that* loss!

## How to Decide Between Storage Bags and Bottles

There is some controversy over whether the plastic storage bags specifically designated for pumped milk storage that are sold on your grocery shelf are safe for storing milk. Some experts believe that polymers (chemical compounds) from the plastic can leach into the breastmilk. In addition, the bags are thin, which causes them to tear easily, and porous, which could allow bacteria to get in. But freezer storage space is usually an issue for most women, so the bags are convenient. If you have a large freezer, though, and can spring for a lot of extra bottles, that's a better option. Use small (four- to six-ounce) glass or hard plastic bottles (glass is better than any kind of plastic). Put a piece of masking tape on the bottles and label all milk with the date that you pumped it. Some lactation consultants will tell you to note on the bottle any strange food you've had that day in case your child shows an allergic reaction. I'll bet these same lactation consultants keep their shoes in their original boxes and hang up all of their clothes. Another suggestion is to put your milk into a clean ice tray, freeze it, then transfer the frozen milk in small

1-ounce cubes to a plastic freezer bag. Just don't use those ice cubes in your guests' Martinis.

If you're comfortable with the idea of storing your milk in the plastic bags sold in your grocery store, buy the four-ounce bags. Don't fill the bag completely; allow room for the milk to expand as it freezes. Put about three ounces in a four-ounce bag. I used little wire twist ties to seal the bags. Then I stored them upright in a cardboard box in the freezer. I found the twist ties easier to use than rubber bands because they were easier to undo, and I had a lot of them lying around so I never had to hunt for one.

You can also purchase thick plastic breastmilk storage bags, which are less permeable and supposedly less likely to leach polymers into the milk. Breast pump manufacturers sell these. But these bags cost about forty cents a bag. Write the date on the end of the bag, away from the opening. Use pencil so that the ink doesn't leach into the milk. Most manufactured breastmilk bags have a surface to write on. If there isn't one, write the date ( in pencil again) on masking tape, and attach it to the bag.

## Which Milk Should Be Given First?

Most lactation experts will tell you to give your baby the freshest milk you have available and save the frozen milk for emergencies. That means, milk is best by breast, then freshly pumped milk, then refrigerated pumped milk, and finally frozen pumped milk. But when you resort to refrigerated or frozen milk, use the older milk first, so that you can use it before it spoils.

## How to Defrost Milk

When you need to defrost frozen breastmilk, don't microwave it. That's the biggest rule. Microwaving milk changes its composition, and can cause hot spots that could scald your baby. The way to defrost breastmilk is to put it under warm tap water or "float" the bottle or bag of milk in a cup. Babies don't necessarily need very warm milk. They'll drink it at room temperature. Remember, when they get it directly from you, they're drinking it at your body temperature, which is considerably cooler than heated formula.

If you're on your way to work and you're afraid your caregiver might start getting the baby's meal ready at the last minute, you can take bags out of the freezer and leave them to thaw overnight in the refrigerator. That way, when the caregiver goes to heat the milk, it's a one-minute wait for the baby versus a five-minute wait. Shake the milk to redistribute the fat, but not too much. You don't want to make butter or whipped cream.

## Don't Be Afraid to Toss It Out!

As difficult as it is to throw away breastmilk, don't refrigerate whatever your baby didn't drink and give it to him at the next feeding. There are bacteria in the baby's mouth, and once he's used the bottle, bacteria could grow in the milk while it sits in the refrigerator. It's a good idea to only defrost what the baby will drink. Whatever he doesn't drink should be used as food for the pipes in the kitchen sink. Be sure to tell whomever is feeding him not to force him to finish the bottle, even if there's still an ounce or so left.

Taste the breastmilk if you're not sure. It's supposed to taste sweet. If it's spoiled, it'll taste sour. Poor Helen, the one who was so proud of her frozen milk store, had to dump a whole batch of it out because it smelled funny. She dunked one finger in, tasted it, and burst into tears. It had gone bad.

It might be worth it to you to invest in a special pump tote bag. This is disguised as a gym bag and sold through the manufacturer or through pump rental stores. You can put your sterilized bottles and pump parts in a plastic bag. Look for one that has a "cooler" section to store the milk after you've pumped.

## How to Hand Express

If you get good at hand expressing your milk, I'm told it is an easy, inexpensive alternative to pumping. It will also work if you don't want to rent a pump, or you've forgotten to bring your breast pump along on a business trip or on an outing without Junior. I wanted to pump and be done with it. But many women say hand expression is just as fast, and you don't need any special equipment other than your hands and a plastic bowl. This skill came in handy for Nancy, a new mother. She was in law school and living in "married student housing." One day, she heard pounding on her door. Her upstairs neighbor, a Ph.D. candidate in the middle of dissertation hell, was flushed and agitated. "Do you have any milk?" he begged. The professor who was his adviser and would ultimately be the person to bestow or deny his degree had dropped in unexpectedly for a chat and some coffee. "He takes milk! Milk!," he kept insisting. "Do you have anything? Regular, skim, 2-percent, 1-percent, powdered, condensed, canned—anything at all?" Nancy shook her head, and then remembered one kind of milk she did have. "Well, I do have some milk." When she pointed to her breasts, her neighbor didn't hesitate. "Fine. That's fine," he said. She disappeared and was able to hand express some breastmilk. Minutes later, he hurried upstairs with a half cup of breastmilk. His professor told him over and over how "great" the coffee tasted. Maybe that "great" coffee was the reason he got his Ph.D.

While you're dealing with engorgement, it's good to learn how to hand express your milk. It is not hard, but you have to be someone who is comfortable touching your own breasts. If you faithfully do your monthly breast exams, you might be good at hand expressing. I was initially as impressed by women who could hand express as I was by women who could diagnose a faulty carburetor. But then I saw it done correctly, and I understood why I was unable to get any milk when I first tried hand expression. Chele Marmet, who gets the credit for inventing the most widely accepted hand expression technique (naturally, it's called the Marmet Technique), tells me it's not only possible for most women to hand express, but once you get the hang of it, it's as easy or easier than using a pump (the one thing it isn't for most women is faster). I've personally seen Chele squirt an entire class full of nurses when she was demonstrating hand expression on a new mother. No one got splashed, though. (Nurses have developed amazing reflexes to get out of the way of oncoming bodily fluids.)

## Step By Step for Hand Expression

First, put your thumb above your nipple at about 12:00 o'clock and your first two fingers at about 6:00 o'clock below your nipple. Keep your hand about one to one and one-half inches behind your nipple. You want to form the letter C with your hand. Don't cup your breast as if you are holding and guiding it toward your baby. Instead, push your fingers straight back into the chest wall. Don't spread your fingers apart. To get milk, gently roll your fingers forward at the same time, like you would to make a complete fingerprint. If you've never been fingerprinted, you may not know what that motion looks like. You need to press your fingers in and roll your fingertips along the skin as though you were trying to touch your thumb on the top of your breast to your fingers under your breast. But don't squeeze your breast (which could bruise your skin), slide your hands along it (hard enough to cause skin burns), or pull at the nipple (which could damage the tissue). You want to use a rolling motion to compress and empty the milk reservoirs.

To remove milk from all reservoirs, you will want to move your hand around your breast and do the same compressing motion, turning your hands as though you were rotating around your breast (for once, it won't matter if it's clockwise or counterclockwise).

When you hand express, you will need to catch your milk in a wide-mouth plastic bowl, like the kind your mother used to feature at her Tupperware parties. Your milk will be coming out of between ten and twenty holes, not one big hole in the center of your nipple, and after all that work, it'd be nice to catch a little bit of it.

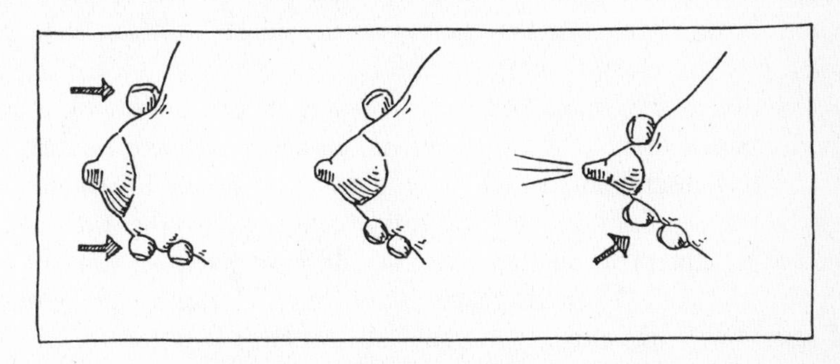

Manual expression: Think: position, push, roll, repeat.
Step 1: *Position* your thumb and first two fingers about 1–1.5 inches behind the nipple, and *push* straight back into your chest wall.
Step 2: *Roll* thumb and fingers forward, compressing the breast tissue.
Step 3: Finish your roll and squirt! *Repeat* until you've expressed as much as you can.

## How to Help Your Milk-Ejection Reflex

Remember that you need to stimulate the production of the hormone oxytocin to turn on your milk-ejection reflex. To help get the milk to squirt, you should gently massage your breast, using the same kind of motion you use for your breast self-exam. Then, stroke the breast area from the top of the breast to the nipple with a light touch, using your fingertips. This light massaging and caressing sets biology into motion and lets your breast know it can now eject milk. Because you're massaging and using your hands, you might have more success hand expressing milk than with the plastic shield of the pump. Plastic wasn't around when the human brain was evolving, so you are programmed to react to the human touch (your baby, your hands), not to a machine.

Next, shake your breasts while leaning forward so that gravity will help you get your milk out. It'll take you five to seven minutes to express milk from each breast, thirty seconds or so to massage-stroke-shake, another three to five minutes to express from each breast again, massage-stroke-shake, then two to three minutes to express from each breast a last time. You won't have to stick to these times if your milk supply is well-established and hand expression comes easy to you. Keep expressing until the milk slows down. Squirt to the last drop, that is.

## What's Safe For Me to Eat and Drink?

I had a conversation with a woman who'd adopted a child. It is still one of the most bizarre conversations I've had on the subject of breastfeeding. She insisted that the ancient Chinese rice formula she'd made for her daughter was superior to breastmilk because, according to her, breastmilk is full of "environmental toxins." But then she did an about-face and told me she'd been terribly disappointed that she couldn't find donor breastmilk when her baby was small. I told her I was sorry I hadn't known her then, because since our daughters are the same age, I could have given her some of mine. "Oh no," she said. "I wouldn't have taken yours." I tried not to be insulted and said, "Well of course, you could always have it tested for H.I.V. or hepatitis B" (neither of which I have). "But what about your *mysticism*?," she said. "I don't know what kind of mysticism you have in your milk." Okay, she had me there. No, I don't know how to test for the mysticism in my milk. I just hope for her daughter's sake that her baby came with the right mysticism in her DNA.

Out of this conversation comes only one salient point: many mothers are worried about what's in their milk because, let's face it, we no longer live on the same planet that the Indians inhabited. But, in spite of the fact that there are many environmental pollutants, this woman was wrong about her ancient Chinese concoction. There is nothing you can make, regardless of the health store in which you shop, that is superior to breastmilk. Studies have shown that environmental toxins don't usually interfere with your ability to produce good, safe breastmilk.

On the other hand, there are ways to keep your milk as safe as possible. You can try to be conscientious about what you put in your mouth. Try to find organic produce. It can be more expensive and harder to find, but it is grown without pesticides, which means you and your baby will be ingesting fewer chemicals. If you believe you've been exposed to a harmful toxin, you can contact your state department of health and get your milk tested.

## A Balanced Diet

You don't really need to do anything regimented; just try to eat things in moderation. Rotate all of your less-than-healthy foods. That means, allow yourself french fries (if you have to have them) once a week. You can probably eat one "bad" thing a day (but not too much of it) and still be okay. Eat as many "good" things as you can in their most natural packages (fruit in its original "wrapper," whole grains, beans, and so on). Stay away as much as you can from manufactured, canned, refined, and processed-to-within-an-inch-of-its-life-and-dyed-red-#700 food.

Try to get at least five servings of fruit or vegetables into your body every day. My younger brother used to make us cut up his vegetables very small. Then he would swallow them like pills. That's one way. If you don't want to breastfeed because you hate eating vegetables, figure out the vegetables you will eat. Salads? Fruit? Potato? Carrot juice? Okay, canned corn.

Even if your diet is like the diet of a seventh-grade boy who buys his lunch at a vending machine, breastfeeding is still worth doing. The milk of starving women has been compared with the milk of prosperous Swedes. It wasn't that different. I tell you that piece of information not to encourage your bad habits, though. There's only so much testing science can do. Nobody disputes that "you are what you eat." Try not to be a Twinkie.

Furthermore, very soon you'll have a toddler who will want to eat everything you are eating. Children seem to come with a sensor that drags them toward any food that's bad for them. My daughter never had candy, yet she knew what candy was. If there was any candy, anywhere in the house, no matter how high the shelf, she'd find it. I was pretty good about my diet when she was inside my womb. When I was breastfeeding, I was a little more lax. Finally I went back to my old ways. But when she wanted what I was eating, I decided to keep the junk food in my house to a minimum. *I* could eat the faux-sour-cream-and-onion potato chips, but the idea of her little stomach churning up all that fat, starch, and salt made me sick. Particularly because it seems that toddlers take in about six ounces of solid food a day, and if those six ounces happen to be empty calories and saturated fat, what's it to them?

I couldn't completely kick my addiction to fat, salt, and sugar, but I toned it down a little. If you start working on your diet, not to lose weight, but just to keep yourself healthy, your baby will learn healthy habits from you. Do not go on a crash diet. It will affect the quantity and quality of your milk.

## Alcohol

Sorry, the party is still over for you. You can't go back to drinking alcohol in quantity just yet. Some doctors will tell you the occasional glass of wine or beer is okay. In fact, some doctors even used to tell women to drink a glass to relax and help their let-down response. When Victoria was given this advice, she took it a little too literally. "I was drinking a glass of beer before every feed—that meant eight to ten glasses a day!" That was more than she'd ever drunk and way more than her doctor had intended (he meant a drink every other day or so, not a drink at every feeding).

Other doctors think any alcohol is bad if you're breastfeeding. My doctor cautioned me not to drink, and I decided to follow this advice, at least for as long as both babies were drinking breastmilk exclusively. I got a little looser (no dancing with lampshades on my head—just a glass here and there) when they got bigger and older and there was more to their diet than breastmilk. Alcohol and other toxic stuff likes to hang out in fatty tissue. That's what your breast is largely made of. Research has shown that the amount of alcohol in your blood, say it's .1 percent, matches the amount in your milk, which then, will also be .1 percent alcohol. That much alcohol is a lot for a baby. Way too much, experts say. That's when the Breastfeeding Police can pull you over and give you a ticket for drunk milking.

The bigger you are, the faster you can metabolize alcohol. A general rule of thumb is it takes somewhere between two to three hours, depending on your size, to metabolize each drink you take (one drink is considered to be 12 ounces of beer, 4 ounces of wine, or 1.5 ounces of liquor). Two hours for a 120-pound woman (yeah, right—who weighs 120 after childbirth?), and three hours for a 160-pound woman (no comment). If you have more than one drink, you'll need to multiply those numbers.

Babies' livers don't mature until they're about three months old, so damage is probably greater for a younger (under six to twelve months) infant. They metabolize the alcohol at about half the rate an adult liver can, so the alcohol is in their system longer. And if you're breastfeeding and haven't started menstruating again, your rate of alcohol absorption will be even higher.

In a study published in the *New England Journal of Medicine*, the motor development of babies whose mothers had one drink a day for the first year was "significantly lower" when their babies were twelve months, when compared to babies who were not exposed "similarly" to alcohol.

The researchers recommend eating before and while you drink, limiting the number of drinks you have, drinking drinks low in alcohol and diluted with water or juice, measuring, not eye-balling liquor, drinking slowly, and waiting two to three hours per drink before breastfeeding (that means you'll have to pump ahead of time so your baby has something to eat).

Some doctors aren't that concerned about women who drink small amounts of alcohol and breastfeed. For some people, alcohol is tough to give up. If you are tempted to quit breastfeeding because you want to have a little alcohol every now and then, your baby will be much better off getting breastmilk, even if it has a little wine in it. But alcohol *does* affect the baby's central nervous system. The amount you drink will directly relate to the alcohol's effect on your baby, so keep it light.

You will have to make your own decision after consulting with your doctor. Check with your pediatrician and find out whether he or she believes moderate consumption of alcohol will have any lasting effects on your baby. But above all, understand what *moderate* means for a nursing mother. The use of the word *moderate* is what makes Dr. Gordon skeptical about advising breastfeeding mothers they can drink "moderately." "Usually, when people say, 'a beer or two,' they mean a six-pack. To me, 'moderate' means a drink or two a week."

If you do drink too much, say on New Year's Eve or on a birthday or anniversary, you can pump your milk and toss it out. Doing this once will likely cure you of drinking too much. It'll hurt to throw away your milk, but it's better to feed your baby stored breastmilk or even formula than to give him shots of breastmilk laced with tequila. Even if you've simply had too much wine at dinner, it's best not to take a chance. The rule is pump and dump. That wicked hangover will be even more punishment.

One woman complained to a lactation consultant that she couldn't get her breastmilk to freeze. It turns out the mother drank vodka. A lot of vodka. If your breastmilk won't freeze, you are drinking way too much. Your husband or partner can help keep you on the straight and narrow. You can tell him all the things you know about alcohol. It is, after all, his kid, too. Tell him so that he can discourage you when that frothy, ice cold beer is calling your name or that inviting glass of Chianti (for those of you who still drink it after *Silence of the Lambs*) wants to sit at your table. Every time I even looked at a glass of beer, my husband told me that when Olivia has trouble learning to ride her two-wheeler, we'll all know whose fault it was. It didn't seem worth it to me.

### Caffeine

Caffeine was another story. I drank decaffeinated coffee all through my pregnancy. I'm the kind of person who'll spend $3 on a cup of coffee as long as it has an Italian name, so weaning myself off that daily shot of espresso was hard. After nine months without, I could have accepted the caffeine deprivation. But one day, when my daughter was a few weeks old, I woke up exhausted after a night of endless feedings. I really wanted a hit of caffeine. So, I made the mistake of having a strong cup of coffee. Like alcohol, caffeine also ends up in your milk. You get a rush, your baby gets a rush. One daughter was not fond of caffeine. It made her irritable, which means I had an even longer day with a crying child who couldn't be consoled. I went back to decaf. The same is true for some babies and chocolate or Coca-Cola (and anything else with caffeine). But experts say at a cup a day, coffee is compatible with breastfeeding.

## Food Allergies

If your baby seems crankier than usual and he's not sick, it could be because you ate something that doesn't agree with him. Some babies will react to spicy foods. Don't chalk it up to colic if your baby has a bad day; it may just be a bad day. On the other hand, it may be because you ate something that's now giving your child serious gas pains.

Keep track of what you eat. If you've eaten something unusual and your baby seems fussier or gassier than usual, the new food could be the cause. (See Chapter 7.)

## Tobacco

If you're a smoker and you can't stop smoking that one last cigarette, as long as you keep consumption down, your baby is better off if you breastfeed than if you don't. Obviously, your baby is best off if you don't smoke at all. Smoking has been shown to greatly decrease milk supply. Also, no matter what, you should never smoke around your baby because you'll cause him the same respiratory problems you'll eventually cause yourself.

But the benefits of breastmilk, even from a mother who smokes, usually far outweigh the liabilities of artificial baby milk. Try to cut back if you can't quit altogether, and check with a medical expert, being truthful about how much you smoke. If you feel uncomfortable talking to your pediatrician, make an anonymous phone call to one of the nursing organizations listed in the Appendix.

## Marijuana and Other Recreational Drugs

Does anybody smoke marijuana anymore? Does anyone admit to inhaling?

If you do, stop while you're breastfeeding. Marijuana can affect your milk supply and has been shown to alter a baby's brain growth. One evening, when I was at a party at an acquaintance's home, I was shocked to find her on the back porch, smoking marijuana with her brother. I had just seen her breastfeeding her three-month-old. Up until that point, I'd only known her to be a sweet, concerned, seemingly intelligent mother. I asked her about it, and she said, "At least it's not alcohol."

Marijuana is not a harmless substance. Using anything that alters the brain growth of an infant is not a good idea. Another recent study indicates that children born to mothers who smoked marijuana heavily through their pregnancies have trouble with sequencing and decision making later in life. The world is hard enough without further compromising your child's future.

Do not take *any* other recreational drugs either. In fact, don't take anything that has not been approved by your doctor.

## Prescription and Over-the-Counter Medications

Most medications have never been tested in breastfeeding women, for obvious reasons. Would you volunteer to take a drug while nursing an infant just to find out what the side effects were? That's the problem. Unfortunately, this has led to the old "cover your butt" rule of thumb, which means that many drug manufacturers caution pregnant or lactating women not to take certain drugs. The caution doesn't necessarily mean that these drugs are harmful, just that the drug manufacturers would prefer to be safe than sued.

If you must take a drug that is incompatible with breastfeeding, ask your doctor if there are any alternative drugs that may be safer to take while you're breastfeeding. If possible, delay taking a drug. Or you could do what Sindy did. She had a serious asthma attack that put her in the hospital. When the doctor told her she could not breastfeed her daughter for two weeks, she pumped every day. "I cried every time I pumped the milk and dumped it out. But when the two weeks was up, she had no trouble going right back to my breast."

Many doctors are conservative and advise women not to take anything that could pass through the breastmilk while they're breastfeeding. But some drugs end up in breastmilk in minute quantities. Depending on the drug, this may or may not be a problem. You will need the help of a professional to help you assess what's safe and what's not for your particular situation. If your doctor can't tell you which specific drugs are definitely harmful or seems to have a "no drug policy" period, get a second opinion, particularly on a medication that you need, if it's causing you to think seriously about weaning. An important rule of thumb if you do have to take medication: if it's a short-acting drug (like an antibiotic), take it immediately *after* feeding your baby. Long-acting drugs (like over-the-counter twelve-hour cold remedies) are more problematic because they were designed to stay in your system. Ask your doctor when to take them to minimize their risk.

Make sure you don't even take over-the-counter medication without first reading the packaging and then checking with your pediatrician. Pharmacists are a big help, too. They can tell you what the drug manufacturer recommends, even though the drug company may routinely say, "Not for pregnant or lactating women." For more help, call any one of the drug information hotlines listed in the Appendix.

### Safe Medications

The American Academy of Pediatrics considers the following drugs usually compatible with breastfeeding:

- acetaminophen (brand name: Tylenol)
- many antibiotics, but be on the lookout for thrush or diarrhea in your baby
- anticonvulsants (with the exception of Primidone, which should be given with caution)
- aspirin
- codeine
- decongestants
- ibuprofen (brand name: Advil)
- insulin
- naproxen
- quinine
- thyroid medications

### Unsafe Medications

Don't breastfeed and take any of the following drugs:

- bromocriptine (Parlodel), for Parkinson's disease
- most chemotherapy drugs, for cancer. You're taking them to kill cancer cells, but they kill healthy cells, too

- ergotamine, for migraine headaches; causes vomiting, diarrhea and convulsions in infants
- lithium, for manic-depressive illness
- methotrexate, for arthritis; can suppress baby's immune system
- all street drugs: cocaine, crack, PCP, amphetamines, heroin, and anything else you can think of that you can buy in bags from people looking over their shoulders

### Birth Control Pills

Taking birth control pills or other hormones can lower your milk supply. Wanda says she began taking birth control pills again when her daughter was three months old and soon discovered she had stopped producing milk. "I was mad that no one had told me this," she says. "I certainly could have waited to take the birth control pills."

### Antidepressants

Denise began taking Prozac to help her through PMS depression that "made me want to jump out the window." She had just begun to feel the pleasant effects of the antidepressant when she found out she was pregnant for the second time. "I went off it immediately, but boy, did I miss the Prozac during my pregnancy, which for me, means nine months of PMS." Her doctor recommended that she not take Prozac again until her child was weaned. "I had bad postpartum depression and kept opening my medicine cabinet and looking longingly at the thing I knew could fix it—the thing I couldn't take." She breastfed her son until he was a year old.

Denise says, "I agonized over what to do, but the truth is, I was nearly suicidal, and he wasn't ready to be completely weaned." She began taking a mild dose of Prozac and slowly weaned Max to just one feeding a day. "My doctor seemed to think this was safe, and it was certainly better than the alternative I'd considered." Gradually, she weaned her son.

There is very little hard data on the safety of antidepressants for breastfeeding mothers. Doctors and the San Diego drug hotline urge women with depression that isn't completely debilitating to stay off most of them while they breastfeed, though if this is really a problem for you, consult an expert.

That's because most antidepressants have been ruled "unsafe" for breastfeeding women. Again, as with many drugs, it is ultimately a decision mothers have to make with medical guidance: which is the lesser of two evils? The symptoms or the cure?

## Dosage

Dosage is one of the critical things when deciding whether a medicine is safe. How much is getting into your breastmilk, how often is the baby feeding, and how big is the baby? Those three factors combined with the degree of necessity of the drug, and the particular drug itself, are the factors you need to weigh when deciding whether to take a medication and breastfeed, wait, or wean. There are medications that you cannot do without and that may interfere with your ability to breastfeed. You need to weigh the pros and cons in consultation with a knowledgeable professional who also understands the value of breastfeeding before you decide to stop breastfeeding and start taking a drug, or continue breastfeeding and put off your need for whatever it is you've been advised to take. No matter what, check before you put it in your mouth.

## Chapter 12

# Leaving the House and Taking Your Breasts with You (Otherwise Known as Working)

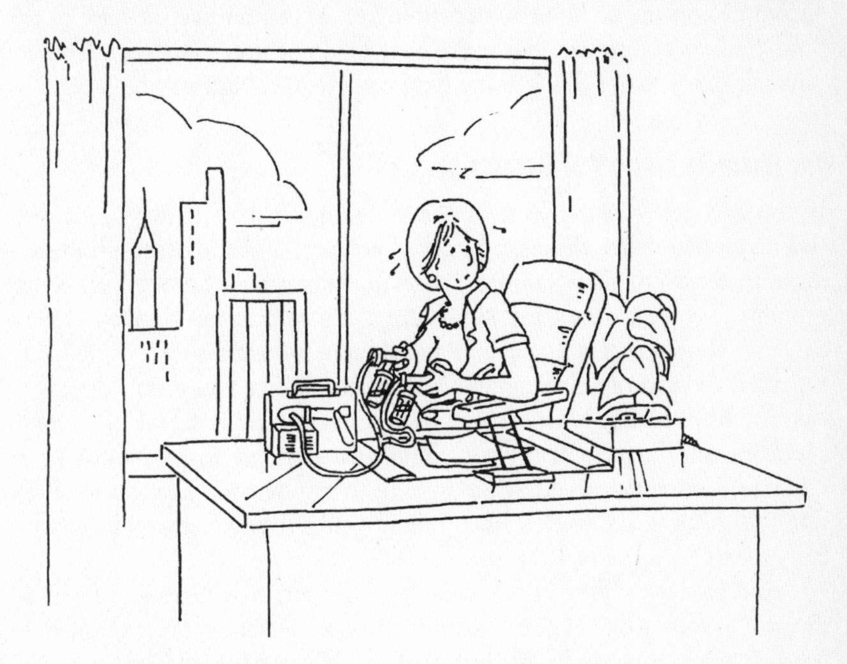

Nowadays, Women:
Matriculate
Educate
Administrate and
Legislate.

They also:
Menstruate
Gestate...and
Lactate.

— SANDRA JANSEN

## "I used to be a professional. Now I'm a professional cow."

Give yourself time to adjust if you're home for awhile. There are precious few times in life when you can stop the world and get off. One of those times is when you have a baby. Even all of your hard-core ladder-climbing friends will indulge you and fall all over themselves to get a look at your baby.

The hard part for you if you're used to accomplishing a lot is that all of a sudden, you'll be doing nothing—and everything. You won't be getting paid, and you will have nothing but an exhausted baby and body to show at the end of a hard workday. But the payoffs to this work are there. They're huge—and they're subtle. You and your baby are getting to know each other, and you're likely falling in love. This is a lifelong relationship.

If you're still trying to use your day "wisely," understand what mothers do: they keep the world going 'round. They're the ones with the real accomplishments, or failures, depending on how attentive they are to their tasks (fathers count, too, but we're busy talking about you now). Convince yourself that you are doing something worthwhile, because you are.

## Try Chanting While You Breastfeed

If you can get into the Zen of breastfeeding, it'll be easier to sit down when you have dirty dishes, a hundred errands, and seventeen phone messages to return. This is good practice for your brain. Sometimes, being a mommy is—geez, dare I say it?—boring. It's helpful for your child if you can put your worries aside in a big imaginary glass bowl while you're together. Instead of thinking about all of the things you didn't do, should do, and have to do, look at your baby's sweet little rosebud of a mouth. Hold his tiny fingers. Brush your hands through his wispy hair, if he has any. Stop worrying about what's going to happen to your career if you don't go back in six weeks. Keep telling yourself your baby will only be a baby for a few years of your life.

And stop worrying about what will happen to your baby when you do go back to work. Give yourself a break. Working everything out is hard. It takes time and usually help from other people. Give your baby the time you do have right now instead of worrying about the time you won't have later.

## Don't Commit

If possible, try to commit to as few things postpartum as possible. If your employer insists you go back to work in six weeks and you need to go back, then you'll have fewer options. Kendra's boss said to her, "Listen, if you want to take the year off, the job will wait." Kendra, who admits to a certain paranoia in her competitive field, says she believed at the time her boss "wanted to get rid of me," and she brushed off his suggestion. When she quit her job a year later to take part-time work and stay home more, she laughs at her preoccupation with work. "I really could have taken the year off. He meant it." But working out things at work and at home takes time, usually a lot longer than six weeks. You'll eventually figure out what works for you. Don't be upset if you don't have it all together when your maternity leave is up.

Steer clear of promising to type four hundred letters, complete that book, computer program, sewing project, screenplay, tax return, interior design, or whatever other project is incomplete. If you have something hanging over your head that has to be started as soon as the epidural wears off, you'll be under more pressure. And pressure is what you don't need.

"Many women don't understand they are at the most vulnerable period in their lives," says Judy Chapman, a lactation consultant. You still have raging hormones, you're not sleeping, you're caring for an infant—which is like digging ditches in terms of how physically tired you'll be—and depending on your particular partner, you may feel very lonely. If you're home all day, and you're used to sharing news of your day with your husband at dinner time, he might not be able to relate to what you're now interested in. "I had a long conversation with another mother about her sore nipples," Cindy says. "Was it thrush, was it eczema, was I just positioning her wrong? My husband fell asleep while I was talking to him about it."

I know you're also used to doing something. If you need to, do what Marian, our friend the list-maker, does. "I make a list of fifty things to do by the end of the day. And by 6:00 p.m., I'll be able to cross one thing off." There you go. One thing down, 49 to go . . .

## Getting a Milk Supply Going

I began pumping about three days after my daughter Olivia was born. This was early, but I had to go back to work in six weeks and my goal was to fill a freezer. Some lactation experts suggest you wait three weeks before regular pumping until your milk supply is established and you are not engorged. But if you know you have to go back to work soon after your baby is born, there's really nothing wrong with pumping once your milk has come in.

## "When Should I Pump?"

You will likely get the biggest supply of milk in the morning because you've been resting and because that's a big feeding time for your baby. The worst time of day will likely be in the evening. Some experts will tell you to first feed the baby, then pump the excess. Some tell you to pump, then feed the baby the excess. I was always concerned that there wouldn't be enough for the baby, though this was based not on science but on my Italian heritage that requires forcing food on people. I fed her, then pumped. There always seemed to be plenty, once my body got used to the idea that it had to make milk twice: once for her, once for the pump. It usually takes a few days for your body to adjust, and it's best if you can pump at regular times so that your body has an easier time adjusting. My all-time pumping high was eleven ounces. Don't ask me how I managed that. That number still looks impressive as I write it. Most days you'll get between one and six ounces.

Each day, I pumped before I left for work and put a bottle of pumped milk for my daughter in the refrigerator. If I couldn't come home at lunch, I'd pump, bring that bottle home, and store it in the refrigerator for the next day. She had breakfast and lunch in the refrigerator waiting. Since I usually left her four ounces, came home at lunch and brought home about four pumped ounces at the end of the day, I had plenty of milk and didn't have to resort to formula. I figured it would take her months to get through my milk supply in the freezer. I was correct.

"I only got two ounces!" Jane wailed on the phone to me. I'd made the mistake of bragging about the number of ounces I made every morning. Two ounces is perfectly normal. You're doing fine if that's what you're getting. Also, remember as the day wears on, it will get harder for you to get milk out of your breasts.

But if you pump every morning beginning the first week, by the time you go back to work, you'll have somewhere between forty-five and a few thousand ounces. This gives you a head start so that each day, you can bring home the milk you pumped during the day at work, add that to the stock, and have plenty of back-up milk in the freezer.

## From Professional Cow to Professional Working Cow

Before you go back to your job, come up with a plan that will work for you. The important thing is to try to be flexible. This doesn't necessarily mean you'll be stuck expressing in a broom closet, though I have talked to women who did end up pumping there. Going home at lunchtime or having someone bring your infant to you is a good option, but may not be practical for you. However, don't rule it out. Remeber the times you've taken a job because you needed the money, and it turned into something wonderful? You can work out a lot of solutions to your baby/work paradox that you never dreamed were possible. You might plan to pump for a while and see how it goes. Don't ask your boss for everything up front, but know as you go along that it is almost always easier for companies to accommodate good employees minimally than it is to recruit and hire new people (even in very competitive fields). If you're good at what you do, you stand a good chance of bending some rules.

I lived fifteen to twenty minutes away from my office, depending on traffic. For months, I dutifully pumped at work, then shoved down a sandwich at my desk and worked until I could go home. I remember feeling upset because I was stuck by myself pumping. I missed my baby, and though I knew I was doing a good thing for her, sitting there trying not to splatter my suits with milk was not how I'd envisioned motherhood and career meshing. Then I realized that even with the thirty- to forty-minute roundtrip commute, I could still squeeze out twenty minutes with my daughter in the middle of the day. That was better than no time with her. I started going home for lunch. Sure, I pushed the envelope. After five years of never taking lunch, I figured no one would shout at me. Okay, so, I stretched some lunches out a bit and I didn't make lunch dates anymore, but I did get to go home regularly.

Don't rule out going home, unless you have a very long commute. If there is any way to swing this, it's nice for everyone to get together, and it's ultimately easier than pumping. If the trip from office to home is more than fifteen minutes, you'll have more trouble getting there and back in a one-hour lunch break. But you could offer to come in earlier or stay later in order to take a longer lunch break.

## If Mohammed Can't Go to the Mountain . . .

Maybe the baby can come to you. Rebecca, a nurse, went back to work when her daughter was eight months. Because both she and her husband worked twelve-hour shifts, three days a week, they were able to rotate child care, and baby Francis always had either Mom or Dad home. The only problem with Dad's shift is that his did not come with breasts. For a while, Rebecca's husband would bring Francis to work during Rebecca's dinner break at the hospital. If it was a busy night and there were no spare rooms, Rebecca would meet them in the car and get to spend some time with Francis, who was happy to breastfeed anywhere, even in the front seat of a Chevrolet.

"Errr-errr, errr-errr, errr-errr." This is the sound your colleagues are going to have to get used to. It is the sound of a milking mother. Contrary to every article I've read on the subject about how employers bend over backwards for breastfeeding women, this was not my experience. There are some businesses that have rented or purchased pumps and set up a room for women to do their business during breaks and lunch. If you work at a place that does this, fabulous. You don't need to read this section. If you don't, welcome to the real world.

Sandra Jansen, R.N., tried to get corporate America interested in setting up pump stations for women by pointing out studies that showed businesses saved money in the long run because breastfeeding women were on the job more days—they needed fewer days off to care for a sick infant. But as soon as Sandra started talking to Human Resources or Personnel, the roomful of executives turned into third graders. "Do we get a free demonstration?" one man once sniggered, pointing at Sandra's chest. Many executives told her that women in *their* company "don't do that." These were the same companies that wouldn't install tampon machines in their bathrooms. Apparently, their female workers didn't do that, either. But when Sandra insisted that they tour the halls and actually talk to some of those females, the executives were shocked to find out that many of those dedicated, genderless employees were (horrors!) secretly pumping at work!

## Don't Ask, Don't Tell?

One prominent doctor advises working women to have a discussion with their employer about their plans to pump at work. I'm not sure I like this advice. I certainly didn't take it. I really didn't think it was my boss's business, and I would have been very uncomfortable having a conference with her about my plans to use my own lunch hour to pump. I didn't tell her on the days that I drank too much coffee that I'd be using the bathroom frequently that day, so why did she need to know I was pumping?

If you're lucky enough to control your own breaks, you won't necessarily have to let your boss know in advance you plan to pump. You should be able to pump without having to inform everyone in the building. But you may not be able to.

If you are an hourly wage earner, work in a factory, or work in a place where there are strictly mandated breaks and lunch hours, then you will have to enlist the help of a (hopefully) sympathetic supervisor. You will need to pump at regular intervals that may or may not initially coincide with your breaks. If there are ninety minutes until lunch, but your breasts are becoming engorged, you need to pump now, not in an hour and a half. Tell your boss you'll be flexible and make up whatever time is lost, though you should easily be able to pump during fifteen-minute breaks if you use a dual-action pump (and get both breasts at the same time).

### Getting over Your Self-consciousness

I was self-conscious about pumping. There was something distinctly weird about any of my colleagues knowing that I was breastfeeding. I called my breast pump the "stealth pump" because I literally felt like I was sneaking around when I needed to pump.

I was only truly embarrassed once, when a group of county sheriffs surrounded me and my bag after it failed a metal detector test at the entrance to a courthouse. "What's in the bag, Ma'am?" one sheriff growled, his hand on his holster. "It's a pump," I stammered. Of course, all four men now had their hands on their guns. "What kind of pump? Hmmmm??!! A 12-gauge? Huh? Speak up!" I got slightly hysterical and said a little too loudly, "A breast pump! Okay? Are you happy now?" I think they must have felt bad about the shakedown because they vacated their private lounge area and let me pump in privacy.

Nancy is a single mother of two and when her children were babies, she worked as a lawyer in a prestigious firm. Lucky for Nancy she had her own office, so she could pump in privacy—or at least she was blessed with the *illusion* of privacy. By the second or third time she'd pumped, all of the men in the office had stopped working and were crowded around outside her office door taking bets on what she was doing inside. "They thought I brought a vibrator to work so that when I had to write a particularly stressful brief, I used it to calm myself down." When Nancy realized that potential associates and new employees were passing her door as part of their introductory tour around the office, she decided to break the news that what she was doing wasn't nearly so interesting. "They all nodded and shuffled away from the door looking embarrassed. But they still liked to tell the new associates I was using a vibrator," she says.

## Stay Relaxed

I often felt squeezed when I was trying to find fifteen calm minutes in my day to have a milk-ejection reflex. It's not so easy when you're pacing with your chest naked, telling your breasts "C'mon," listening to phones ringing in the background, and your fiftyish boss, who isn't crazy about working with "girls," is asking everyone, "Hey, has anyone seen [fill in your name]?"

For a while, every time I went to use my breast pump, it seemed that I had an awkward conversation with someone. "Where are you going?" "When will you be back?" "Well, what is it you have to do? We could just talk about this while you're doing it." Finally, it seemed easier to just tell the truth. No matter how little I said, it was usually more than most people wanted to know. (It was also the best way to avoid future personal questions.)

Michelle says a coworker, who had an older baby, paved the way for her, scouting out all of the places she could pump at work. But Michelle had another problem. Her job frequently took her to other offices. "My friend knew every bathroom with an outlet, every friendly secretary, every broom closet. I'd just ask her before I had a meeting somewhere else, 'Where did you pump?'" Michelle and her friend developed a funny euphemism for pumping. They call it *farming*. Michelle tells her secretary she has to "go to the farm." Everybody knows what she's up to, but she doesn't actually have to say what she's doing. Sort of like saying, "I'm going to the restroom" instead of something more specific. Nobody bats an eye while she's "down at the farm."

## Finding a Little Privacy

### Beg, Borrow

If you don't have a private office, maybe some friendly member of your staff will give up his or hers during lunch. I sat at somebody else's desk, put the machine on the floor, and spread out the Lifestyle section of *USA Today* to read while I pumped. You'll get frustrated on a dual-action pump trying to read a book because you will have to turn the pages with your elbow, keep both suction cups on your breasts, and since you're in a borrowed office, avoid spilling breastmilk on the vice president's leather blotter. I always brought along a paper towel or napkin because some people are a little squeamish about body fluids, even a sweet, harmless one like breastmilk.

Pumping in the bathroom personally made me sick, but then we had a lax cleaning staff. There was no place to put the pump except on the floor.

The worst thing was trying to juggle sterilized bottles without touching anything. Plus, I often would hear footsteps, then see a pair of shoes pause awkwardly outside my stall. I knew they were wondering what kind of equipment I was using on myself. Finally, our production manager took pity on me and offered me her office during her lunch break. It was the only one with a lock because it had the personnel records. Too bad I had both hands full, or I might have been able to digest enough information on everybody to become successful at blackmail.

### Batten Down the Hatches

Do not ever get yourself set up to pump without first making sure the lock works or bracing furniture against the door. In offices, there are always people who will barge in, and, as liberal as I am, I still think it wouldn't have been a career enhancer if my executive producer had seen my breasts attached to a milking machine. You can get away with an unzipped fly once or twice, but full frontal nudity....

### Get Batteries

Another tip: if you rent or buy a pump, make sure you get one with a battery pack so you won't be stuck searching for outlets. Many bathrooms in airports and offices don't have outlets in them, and when they do, somebody has a curling iron plugged in. I rented a pump without an optional battery. I was on the road a lot, and I can't even count how many fast-food restaurants, cafés, and family-style diners had bathrooms without outlets. One time, I was in a very rural section of northern California that had small towns every half an hour. The crew and I were already late for an interview, but my breasts were getting dangerously full. I didn't know the crew I was working with and didn't tell them why I had to duck into the restroom of every fast-food restaurant within a fifty-mile radius of our ultimate destination (the home of a man suspected of murdering his wife—not the kind of place where I wanted to take time to pump). Finally, I was so frustrated at the wasted time and my impending breast explosion that I finally blurted out what I was looking for. The crew sighed with relief and told me they thought I was some kind of an addict. I was. I was addicted to that machine.

## Male-Dominated Fields

Susan pumped for months and months. No one at work had any idea. But then one day, Susan, who had recently been promoted to sergeant and was the only senior female in her division of the Los Angeles Police

Department, was shooting the breeze with her sergeant colleagues. One said, "So how's the baby doing on formula?" Susan paused as the seconds ticked by, wondering what to say. It was the first time anyone at work had asked such a direct feeding question. Susan had the same policy as the military has toward gays: "Don't ask, don't tell."

"But I wasn't going to lie," she says. "I told them, 'She's never had formula.'" There was an even longer pause as the men with children took this in. Then Susan's supervisor, a gruff, no-nonsense cop, burst out, "Good for you! That's great." Susan says that to her surprise, all of the men beamed at her. That reaction was followed by some blushing and a quick change of subject. "But I knew they were all wondering, 'How does she do it at work?'"

If you don't work with other mothers, or you work with women who bottle-feed their children, you'll find that for once in your life, you may have more in common with men—men whose wives breastfed, that is. I had long conversations with cameramen on the road. One even offered to stop by his house while we were shooting in Tucson to pick up spare parts for my breast pump since I'd (once again) left my parts on my kitchen drainboard in California. Fathers of breastfed babies are more comfortable with the topic, and they'll know to steer clear of unmarked bottles of white liquid in the office refrigerator.

## I Feel Guilty

A lot of women want to or need to return to work after their baby is born. I'm not here to tell you not to. I went back to work full-time when my first daughter was four months, quit when she was fourteen months, worked again when she was eighteen months, worked part-time, quit, wrote a book, and went back to work, quit, had another baby, started another book. . . .

Motherhood and a career create the ultimate paradox. You may never feel 100 percent comfortable in either role again. When I'm working, I worry about the quality of my daughters' lives. When I'm home, I worry about the eventual quality of my life if I don't keep my career moving forward. The time you'll spend nursing your child is a snap of your life's fingers. It won't seem like that at the time, but the time you put in when they're young is an investment that you'll reap the benefits of when they're older. Studies have shown that in spite of the fatigue, working mothers wouldn't have it any other way. There is a great deal of satisfaction in breastfeeding when you are also a working mother.

When somebody at work would ask me a direct question about whether I'd bottle-fed or breastfed my child, and I said that I was still breastfeeding, I'd get this weird look that said, "Poor you! What's it like to be without a life?" I wasn't a saint. In fact, I felt like a very bad mommy to be putting on grown-up clothes and leaving my sometimes wailing infant in the arms of her caregiver. My husband's business took an unexpected hit the year my daughter was born. We needed the money. It was as simple as that. And I needed to feel less guilty about leaving her. Breastfeeding actually helped ease some of the guilt for me. The caregiver could not breastfeed her. Her daddy couldn't do it. The only one in her life who had that unique connection to her was me. And I was glad of it. And no matter how difficult it can occasionally be, most working mothers feel the same way. "I had to be gone," says Claire. "But in a way, I was with my son every time he ate. That was very comforting for me because I was still giving him something no one else could."

You are perfectly normal if you feel sad, conflicted, anxious, and guilty. But if you blame your conflicted feelings on breastfeeding, you'll find that even if you were to wean your baby, you'd still feel conflicted. No doubt about it, babies need their mothers, and mothers need their babies. But you also need to eat and have a roof over your head. If your child care arrangement is a good one, you'll feel less anxious, though you'll likely miss your child just as much. Breastfeeding does bring you closer. I don't know a mother who doesn't want that.

## Do Working Women Breastfeed?

Someone said to me on a radio talk show that I was a guest on, "Working women don't breastfeed." Actually, a higher percentage of working mothers than stay-at-home mothers breastfeed. But a higher percentage also quit after six months because they don't want to pump. You can work and continue to breastfeed. Like everything else in your new life, you'll need to do a little planning to accommodate your date with your breast pump or wait until your body is better prepared to produce milk on your schedule before you're able to completely stop pumping.

"I really don't want to pump at work," Sarina said a month before her maternity leave was up. Yes, pumping is a pain in the neck. But it's not that big a pain in the neck. If your baby is very young and eating every two hours, when you return to work, your body is programmed to produce milk that often. That means pumping two to ten ounces four times a day.

If this seems overwhelming or impossible, you'll need to slowly train your body to make less milk. Maybe you can fit in one pump break during lunch. As the work week went along, I found myself pumping less and less often. Over the weekend, my daughter Olivia was breastfeeding every two hours again, and there was always milk for her. Of course, Monday and Tuesday, there was a little too much milk.

You probably won't be able to train your body for specific pumping times until your baby is at least four months.

You can eventually train your body not to make milk at the times your baby used to be feeding. You simply start dropping one of your pumping sessions every few days (do it slowly to avoid getting engorged). This is to help you avoid having to completely wean your baby because, for whatever reason, you aren't pumping. Some women elect to continue to breastfeed in the morning, in the evening, and during the night. Your body is able to do this, though there may be a lag time between your desires and your body's ability to conform to them. Even if you think you can only get in one pump during your work hours, this too is better than no pumping at all. Lactation consultants used to say it took three to four days for your body to catch up with an increased or a decreased demand for milk. But new research seems to suggest your body is smarter than that and figures out, feed by feed, how much milk your baby is demanding. How much milk you make and how frequently also depends on your milk storage capacity, meaning roughly the size of your breasts. What works for your small-breasted friend might not work for big-breasted you and vice versa (though some small chests can hold a lot and big ones have a small capacity). You'll have to figure out based on your body, how often you need to pump, but don't be surprised if you make different amounts every time you pump. Also, if you've dropped a feeding and need it back, it'll only take a few days before that's part of your body's schedule again. Ultimately, breastfeeding should make your working life easier, not harder.

I pumped for about the first year, but after the first few months, I never found the time to pump more than once a day. During the transition, I did find times when I was engorged, and it wasn't pleasant. But my body eventually stopped making the brunch and late lunch meals and just made the lunch buffet of eight ounces or so.

## It Keeps Your Baby Healthy While You're Away

One of the wonderfully beneficial side effects of breastfeeding for working mothers is that on average, their children will rarely be sick. Leaving a healthy baby to go to work is bad enough. But imagine leaving your baby when he's crying, his nose is running, and his temperature is soaring. Being sick is a big deal for babies. (If your husband is a baby when he's sick, then you know all about this.)

## Breastfed Babies Can Still Get Sick

If you're pumping at work, your baby is getting breastmilk, but he's not getting all of the benefits. Remember when I talked about that study that shows mammary ducts seem to be able to analyze the germ that your baby's been exposed to and come up with germ-fighters manufactured on-site? This protective response won't happen with a breast pump. It only happens if the baby's mouth is in contact with your breast.

That doesn't mean you should stop pumping or expressing. Your baby is still getting plenty of things to strengthen his immune system through your breastmilk. The honest truth is I pumped at work because I was already overwhelmed by guilt, and it made me feel better to think that even if my baby couldn't always have me, she could still have my nutrients.

## Finding a Caregiver or a Daycare Center

The first caregiver we hired couldn't have been nicer when we interviewed her. Great resumé, good references, spotless record. But by the second day, we got to see another side of her. I came back in from my car because I'd forgotten something and saw her expression. She was sighing and acting like a storm cloud as she was changing my daughter's diapers. When I tried to talk to her, she blurted out, "I really don't like children." Ooops.

A good test if you're looking for a daycare center for your baby is to see how receptive the caregivers are to a breastfeeding mother. If they tell you that you can breastfeed at the facility, they'll accommodate pumped breastmilk, and they'll take your phone call when you need to tell them you'll pick up your baby in an hour and want to breastfeed him when you arrive, you are probably going to be in good hands.

Hopefully, it's a center whose caregivers will follow your careful instructions about when to stop giving bottles so that as soon as you get to the center, or home, you can breastfeed your baby. This may require some flexibility if you have a job where you can't always predict when you'll arrive there. You don't want a starving baby. But you don't want to end up with overfull, painful breasts while your baby burps up pumped milk and couldn't be less interested in more food.

When Maria was checking out daycare facilities, she was interviewing the director, who told her, "Most of our mothers just find that breastfeeding and working is too much stress, so babies here are fed formula." Whooop-whoop! Breastfeeding sensors going off. Maria excused herself immediately after those comments and eventually hired a woman who came to her home every day. She says, "I decided one-on-one was a much better arrangement for my daughter anyway. Yes, it's expensive. But she's precious to me, and if I'm going to spend my hard-earned money on something other than the rent and the power bill, it might as well be on her."

## Your Daily Routine

### Mornings

Your life will be easier in the morning if you breastfeed your baby in bed, then pump, then shower and get ready. Do your make-up and hair, maybe even put on your pantyhose, but don't put on your clean work outfit until you're walking out the door. Wait, sorry, I forgot about the neighbors. It's probably better if you get dressed before walking out the door. Until then, wear a bathrobe. That way, you can hold your baby and laugh when he spits up milk, instead of cursing your dry cleaning bill.

### Don't Rush

Try to give yourself enough time. If you're racing around and you throw your baby into the caregiver's arms as soon as she walks in the door, everyone, including you, will feel stressed and rushed. If you have in-home care, have the caregiver arrive a half hour to an hour before you have to leave. That way, your baby will have a transition period before Mommy goes. It'll also give you a chance to search for your pearl earrings, put on your bra without somebody hanging on, and swig your orange juice.

If you have to drive your baby to daycare, getting ready may be a little more complicated. Maybe you can breastfeed your baby in bed, then give the baby to your husband to keep warm on his chest. If feeding time works out right, you can get up a half hour earlier so that you can get ready without having to hold the baby while you blow-dry your hair. Also, this gives your husband some quiet time with a sated, contented baby.

If you're pumping in the morning to leave an extra bottle, you'll need to set aside time for this, too. Open your newspaper, sit down in a quiet place, and read the paper while you pump.

April swears the nursing bras on the market that allow you to fit the pump attachments on your breasts and let go work! She and Dorinda, who's matched this feat, say that this particular bra with the flaps in the front can be maneuvered so that you fit the plastic pump cups on your breasts, turn on the pump to create suction, and then arrange the bra flaps so that the material holds the plastic in place instead of you. Fool around with this. Maybe this method will work for you. There will soon be a new bra designed to give you that "Look Ma, no hands!" feel. It holds the plastic so you don't have to.

You can also arrange it so that you give your baby one last feed at the daycare center, or at the caregiver's house, if there is a quiet area. You don't want to be breastfeeding at a center while seated at a desk built for a two-year-old with other parents rushing around you shouting their good-byes. If you're comfortable breastfeeding in your car, you can also do that in front of the facility.

Pumped milk going along to daycare needs to be refrigerated unless you pumped it that morning and you expect your baby to drink it within six hours of pumping. Remind whomever is feeding the baby to throw out unfinished milk because of the risk of bacteria growing after the baby has used the bottle.

## Most People Will Admire Your Commitment

It is very hard to be a working mother. Our culture hasn't yet figured out quite how to keep all of the balls in the air. But for the most part, people at work who knew I was breastfeeding were compassionate and understanding. (Unfortunately, these were never the people in charge, so there was no set policy.) You'll find people who'll be supportive, too.

When you come across disapproving critics, don't let them get you down. I know a woman with three children who's a high-powered advertising executive. When she came by my home to drop off a gift and saw that I was breastfeeding, she was appalled (she was way beyond shocked). "I can't believe a woman like you would breastfeed!" she said, in the same tone you'd say, "I can't believe a woman like you would advocate baking sugar cookies instead of getting a college degree!" I didn't know that she had formula-fed all three of her children and gone back to work within weeks of their births. Our friendship quickly died after this conversation. She couldn't believe I would. I couldn't believe she wouldn't.

As difficult as it will seem at times, you can be a good parent and a working parent. But you'll have to work harder. It's like holding down two full-time jobs. Breastfeeding is something that you can do for your child for as long as you feel you are able. No matter how long you do, you will have given you child something that no salary could ever buy.

# Chapter 13

# Daddy's Turn: So *That's* What They're For, Too!

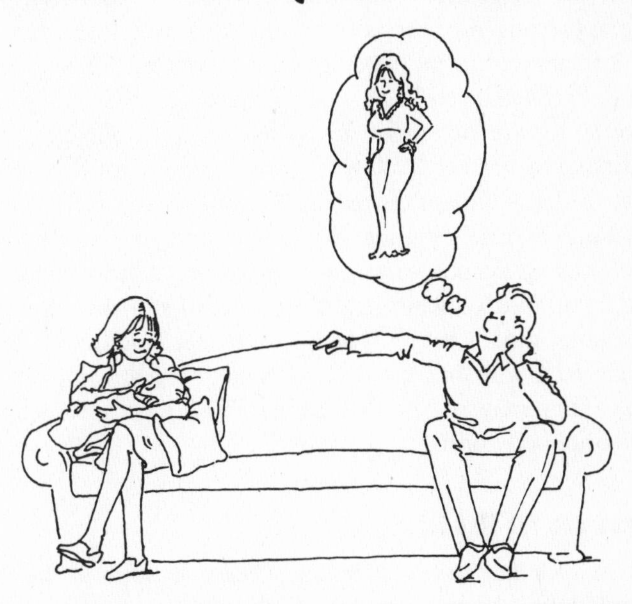

*America:* Tits is the most commonly used . . . [slang word] for breasts. If you want to stand out from the crowd, try melons, honkers, hooters, knockers, tatas, jugs, boobs, bazookas, bazoomas, bazoombas, funbags, love mounds, and headlights [as in, "yours are on"].

*Great Britain:* Thrupenny bits, Bristols, Manchesters, Jerseys (as in City-titties), love boats, cabman's rests, BSH (British Standard Handfuls), catheads (a type of biscuit), pillows, puppy dogs, horror show groodies (from *A Clockwork Orange*), team [as in "great team, wonder if she needs a coach"].

*France:* Nenes, nichons, flotteurs, nibards, doudounes, blobloches and Les Tetons [as in "Grand"].

*Italy:* Le tette, menne, minocchi.

— Annalisa Barbieri, *The Independent*— October 29, 1995

Ever wonder why men have so many names for your breasts? Because they like them, that's why. And now, you've gone and given them to someone else. This is perhaps the biggest transition your husband or partner will have to make. That private little playground he may or may not have used is no longer his. Some other kid is hogging all the swings.

## Dealing with Your Partner

If your partner seems neutral, lukewarm, or even negative, it's normal. It's partly because your breasts aren't his anymore. But that isn't all. Some men, it turns out, are prudes. They think it's indecent, immoral, or at the very least unappetizing for breasts to be used this way. I heard two salesmen on an airplane discussing whether they should turn a woman in for breastfeeding. "Is that legal?" one said to the other, then pulled out his reading material for the long flight. Yes, of course, it was *Playboy*.

Your husband or partner is allowed to have ambivalent feelings. This is not an indicator that he doesn't love you or his new baby. He's sharing you for the first time, and he's sharing an intimate part of you. And he's not the one who's been pregnant, so warm-up time takes a little longer.

Remember the doctor who taught his medical students about breastfeeding by saying "What's baby's is baby's and what's Daddy's is Daddy's" while pointing to a woman's breasts on an anatomy drawing? Men may feel this way. They may not be that happy about having somebody else near their favorite body parts.

## The Good News and the Bad News

Your partner is your key to breastfeeding success. In spite of the fact that you're the one doing the breastfeeding, husbands and partners play a key role in whether you start, continue, or stop breastfeeding. In a study done with 268 expectant mothers and fathers published in *The Journal of Family Practice*, more mothers than fathers preferred breastfeeding as their feeding method (69 percent versus 58 percent). Only 54 percent of couples both preferred breastfeeding. Many of the fathers who said they preferred formula also had misconceptions and some negative attitudes about breastfeeding (but not about breasts). This study also established that women are not able to "accurately predict their partner's attitudes and opinions regarding breastfeeding." Bottom line, if your partner doesn't seem keen about it, you can help him the same way you helped yourself. Give him information, time to digest it, a little understanding, and some room.

## Why Wouldn't Men Want Their Children Breastfed?

Walter sabotaged his wife. He admits it now that his daughter is five—and he has his wife back. Whenever Zoe breastfed Erin, Walter would pick a fight, give her the silent treatment, choose that particular moment to ask her to help him hunt for a sock, or ask her how long she intended to breastfeed. "It became a battle," Zoe says. "He'd seen his brothers and sisters fed with a bottle—then all of his nieces and nephews fed the same way. Always plugged up and propped someplace. I think he was essentially jealous of the attention Erin was getting."

Zoe made Walter read a research article about the benefits of breastfeeding, and suddenly, the struggle was over. "He obviously loved her as much as I did, and he wanted her to get all of this great stuff from breastmilk. He realized that it was all just a big adjustment period, and he backed off."

Some husbands are put in the position of having to defend their wives, and they find themselves resenting it. Steve, who had a baby with his second wife when both were in their forties, says his mother didn't like the idea of breastfeeding. "I think it's just distasteful to her." Jane, Steve's wife, is an independent, smart television anchor, who was not about to back down when her mother-in-law turned up her nose at such a plebeian pursuit.

Steve admits he may even be carrying around some of his mother's generation's prejudice. He was bottle-fed. Since Steve travels for business, he says that he often sees "these earth mothers" in just the places they can be expected to be found: Berkeley, Greenwich Village, and Colorado. "It bothers me to see other women doing it, especially if it's not a baby."

Tim, a radio shock-jock, isn't bothered by much, and his regular stock and trade on his morning show is breast jokes. But he was bothered by his beautiful wife's transition from model to nursing mother. However, even he rose to the occasion when an elderly man in an airport told Tim's wife, who was discreetly breastfeeding, "Don't you be doing *that* here!" Tim's wife tried to ignore the man, but when he came close to her and waved his fist at her, Tim borrowed her breast from his infant son, and squirted the man with breastmilk. That is certainly *one* way to handle it.

## "But We Had the Perfect Relationship Before"

If you had a wedding, even if it was "the perfect wedding," you might remember how all of the families' old rivalries, bitter struggles, and unresolved crap kept rearing its head when you were just trying to decide between chocolate and lemon cake. The same thing happens when a new baby comes into the picture, because it is so stressful. All of the stuff you and your husband or partner have ever had a fight about will suddenly be back. You'll be battling fatigue, overstimulation, a huge change in your life, and most of all the sudden appearance of a third person who's around all of the time and demands every nanosecond of your time. You are caring for someone who is essentially bedridden and needs help doing everything. Lucky for us that babies come in small, cute packages. The bottom line is if all isn't bliss at your house for the first few months of the first year, it doesn't mean you're headed for a divorce or a break-up.

## "Could We Schedule Some Spontaneous Time?"

*Planning* is essential with a new baby and it may be a new concept for you. If before your bundle of joy arrived, you'd had sex when you were in the mood, read the paper when it arrived, and dashed off to see a movie as soon as it was premiering, guess what? Now you have to plan like you're a general readying for an invasion.

Breastfeeding throws an additional wrench into this planning during the early months because you can only be away from your baby, or breast pump, for relatively short periods of time.

Michelle says she and her husband finally gave up trying to be social for a while, unless they were visiting somebody who had a baby and could relate. "We were late to everything, left early, and spent the entire time in a back room dealing with the baby. Finally, we decided it wasn't worth it, and we stayed home until Jenna was bigger."

## Ways to Convince Him to Share

My husband had not been breastfed. His sister did not breastfeed her children. I believe he was somewhat neutral on the topic until he found out Michael Jordan was a breastfed baby. Actually, as soon as he found out some key facts, like the part about how breastfed babies are ahead developmentally, cognitively and may even get more IQ points, he was very supportive. He learned that breastfed babies are on average much healthier. Since he has asthma and terrible allergies that have dogged him his whole life and wrecked his athletic career (we're talking Pop Warner football, not the '49ers), he was overwhelmed at the idea that he might not necessarily have had the same health problems if he'd been breastfed. That made him a strong proponent.

At the same time, your husband just may not be as enthusiastic or as interested in breastfeeding as you are, just as he may not have wanted to feel the baby move each of the 5,098,482,017 times he kicked. That's okay. Andy supports Dorinda's decision to "do it for as long as she wants." Andy says he doesn't care how long she does it and professes not to care whether she does it at all, though he does know some of the health advantages and he says he has "great respect" for his wife because she got through some early problems and kept breastfeeding. Dorinda is resigned to Andy's declared neutrality. "I said we would renegotiate when the baby is six months."

Laura, who has two children, daughter Lizzie and son John, says she hovered too much over her husband, and that was what was interfering with their relationship, not the breastfeeding. "I'll admit, I was a fusser," she says. "I'd see him doing something, changing, rocking, holding, and I'd have to say, 'You're not doing it right!'" She says she was trying to let her husband do everything but the one thing he couldn't do, but it wasn't easy. She couldn't keep from giving him instructions and supervising his every effort. One day, her well-mannered, helpful mother, who had been silent until then, gave Laura a golden piece of advice. Her mother made her a nice cup of tea, sat her down, smiled at her warmly, and said, "Laura, I have an important thing to tell you—*shut up*."

Most men (even really nice men) whose wives have breastfed have had mixed feelings about it. "I want to breastfeed," Rob, a warm, soft-spoken dancer, whose partner is expecting a baby, told me. I started to explain that in some African tribes, men who are unable to hunt stay in the village and care for the infants. They will put the babies to their breasts to soothe them, and because men are mammals too and have mammary ducts, this constant stimulation will sometimes cause these men to lactate. Yes, you read that right. They will make some milk. But in the middle of this lengthy explanation, Rob said, "No, no. I want to be the one *on* the breast, not the one *with* the breasts." A lot of men feel this way. That was their special area before the baby came along.

Women can have mixed feelings, too. I remember thinking about the children's story *Heidi* one day when I was watching my daughter. Clara is all messed up because her father saved her instead of her mother when their boat tipped over. I kept imagining myself in rapids with the ability to save only one member of my family: my husband or my baby. I felt so guilty knowing that my first instinct was always to imagine grabbing my child. I have never told my husband this, and it is one of the reasons why the three of us have not been on a boat together.

Men sense your protective feelings toward the baby. *They* used to be that important to you. Before the baby, you'd have rescued *them* from the rapids first. And now, there's someone between you. Some men feel very left out. (Actually, it's highly likely your husband's first instincts would be to grab his child, too. That's why Clara survived.) Even if you're so wrapped up in your baby you can't remember who donated the sperm, try not to leave your partner out. He needs you, too, and he needs to develop a separate but equal relationship with your child.

Jane didn't tell her husband Steve that no one in her life had ever made her feel as loved, special, indispensable, and warm as her daughter, Alyx Anne. She was wise not to. It's better not to tell your husband if suddenly you feel like you love your child more. You will and you won't. You'll love differently, and depending on who's driving you the craziest, your feelings will swing back and forth.

Men can feel left out of the parenting process if you insist on doing all the changing, cooing, holding, bathing, burping, and cuddling. They know you have to do all of the breastfeeding. They know that your breasts now have a different purpose. That's a hard adjustment. "Yeah, I missed her," says Nathan. "We had had such a great sex life, and suddenly, not only did Viv have no time for me, I had no access to her body. Only the baby did." But men sometimes hesitate to share their thoughts with partners because women sometimes take it as a statement of feelings about the child. "I kept wondering, 'Is he jealous of his son? Doesn't he love his son? Why is this an issue?'" Elaine says. But it doesn't have much to do with his love for the baby. It has to do with his love for you. That's a good thing, not a bad thing. Both partners have to recognize that this new craziness and possible loss of sexual intimacy is a temporary condition as long as you're committed to being partners.

## To Have and to Hold, in Poopy Diapers and in Health

Men initially may feel that they're not that important in the baby's life. After all, if you're breastfeeding, you are necessary for the baby's survival. His father isn't, at least not yet. "The truth is," Michael says in a near whisper, "I really felt left out that I couldn't do that (breastfeed)." When his first son was born, he says of the new "breastfeeding couple," wife Cheryl and son Jared, "I saw what an intimate bond the two of them had, and I could do everything else. But that was the thing he liked the most. And I couldn't do it."

My four-year-old daughter met me at the door one night after I'd left Dad home to baby-sit her and the new baby, Julia. "The baby doesn't like Dad," Olivia said soberly. "He doesn't have breasts." She didn't know that when she was a baby, many times, her father looked down forlornly at his hairy chest and said, "It's not fair. Why don't I have something that calms her that quickly?" Actually, sometimes your baby might root around on her father's bare chest. Olivia did this a couple of times, then spit out nipple and chest hairs with a loud, "Phew-twohhhhh" sound and a horrified expression on her face as if to say, "What the heck was that?"

There are many, many ways your husband can bond with your baby that do not involve feeding. And that does not mean handing the baby off every time he or she needs a diaper change. You need to share the pleasant parts, too. You're no more capable of handling a squirming baby if you have no experience with babies than your husband is. In fact, your husband, if he happens to work with his hands as, say, a mechanic or a brain surgeon or pianist, might even be more comfortable holding the baby than you are initially. My husband gave Olivia her debut bath because he can take apart a motor and put it back together without dropping and losing important parts.

Men also have a tendency to be solution-oriented. A lot of them are just waiting to be told what you need. Laura counsels new mothers to begin sentences with, "Honey, I'd love it if you could . . . " Fill in your request: "Hold the baby.' "Let me sleep." "Get rid of your mother."

Nurses at a southern California hospital still laugh at a proud new father, who got his daughter to latch on to his "breast" after he saw his wife nursing. He wanted to try it, too. "He was bare-chested, walking down the hall of the maternity ward with his daughter 'breastfeeding,'" laughs one nurse. "He was so proud of himself. He kept saying, 'Look! I'm doing it too!'"

Howard Stern reportedly shaved his chest to see if he could get his baby to breastfeed. While your partner probably won't think this is such a neat idea, he does need to support what you're doing with your chest.

## "I'm Not Gonna Try It! You Try It!"

Husbands and partners are curious. They may even be interested in trying the milk. I hope that doesn't sound gross to you. I overheard my husband explaining to a male friend who'd come by for a business meeting the reasons why I was breastfeeding. Then I saw him sneaking into the kitchen and filling a shot glass with breastmilk out of the refrigerator. I didn't want to scare them, so I didn't make my presence known, but I did keep eavesdropping. I overheard a discussion between them that went something like this: "I'm not gonna try it. You try it!" "No way, I'm not gonna try it—you try it." That exchange followed by scuffling noises, an audible slurp and a long pause. "Hey, it's good! Tastes like vanilla ice cream!"

Patrick, a twenty-three-year-old aspiring law enforcement officer, didn't have the same reaction, but maybe it's because he didn't drink his cold. "It's gross. It tastes like warm skim milk."

## Other Ways to Share the Fun

Wanda, mother of Taylor, says her husband wanted to try hand expressing and eventually got good at it. Enlisting your husband's help might not be the most comfortable solution for you, though. I love my husband, but there are two things I wouldn't allow him to do: remain in the bathroom while anything complicated is going on or milk my breasts. But Wanda and Gary are two of the most well-adjusted, least squeamish people I know. Gary is a trouper in every department, and both he and his wife have wonderful senses of humor. Gary, big city executive, thought it was funny to be back to his farm boy roots, once again working on a farm.

My husband sometimes sat and talked to me while the breast pump whirred. After eight years of marriage, he's seen me looking as pitiful as I can look. (During my first delivery, he spritzed the room with breath freshener because he told me he has a "strong gag reflex" and the sights, sounds, and particularly the smells of birth were getting to him.) He laughed the first time he saw me attached to the pump and said I reminded him of his first field trip, to a dairy farm. I couldn't get mad because in this case, truth was a defense. Besides, he says he meant it in a "complimentary" way. But he never got as excited as I did over how much milk I could make.

Sometimes when I was breastfeeding my daughter, I would set up next to my husband while he paid bills, read or watched football. It was nice just to be near each other.

Think about all of those goofy articles you've read in women's magazines about spicing up your love life. Don't forget that even though you've made a baby, you might still want to have a little recreational sex. "You mean I have to do it again?" April says she told her husband the first time he hinted he wanted to have sex after their daughter was born.

Yes, you have to do it again. Maybe not right this second. In the meantime, pretend that you are feeling all of the feelings you'd like to be feeling. Like tranquillity, for instance. Buy some inexpensive candles. One night, turn off the overhead fluorescent, and light the candles. Put on some nice music. Work to make the home environment pleasant for yourself, your husband, and your baby. Not everything has to lead to sex.

April says the first time she and her husband tried to have sex was six weeks after delivery. "We finally got the baby to go to sleep, then we snuck out to the living room." April says they'd gotten spoiled during their attempts to conceive and, of course, during pregnancy. They hadn't had to hassle with birth control. "We'd never had to do this planning thing before. We hadn't used birth control in so long. Here we were fumbling with all of these boxes of KY jelly and condoms, like we were about to do a craft project." By the time they'd gotten ready, "we were sitting there stark naked, and I said, 'Are you into this?' My husband said, 'Not really.' We started laughing, and we laughed and laughed. We ended up just cuddling on the couch together and talking."

## Trade Favors

Do nice things for your husband, whatever little things you can manage. And he just might do nice things back. My husband likes motor sports, so one night when he worked late, I taped everything on television that featured wheels and a motor. When he came home, I gave him the tape with a ribbon wrapped around it.

Instead of making a list of all the things he doesn't do, stop yourself and remember all of the things he does do. Wait until you're in a pleasant mood before you bring up whatever it is you'd like him to do. For example, suggest, "I'll pay the bills if you'll do the grocery shopping this week." Whatever. It also usually works better if you can offer a choice. "Do you want to finish the dishes or get the baby ready for bed?" That way, you aren't ordering him around and he won't be resentful.

If you've ever been around an incredibly crotchety person for any length of time, then you know what it's like to be near someone who can ruin your day with a few words. So try not to speak angry words hastily. Yes, I'm suggesting that *you* might be a little crotchety, not your partner. You're not a bad person. You're a tired person with a new baby. Your short temper is normal, but it can be hard for your partner if you are insensitive. Everything has changed for him, too. You will eventually go back to being yourself, but he doesn't know this yet.

## Include Him

Because men like to fix things, he may feel totally overwhelmed and withdraw because he can't fix all that's wrong with you. You have to heal physically, you need sleep, and your hormones are wacky. There's no easy way to fix all that's wrong with the baby, either. Once the diaper's changed, it's time to be fed, or changed again, or rocked, or put to sleep, or changed or fed. So find something for him to fix or to do. Have him fix the broken spring on the crib.

Force yourself to make some time for each other, alone. Somehow, this falls to the lowest rung on your priority ladder, even below rotating the mattress. While it's lovely to do things together as a family, you need to continue to have a relationship with each other. Try to arrange for a sitter even one night a week or month. My husband and I would go watch a movie and then sit for a while and have a cup of coffee. The first time we did this, I remembered why I'd liked my husband so much in the first place. We'd been so busy arguing over who forgot to buy diapers, change the baby, and pay the water bill that we weren't having a whole lot of fun being married.

## Sleeping Arrangements

Money will always be an issue. So will in-laws. But sleep doesn't have to be. Patrick says the worst part about long-term breastfeeding for him was that his daughter ended up sleeping between him and his wife Michelle every night. When I asked if they still had a sex life, he laughed. "Yeah, we sneak around. Brooke falls asleep in our bed, then *we* go into *her* bedroom." While Brooke lies spread-eagled in her parents' king-size bed, Patrick and Michelle work to get all of their limbs on top of her small bed. I didn't ask if they both fit into Brooke's crib before she had the big-girl bed.

Sleeping with your child long-term might not be the ideal arrangement for one or both of you, but a lot of couples do it. Not many feel comfortable admitting it, since America frowns on this (though there is no research that has ever indicated it is harmful and other countries have no problem with it). Patrick and Michelle got married after daughter Brooke was born. They never had a honeymoon. Brooke slept with her parents and Michelle told Patrick that she would stop breastfeeding when Brooke turned eighteen months. At eighteen months, Brooke was still sleeping with her parents and Patrick says, "I started getting a little annoyed."

Most women whose husbands ask will give a low estimate. Like when you're trying to talk your husband into clothes shopping, you say, "I just want to look for a minute." You might tell him you're only going to breastfeed for a few weeks, or a few months, or a year—whatever feels like the bare minimum to you. Your partner may forget that you set up an arbitrary deadline. Or he may not, and you'll have to talk to him about it. Patrick says he secretly wishes his wife had stopped breastfeeding his daughter at the end of her first year. What he misses most is the ability to go out together or go camping overnight.

You will need to include your man when you're sorting through the sleeping arrangements. It's easy to fall into the family bed routine, but if it's not working well in your marriage, you may need to discuss ways to eventually get your baby back in his own bed. Sleep seems to be a hot button for men for obvious reasons. They're not interested in merely sleeping—they're interested in sleeping with you. And that's a good thing. A healthy marriage ultimately makes for healthier, happier children.

Emphasize the positive reasons to breastfeed. Dylan likes the fact that because of wife Trudy's breastfeeding, "our baby is never sick, which is great because my brother's kid is always sick." But he says he's happiest about nighttime breastfeeding after he's compared notes with some of his peers whose wives don't breastfeed. "They never get any sleep because they're constantly mixing and heating formula. I didn't have to do anything—except share Trudy. But then, she has to share me, too."

## Your Sex Life

I know, sex is definitely at the top of your list right now. Right up there next to cleaning closets and going through boxes stored in the attic. "I'm just not interested," says Michelle, mother of a three-month-old, who was delivered through a C-section. "Okay, one time I was kind of enjoying it, but my incision hurt whether he was on top or I was on top. Internally, it also killed."

### "Nobody Told Me Sex Would Hurt"

Many women are surprised that sex hurts, even after their doctors have told them that their C-sections and episiotomies have healed. But C-sections and episiotomies can take a long time to heal internally. While the exterior cut may be healed, the scar tissue is still sensitive and sore. "Sex hurt for six months," says Brenda, who had an episiotomy. Other women say they feel fine during sex after the first few months.

Hormones that the body secretes for breastfeeding can also make sex a little more uncomfortable (especially in the early months of breastfeeding). "It just doesn't feel the same to me," says Helen, who has a young baby.

Andy says Dorinda was in so much pain the first few times they tried, "It was like that old vaudeville routine, where the guy says, 'Doctor, it hurts when I do this.' The doctor says, 'So don't do that.'" Andy says each time they tried, it got a little less painful for Dorinda.

Lactation consultants recommend two things to help with the pain: use plenty of personal lubricant, such as K-Y Jelly, during sex and do your Kegel exercises a few times a day. Sandra Jansen recommends Astroglide lubricant made in West Hollywood, California. Helen tried it and calls it "a wonderful gucky mess." Don't use Vaseline or other petroleum jellies; you want a water-soluble lubricant. You can also use saliva.

As for Kegel exercises, if you haven't been doing these all along, you should start now. To do a Kegel, tighten the muscles around your anus, vagina, and urethra, squeezing them as you would to stop the flow of urine midstream. In fact, you can do just that next time you urinate so that you'll be able to gauge whether you're tightening the right muscles. The first time you try this, you probably won't be able to stop the flow of urine. But the more often you do Kegels, the quicker those muscles will get back in shape. Don't worry about anyone wondering what you're doing; if you're doing them right, involving only internal muscles, no one can tell. Mary told me she makes herself do Kegels at every red light. "Though I'm doing a lot more speeding through yellow lights, so I think I need to change that," she says. You can do Kegels in line at the grocery store or while watching television. When you are able to stop the flow of urine, your muscle strength is on its way back.

### Hey, a Squirt Gun

The same hormone that causes your body to make milk is also produced when you're having an orgasm. Be prepared to squirt your partner. Gary says he and wife Wanda were completely unprepared for the fire hose that let down during their romp in the hay. "All of a sudden, she just blasted me in the face with milk. We thought it was funny." They grabbed a towel to stop the flow, then continued. Sandra Jansen says she tells couples to expect this, and most men aren't bothered by it. "I had one guy in class who said, "No problem. I'll bring cookies to bed. I like cookies and milk!"

If you find the thought of a possible breast squirt gun not particularly romantic, you can do a few things to minimize the possibility of it happening. You can breastfeed the baby or pump right before you have sex (god willing, your partner won't go to sleep on you) or you can wear a bra and pads to bed (just remember to take out the curlers).

### Honey, You've Changed

While you may be exhausted and in pain right now, your husband may also be exhausted—and in pain for a different reason. Having a baby changes your body as well as your perception of your body and yourself. But he probably didn't gain weight along with you. He's probably raring to go. Andy, a quiet, orderly attorney, pipes up when I mention sex. "Yes," he says. "I'm definitely in favor of it."

But it's not easy to get used to your postpartum body. I just couldn't believe nature could be so cruel. I couldn't wear my old jeans for months and months, and I burst into tears when my husband offered to lend me a pair of his.

Vicky, who is a marathon runner, couldn't adjust to her new body after giving birth, either. "I think I thought I'd have the baby and be back to the old Vicky. When I looked at myself in the mirror, I thought, 'My gosh, where is she?'" Vicky, who had the body of a long-distance runner, couldn't get used to having hips, thighs, a stomach, and a butt, as she puts it. But her husband really liked the changes and just kept reassuring her. Tom says, "Before the baby, Vicky looked like Bruce Lee. I like all the curves. It's fun—almost like having a new partner. I don't care that her stomach isn't flat."

Helen, a sexy musician before giving birth, was horrified at how different her body looked. Her husband, who is younger than she is, also made a few pointed remarks. "He picked up a photo of me in a bathing suit, and said, 'God, you were beautiful.'" But a few weeks later, Eric had stopped sighing and looking at old pictures of his wife. Helen had started to put makeup on and wear some flattering clothes again. She'd also lost some weight. "I was walking in the mall with the baby, and men were turning to look at me again!" she says triumphantly.

### Counseling Helps

What if your sex life was in trouble before the baby was born? Debbie and her husband didn't have sex after her fourth month of pregnancy. "Looking back, I think we stopped right around the time I started to show." Colin was uncomfortable having sex with a pregnant woman, something he now admits. "I feel bad saying this, but I wasn't attracted to her when she was pregnant. Yes, I loved her, but I was afraid of hurting her or the baby, and she was, well hell, she was a *mother*." The two went to counseling after their son was born because their sex life still hadn't repaired itself.

Debbie says, "It took time, but the foundation was there. I tried not to take it personally when he said he went through a phase when he wasn't attracted to me." Colin says the thing that helped the most was the relief he felt when he told Debbie the truth. "In the presence of the counselor, Debbie wasn't as mad as I think she might have been, and I learned that the way I was seeing her was my hang-up." By the time their son was a year old, their sex life had returned to normal. They decided that once a week was a good goal. "But we had to work on getting that languid spontaneousness back," says Debbie. "It didn't just happen."

## Touched Out

Some women complain that they are just "touched out" and uninterested when their husbands want their breasts. "I just think, 'Oh lord, not you too!'" says Melinda. This phase passes, but your husband might feel sad during it. "They weren't his breasts anymore," says Melinda.

Some men just draw an imaginary line around your chest and declare it off-limits. "It took Bob three years before he could get back into my breasts sexually," Trisha says. "He completely avoided them during my two years of breastfeeding my son so he wouldn't 'soil the food source.'" Of course, Bob never told Trisha that this was why he stopped touching her breasts. She assumed it was because he didn't like them anymore. "I had stretch marks," she says. "They're invisible," Bob now laughs. "I never even noticed them, and I wish I'd just told Trisha why I felt weird about putting my hands all over my son's food dish."

Try to talk about your feelings together. Use a neutral third party such as a counselor if that helps. If you don't mind your baby and your husband being interested in your breasts at the same time, work to reassure your husband. If you don't want anyone else handling your breasts, you'll have to reassure your husband that this is a temporary request. And speaking of temporary conditions, you may not want to be touched anywhere for a while. Julie, an experienced mother of two, gave Denise, a new mother, some advice. "She said, 'You know that eight-week postpartum visit where they clear you for sex? Listen to me—tell your husband that the doctor said you have to wait another eight weeks!'"

# Chapter 14

# Weaning: Do I Have To? Will You Ever?

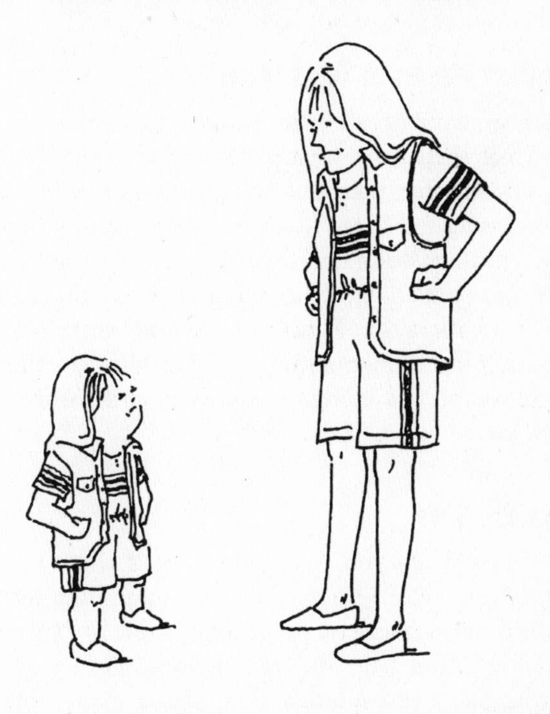

Whether you wean at six weeks or sixteen months, leaving behind this special relationship with your child is hard. Hard for your baby if he isn't ready. Hard for you if you aren't ready and your baby is.

Ideally, your baby will let you know when he is ready to stop. Most babies don't self-wean before nine months. Then, it's anybody's guess. If we let babies decide when they were ready, some would stop at nine months, some would stop at three and a half years, some even older. The average would likely be around two years.

But mothers have reasons for wanting to wean. Some have to. Some want to. Some would like to and then decide it's more trouble to wean than to just keep whipping it out when that certain little person has that plaintive "Gee, I'd really love some milk" look.

### Weaning Too Soon

If you have a newborn, ask yourself, "What's the hurry?" As babies get bigger, they stop breastfeeding around the clock. Once they're also taking in solids (usually by six months), they no longer need to be breastfed more than four or so times a day, though they may ask for it more frequently.

### "My Friend's Baby Weaned at Three Weeks"

Beware of early weaning stories. You will run into women who will swear up and down that their baby weaned himself at a few weeks or months. One woman told me her daughter weaned herself at two weeks. Babies like hers are refusing the breast for some other reason, and mothers can almost always get them back on. They are not weaning themselves. They are distressed over something, either physical or emotional. Babies may be refusing the breast for a whole host of reasons before nine months, but don't fool yourself into thinking they're giving you signs that they want to wean. More likely, they're going on a nursing strike, something that can happen at any age.

### Good Days and Bad Days

There will be days when you think you deserve the mother-of-the-year award and days when you wish you'd done things differently (and you're glad no tabloid show has you caught on tape for their segment on grumpy mommies). You have different moods, and so does your child. Some days will go more smoothly than others, and some times at the breast will go better than other times. You may find that because of some new stress in your life, you feel preoccupied when your child wants to breastfeed. You've started to think about weaning him to try to minimize your stress. But the stress in your life and your breastfeeding your child have nothing to do with each other. And weaning can be a stressful process in itself.

The good and bad thing about breastfeeding is it forces you to be with your baby and do almost nothing else. Sometimes, this can be a little frustrating. If you have a run of feedings during which you wish you were doing something else and you wish your baby was tethered to a bottle instead of to you, allow yourself these feelings. Do not assume that your child would need you less if he had a bottle. He might even need you more.

I went through stages where I really wanted to wean. Each time I would consider it, I would eventually decide against it because the benefits of being able to feed and comfort my daughter far outweighed whatever my current complaint was about breastfeeding.

Quitting completely may leave you ambivalent, though you may still decide you don't want to breastfeed as often as your child seems to want to. But having breastfeeding in your child-calming bag of tricks is something you won't appreciate until you no longer have it. Laura, who weaned John at twenty-three months, said there were many times when she wished she could still calm him by taking him in her arms and popping her breast in his mouth. When little children fall, get sick, or are in very stressful situations, the thing that will calm them the quickest is your arms and your breast. Your breast and the sucking action is incredibly comforting for them.

## Changing Your Weaning Deadline

I think the first time I thought about weaning, my daughter was halfway through her first year. I wondered—now that she was on real food, did she still need the nutrients from my breast? The answer to that is an emphatic yes. Even though your baby is taking in solids, he still needs breastmilk first. That's the food most appropriate for his growing body and brain.

The next time I thought about weaning, my daughter was turning one. I vacillated around her birthday party. So many parenting books and magazine articles tell you that if you go beyond a year, you're doomed to breastfeed for the rest of your life. Not true. Yes, there are some milestones when children may be more likely to wean themselves. But that doesn't mean you can't do it at thirteen months as easily as you might have at twelve months. Yes, at a year your child is learning to walk and talk and yes, this is fun and new. But for many children, nothing, and I do mean nothing, replaces their mother and their mother's breasts. "I thought about quitting when she was a year, but then I wondered why," Joanne says. "I felt like everybody wanted to know, and I thought, 'Why is it such a big deal to everyone else that I am still breastfeeding what is after all, a baby.'" Joanne's daughter Kelly showed no signs of wanting to self-wean, so Joanne kept going. "She was not ready to wean, so would it be easier at thirteen months or fourteen months or seventeen months?" Joanne asks.

Actually, it was much easier at nineteen months. That's when Kelly had had enough and walked away from the breast by herself.

## Stages Where Babies or Toddlers Might Be Willing to Be Weaned

There are several predictable stages in which babies may give signs that they are amenable to weaning. These are only guides, though, and your baby isn't missing the boat if he misses these stages. According to Chele Marmet, babies will self-wean at no earlier than nine months. The next milestone is eighteen months, then two years. Those are the times your baby is *more likely* to initiate weaning, but all babies are different. Don't circle days on the calendar and be disappointed if the dates come and go. On the other hand, if he's just not interested anymore, even if it isn't right on schedule, then he isn't interested (provided it isn't a nursing strike or something else).

## Making *Your* Decision

Many women get cornered and feel pressure to wean, particularly after an aggressive encounter with someone who wouldn't take "I don't know" as an answer for "When are you going to stop that?" To help you decide, ask yourself a variation of the question Dear Abby asks women who think they want a divorce: Are you better off with him or without him? Ask yourself, Are you better off with or without your ability to breastfeed? Sure, breastfeeding may bug you sometimes. But are you better off having breastfeeding in your arsenal, even if you use it sparingly, or not having breastfeeding at all? You also need to think about how your life, health, finances, and other family obligations play into the mix. Whatever decision you make, it should be respected.

## Reasons You Are Considering Weaning

Before you decide to wean, think about why you're weaning, so that you can make your own decision.

### Medical Emergencies

If you are weaning so that you can get emergency medical treatment, such as radiation therapy, for instance, then you have to wean. If you need to get a minor dental procedure done, you can either let the procedure wait or, in most cases, have it done and continue to breastfeed. Many dentists don't know enough about breastfeeding and drugs, so talk to a doctor or call one of the drug information hotlines listed in the Appendix.

### Vacations

You may be thinking about weaning before going on a two-week vacation. But you may have some other options. You could take your baby and a caregiver with you. You could take your pump. You could go for less time. You could change your plans and go when the baby is older. Or you could wean. But plan ahead if you decide to wean. Start weaning weeks before you're scheduled to go. Don't just leave your baby to cope with your being gone and the end of breastfeeding at the same time. You will also find it painful physically to stop breastfeeding cold turkey.

### Working

You may decide to wean because you are working full-time. "It's not the breastfeeding I'm sick of," says Amai. "It's the pumping." Amai's daughter is four months and Amai works full-time. Among many working mothers who breastfeed, not enough make it past six months because pumping is one of those things that eventually doesn't seem as "mandatory" as finishing the report that's due at 5:00 p.m. "It was simply hard to find the time and the space at work," Amai says. After some thought, Amai decided not to wean and learned better ways to accommodate pumping. If you're going back to work, reread Chapters 11 and 12 about pumping and working, and try it. Some women don't mind pumping at all, but it also depends on your work environment.

If you want to wean because you don't want to pump anymore, start by pumping less at work. Your body will adjust to fewer feedings, and maybe you can squeeze in one pumping during an eight-hour day.

There are also ways around having to pump. If your baby is older than three months, you can breastfeed when you're at home with your baby in the morning and at night. Your body will adjust to these spaced feedings in three to four days. At least, you won't have to quit altogether, and your child will still get some of the goodies from breastmilk. This is a practical alternative to lugging around a pump or feeling sad that you're not able to produce any milk anymore.

## Weaning Dos and Don'ts

Regardless of the reason you need or want to wean, you need to do it gradually and with love, and unless you are facing a medical emergency, you can't just stop cold turkey. First of all, you'll be engorged, which is not pleasant. Second, your child will probably be in shock. Your breasts have been most of your child's world. They provide not only sustenance, but comfort, too. Just boarding up shop and telling your child that the dairy farm has closed permanently is not a good way to stop breastfeeding. I remember the time I went to summer camp and was mean to my mom as I got on the bus. I worried for the entire week that I'd get home and find all of my letters still in the mailbox with the words, "moved, no forwarding address." This is what it'll feel like to your baby if you suddenly abandon breastfeeding. You will have moved without him. He will feel rejected, and he won't understand why you've rejected him.

## Figure Out Feedings

Spend a few days keeping close track of your child's breastfeeding pattern. Count up the number and times of feedings so you have a rough idea of when he usually signals that he wants to breastfeed. Before you begin weaning, you should have an idea of how many feedings a day you're doing. For example, if your baby is a year and you breastfeed four times during the day—when he wakes up, before and after his nap, and before bedtime—figure out which session is least important to him. Perhaps he'll take a nap without breastfeeding. This feeding then would be the first one to give up. You need to drop one feeding no more frequently than every four days. So if your baby is breastfeeding four times a day, it'll take you at least sixteen days to wean him. Any faster and you will cause your child unnecessary stress.

Mother nature has also built in a fail-safe to keep you from boarding up the milk factory too quickly. If you wean your child abruptly, you will get engorged and it will be painful. The engorgement could lead to a more severe problem. "I get at least a call a day from a woman with a bad breast infection because she has weaned too quickly," says Sandra Jansen.

## Don't Wean When You're Under Stress

Weaning is stressful for you and for your baby. It's important that you don't wean your baby if other stressful things are happening at the same time, though that's often when most women need to wean. If you're moving, getting divorced, got a bad haircut, or erased the data on your computer's hard drive, don't pick this time of your life to wean. Wait until you're back into your normal routine. You may be disappointed at not being able to wean right at the minute that you want to, but consider the alternative. Or maybe I should say listen to the alternative. Your baby could be crying, whining, pleading, screaming, negotiating or begging.

Does he seem distressed that he can't get near your chest? Believe him. He is genuinely distressed. Miriam's pediatrician told her to just "ignore" Lucas's pleas because he was "having a temper tantrum." Babies and young children breastfeed for comfort, which is a genuine need and shouldn't be dismissed so easily. There is a difference between your child throwing a temper tantrum at the park because he can't have a super-heros candy-coated dripsicle before dinner and exhibiting genuine grief because he's asking to do something he's been doing since birth that's fed him and nurtured him. He's inconsolable because this is a major transition in his life.

## Weaning Young Babies

If your baby is less than a year old when you wean him, you will have to wean him to stored breastmilk or formula; if he's more than a year old (or your doctor has given you the okay), he can have cow's milk. If your baby is younger than three months, he'll probably willingly take a bottle. If he refuses the first few times you try, get a variety of different nipples and try again. If he still won't take a bottle, you might have to wean him to a cup, which means you'll keep breastfeeding until he is a few months older. If you don't necessarily care whether or not he takes a bottle, you can use a periodontic syringe to feed him, but frankly, breastfeeding will be a lot less hassle.

You'll have to do some replacement therapy, too. You'll need to spend more time holding and reading and talking to your baby during the time you used to spend breastfeeding. Take him to the park and let him lie on his back and watch the trees while you talk to him. Let him lie on a blanket in his room and look at your face. Cuddle him and hold him.

When you are trying to wean your baby, don't feed him in the places where you used to breastfeed. He'll immediately make the association and want to nurse. Also, try not to hold your child the way you held him when you were breastfeeding. Guess what happens if you do?

## Weaning Older Babies and Toddlers

Toddlers usually have one or two feedings a day that are sacrosanct. For my first daughter, it was when she woke up in the morning. She would call out for one of us, my husband would usually go and get her, and then she would crawl in bed with us, snuggle up next to me, and nurse. The morning feeding, when I was trying to sneak a little more sleep in, is probably the reason I breastfed her for so long. It took very little effort on my part to keep her happy for forty-five minutes while I slept and she slurped down "number one," as she called it, then crawled over me and had "number two." As she got bigger, I noticed that my tolerance level got lower and lower. I didn't mind as long as it was less than fifteen minutes on each side. Longer than that, and it became irritating. I also started talking to her about the other two times in the day that she'd ask for milk. I told her that I was only going to breastfeed twice a day, then finally once a day. I asked her when she was about twenty-two months which milk she could give up: breakfast, lunch, or dinner milk. She chose dinner, which made sense because the nighttime feeding had always been the least important one for her. If she was at it too long, I'd give her the three-minute warning by telling her that the milk shop was closing soon. It didn't take long before she'd come off my breast by herself without crying or complaining.

When a nosy neighbor wondered when one little boy was going to stop breastfeeding, his grandfather replied tartly, "Would *you* want to stop?" Keep this in mind. Most babies and toddlers will have one favorite feeding. It's usually a feeding that precedes or follows sleep. For most children, it's the just-before-bedtime feed or the just-woke-up-in-the-morning feed.

Claire told me she put a Band-aid on her breast and told her son her breast was "broken" when he was down to one feeding a day. Ellen negotiated with both of her sons. Toddlers start counting early, and she would ask hers how many sucks they wanted. They would come up with a number (toddlers usually pick low numbers, so don't worry about them saying "three thousand"). Then she'd let them suck "four times" or "five times" or whatever they had asked for. My daughter would happily do this too, although the counting went like this: "1-1-1-1-1-1-1-1-1-1-1-1-1-1-1-1-1-1-1-1-1-1-1. 2-2-2-2-2-2-2-2-2-2-2-2-2-2-2-2-2-2-2-2-2-2-2-2-2-2-2-2-2 . . . . . 2½. . . . . 2¾'s . . .

## Weaning an Older Baby Can Be Hard

La Leche League tells mothers who want to wean: don't offer the breast, but don't refuse it.

I personally believe in baby-led weaning, even though my daughter hadn't led the way when I started cutting back on the number of feedings. I started to notice that when she didn't have my full attention, she would want my breast. That was the one sure-fire way she could get me (at least physically) and hold on to me. That's when I started giving her some undivided nonbreastfeeding attention. If you sit on the floor of your child's room and just observe him, he'll let you know what he wants you to do. Sometimes, he's happy just to play in your presence. Sometimes, he'll ask you to read something to him or play something with him. But if he seems especially clingy, needy, and interested in your breast, and you don't think it's because he needs it for food or comfort, try giving him one hour a day of your undivided attention. It takes practice not to talk on the phone, do paperwork, read your own book, or insist on showing him how to play with his toys. But you'll notice a big difference, and he probably won't be as interested in breastfeeding as he was.

I sincerely believe my daughter would have been like the daughter of a woman I know. When her daughter turned four (yes, I realize you are now hyperventilating), Lynn decided it was time to quit and informed her daughter Michelle. Michelle planned her very own weaning party. She drew up the guest list, decided on the refreshments (no, it wasn't one final swig of breastmilk), and with her friends looking on, announced she was weaned. Years later, when Michelle watched the party video, her face darkened and her eyes filled with tears. "Mom," she told Lynn, "that was the worst day of my life." She still missed Mommy's milk.

Another very verbal little girl said philosophically one day, "Mommy, breastfeeding is like smoking: once you start, it's hard to give up." Hard, yes. But not impossible. Wean with love.

Chapter 15

# Toddler Nursing: The Last Frontier

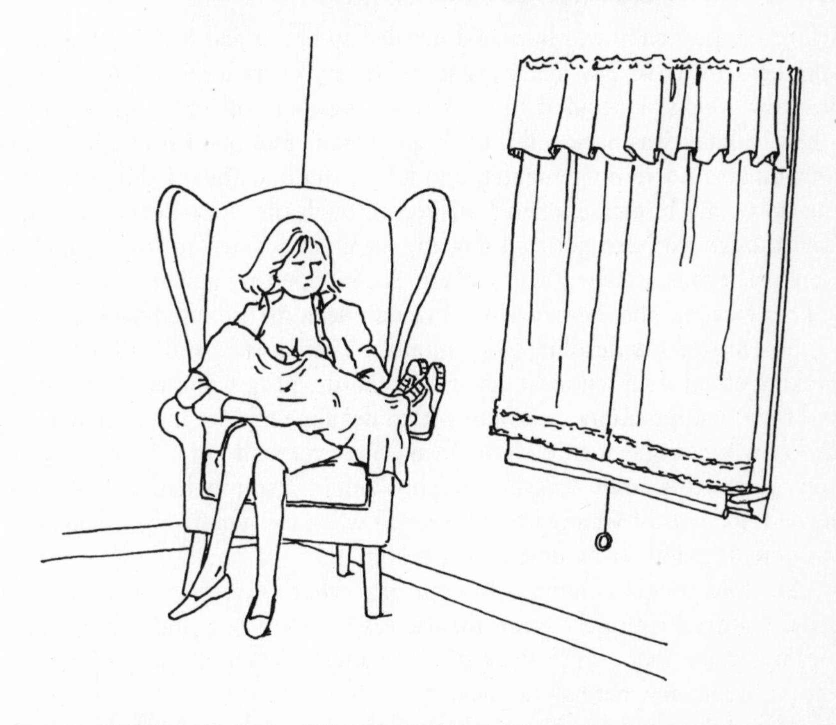

Don't read this chapter until your baby is nearing one year. The idea of breastfeeding a big baby if you've never breastfed a little one or if you are still breastfeeding a newborn may make you feel the way you felt about boys when you were six. "Boys are icky. I'm *never* going to like boys!"

Breastfeeding somebody big enough to walk or talk or both won't make sense to you until your newborn gets bigger. Because it just so happens that even after he's tripled in size, he'll still seem like a teeny, tiny baby to you. A lot of people balk at the idea of older babies nursing. They don't have a problem with infants and young babies, but they have a big problem with big babies. If you're a diligent reader and usually read everything from start to finish, I'm warning you again not to come near this chapter until your child is older. It may seem really, really strange to read about women who nurse babies that can get around and may even ask for "milk" or "chi-chi" or "na-nas," or whatever it is your baby eventually starts calling his milking station.

## How You End Up Breastfeeding a Toddler

Before my first baby was born, I'd decided to breastfeed in earnest until I went back to work. My maternity leave was up in six weeks. But after the first few weeks, I decided to start pumping and collect a milk supply. When I finally was back full-time at about four months, I drove home at lunchtime to nurse my daughter, and it was the first thing I did after setting down my briefcase when I walked through the door in the evening. Even though I'd been gone all day, my daughter seemed to forgive me as soon as she was attached to my chest. She stopped wriggling and fretting and her face had that beatific shine I've only seen on breastfed babies.

So I moved my deadline to six months. Then a year. And without even thinking about it, I ventured beyond my hard-and-fast one-year deadline. And then, I stopped my obsession with a deadline and let my daughter let me know when she was ready to wean. She eventually did. Many of you won't get to this point. I never thought I would. I simply had a child who showed no signs of wanting to be weaned when everybody else thought it was time. It gradually became no big deal to me.

I'm told this is common. In countries where there's no pressure to wean, children routinely wean themselves between one and three. That does not mean that you're stuck breastfeeding your child until he's three. You can wean anywhere along the line.

The sucking need babies are born with goes away at about the age of three. Chele Marmet does point out that in families where allergies are common, children left alone to wean themselves are the most likely candidates to make it to three. This is kind of like your body feeling thirsty after a hard workout. Instinctively, the human body often knows what it needs.

## Toddlers Are Different from Babies

One of the reasons why I continued is because thankfully, breastfeeding a toddler is distinctly different from breastfeeding an infant. An infant feeds regularly, eight to twelve times a day. A toddler may want milk a couple times a day or even more infrequently. Some children will only have a nip every other day or so.

I remember thinking a friend of mine whose baby weaned himself at twenty-three months seemed extreme. No, I'm being kind. I thought of her about the same way I did of Hare Krishnas when I was trying to politely decline their literature in airports. I thought I would never do *that*. Guess what? (No, I did not pass out Hare Krishna literature.)

## Jane and John Q. Public

If you thought society was against breastfeeding an infant, wait until your baby starts to resemble a child. Then the stares from strangers get more pronounced. I was never totally comfortable breastfeeding in public, and I stopped after my daughter hit about nine months and lost the ability to breastfeed discreetly. Although most toddlers are not boisterous at the breast, many have different patterns and habits than infants.

Michelle doesn't mind breastfeeding her daughter, who is two and a half, in public. "I think I'm very discreet," she says. Linda, whose daughter is twenty months, breastfeeds Brooke at home even if she's having company, though she'll only do it in front of close friends. "I made a decision when she was really little that I wasn't going to be forced into another room." Alise was comfortable breastfeeding her son in public until he was two. She is the director of a preschool in Los Angeles, and was firmly committed to what she was doing. But even she started to feel uncomfortable as her son got older. "I was getting such looks of disdain and disgust. At a certain point, even I couldn't take the looks of scorn."

You don't necessarily have to wean your child if you are both still satisfied breastfeeding but you don't like doing it in front of other people. You may end up continuing to breastfeed your toddler only at home. Since your baby will be old enough to understand, you just need to explain that there are new rules for breastfeeding. If he grabs your shirt in public, you can simply tell him gently while removing his hand that that is not okay. Then you can say, "Mommy doesn't want to breastfeed around other people, but she can when we're home." Most toddlers will quickly adapt to this change of rules.

I NEVER in a million years thought I'd breastfeed a toddler. Most women I interviewed didn't, either, because you just don't see it out from behind closed doors in this country. But studies have shown that breastfeeding a two-year-old even once every other day will keep your child far healthier than a child who is getting no breastmilk, because your breasts are still making antibodies specific to whatever germs your baby has been exposed to.

## What You Call It

Be careful with your word choice when deciding what to call *breastfeeding*. Remember that many babies start talking by the end of their first year. If your name for breastfeeding is something you don't want shouted across a grocery store, think carefully before you give your breasts a name. Caitlin thought it was funny to ask her daughter if she wanted "boob." But when Emily started to talk, she would say, "Mommy, BOOB!" If Emily saw any other baby taking a furtive breastfeeding break, she'd point and call out gleefully, "BOOB! BOOB! BOOB!"

I taught my daughter Olivia to ask for milk. When she'd do this in public, strangers would come up to us with pints of milk. That worked for a while, until she learned more words. Then she'd say, "Not that miwk! Miwk from Mommy's breast-es!" Miriam's son Lucas refers to his mom's breasts as "slurpees." He'll say, "I want two slurpees." My daughter also numbered my breasts for a while and would ask for "number one" or "number two."

## "Haven't You Stopped Yet?"

People will be curious and continue to ask you if you've stopped breastfeeding yet. Most of the time, you can guess who'll be shocked or give you a hard time, and who is simply interested. I found it easiest to be vague. Experts will tell you that the weaning process begins when babies first have solids, so you can say truthfully, "I started weaning him when he was six months." You can also change the subject before answering the question or say that you're not that comfortable discussing your breastfeeding habits. I just got tired of feeling that I was being judged by my response, so I stopped answering the question. As your baby gets older, if you don't breastfeed in front of people who don't approve, they'll usually assume that you've stopped and will stop asking.

If you decide to go this long, you're in for a whole lot of pressure to stop. I told people who pressed the issue, like my in-laws and friends (usually when they saw my daughter pulling at my clothes and yelling, "Miwk!") that I've seen four-year-olds with blankets and pacifiers. I wouldn't take away her bottle at this age; or a special toy. Why then, would I take away me?

## Why Stop Now?

There's no firm rule about how long to breastfeed, though I have to say, I'm with people who find it hard to understand women who continue to do it when their child can comfortably digest steak and potatoes and chime in on conversations about local politics. However, I am sympathetic to mothers whose children do it a few times during their day as a source of comfort and even as a source of food. Though much has been written about the nutritive quality of breastmilk sharply declining after a year, for as long as it's been tracked, breastmilk continues to change to supply your growing child with new and fabulous stuff. Science is definitely on your side. The World Health Organization recently released a study that said it's the lucky baby who's breastfed for two years. If you've made it to a year, your child is showing no sign of losing interest, and you don't mind continuing, then keep going. If you're sick of it, and every time at your breast is an uncomfortable struggle, then it is time to gently and gradually begin weaning.

The downside to breastfeeding past the point where you're both attentive to it is that the process can become a pacifier. By that I mean that instead of listening to what your child might really want from you—such as your full attention, a story read, some quiet time, a hug—you may get in the habit of always offering your breast. If your toddler seems fidgety and uncomfortable, regardless of whether or not he's nursing, it may be because he wants something else from you but hasn't figured out how to ask for it. My daughter would try to nurse every time the phone rang. It was my fault for not setting up boundaries. I answered the phone when it rang instead of listening to my child. I took the calls from telephone solicitors, bill collectors, my husband's clients. Finally, it dawned on me that my daughter was having a Pavlovian response to the ringing phone. One day, when I was particularly engrossed in a call, she looked right at me and nipped me. I mean bit me playfully like a puppy. I told her not to bite me, then I thought for a second and said, "Listen, if you have something to say to me, you can tell me. You don't have to bite me." She paused and then she said, "Mommy, get off phone!"

## Biting and Pinching

Biting was a phobia of mine because I remember my mother telling stories about my sister, who had a full set of chompers at three months (or so the story goes). My mother swears my sister bit her hard enough to break the skin a few times (a story I'm inclined to believe since this sister also broke my skin a few times, too). But toddlers with teeth aren't nearly as dangerous as toddlers who watch some of the cartoons on television. Toddlers, even those with a full set of teeth, can't successfully breastfeed and bite you at the same time. They might nip you either when they're falling asleep at your breast and they're losing their grasp, or as a way of getting your attention. But they really do understand when you tell them that it is not okay to bite. If you do get nipped, you will be so surprised, you will likely scream and startle your baby so much, he'll be unlikely to try out this new appliance in the same manner again. If it happens again, you can simply tell him that biting hurts and take away your breast.

Pinching, or twiddling, is another story. If you didn't curb this habit when it started, it will take a while to cure your child of this habit now. For weeks and weeks, I had to tell my daughter several times during each time at the breast not to pinch me. It was as though she needed to "worry" my breast like a blanket when she breastfed.

## Tandem Nursing

Most women don't end up breastfeeding two children at the same time because they wanted to. "I hadn't intended to. My son seemed to be weaned when my daughter came along," Alisha says. "But as soon as I was home with the new baby, he wanted to start again." Brian was fifteen months when his sister Elizabeth was born. "I didn't want to push him away any more than I was, so I just let him," she said. Brian breastfed for another three months until he weaned himself.

Unless you are at risk of miscarrying, you can probably safely continue to breastfeed during your pregnancy. You may notice that your nipples become sensitive again during your pregnancy. Some babies will even wean themselves after about your fourth month of pregnancy because the taste of the milk supposedly changes. But don't count on your child self-weaning during this period.

Once your second child comes along, your body will produce colostrum once again for the newborn. Your older child may even comment on the change in taste and consistency. If you haven't weaned your first baby when your second comes along, now is not a good time, unless you want your children to grow up hating each other. Sibling rivalry is not something most families can get around. You can encourage children to get along by not allowing them to hurt each other, and by encouraging them to solve their own problems. That way, one doesn't become the victim and the other the bully. But your first child will feel some displeasure at a new person competing for Mom's and Dad's attention. (Remember how he always woke up right before you and your husband were about to make love? That's because he was trying to cut down on the competition—and chances of procreation.)

You can gently help your child to understand that the baby's needs are most basic. Maybe you can read a story to your older child or sit next to him while he has a snack and you feed the baby. Some women don't mind breastfeeding two at a time. Once again, you'll have to figure it out as you go along.

Marybeth didn't like the idea of breastfeeding two children at the same time and had a unique solution. She'd take both children to the park during the day. Martha, her two-year-old, had stopped breastfeeding in public a year before, so Martha didn't bat an eye when Jake needed food—as long as it was in a place where Martha didn't breastfeed anymore.

# Appendix
# Resources

## Lactation Consultants

Lactation consultants can be a blessing. But they are not all great. That goes with the territory, right? In what field do you find 100 percent of the practitioners to be perfect? Keep in mind that the field is *not* a licensed profession. Not yet, anyway. Lactation consultants can be found either through (or working in) doctors' offices, private breastfeeding clinics, public health agencies, and hospitals. Most pediatricians, obstetricians, gynecologists, and hospitals can refer you to a good lactation consultant in your area, but there are other ways of finding one if these don't pan out for you.

### Don't Assume They're All Good. Choose a Good One

Be picky when you choose a lactation consultant. It'd be nice if you could find one who is certified. I say "it'd be nice" because I've interviewed and met many consultants who are not certified but are excellent advisors with spotless reputations and years in the field.

You'll know what you're getting without the guesswork if you find someone who has "IBCLC" (International Board of Certified Lactation Consultant) after her name (or his name—there are men who do this, too). That means the consultant has passed a rigorous six-hour exam and has the IBCLCE (International Board of Certified Lactation Consultant Examiners) seal of approval.

Any lactation consultant should have a resume that you can ask to take a look at (this isn't rude—this is business). The resume should list hours of lactation training, coursework, number of hours doing clinical practice (preferably supervised), academic and professional training, and membership in any professional organizations.

Lactation consultancy is a growing and largely unregulated field. It is a new field with few hard and fast rules and regulations, and you may find someone who is not certified (there are only about 5,000 consultants worldwide who are). If your consultant comes well-recommended by a doctor, for example, you might be fine. But pay attention to the advice you get. If the advice doesn't seem to make sense—if, for example, you are encouraged to use formula to "get the baby used to a bottle" or to "just keep trying" even if you're sure there's a problem—seek out someone else.

Your consultant may or may not make house calls. You may have to go to them. But you should find someone who's available for follow-up phone calls. If there is any question that there is something really wrong, get your baby to a doctor as soon as you find your car keys and slip on your shoes.

### Advice by Phone

You can get advice on the phone for little stuff, but that's vastly different from seeing an expert who'll be able to diagnose and usually fix what's going wrong. Use the phone for support, basic questions, and small problems. Most of the time, you can find a lactation consultant who will field your phone calls for free. Some places charge for phone consults, so make sure you ask. The Lactation Institute does phone consults, and although their time is not free, it is very reasonably priced considering their level of expertise. They've seen it all, heard it all, diagnosed it all—and eventually helped most of the mothers who've gone to them after all else failed.

### How to Find a Lactation Consultant

The International Lactation Consultant Association can help you find a lactation consultant in your area. Phone is (919) 787-5181. Their address is ILCA, 4101 Lake Boone Trail, Suite 201, Raleigh, NC 27607-6518.

If you've taken a childbirth class and you liked the instructor, ask her for the name of a consultant she refers mothers to. Some childbirth education centers have consultants on staff.

Your pediatrician, if he or she is knowledgeable about breastfeeding, probably has a consultant that he or she generally refers mothers to. One of the best ways is to call La Leche League for a referral in your area or for basic help on the phone. In most cases, they can tell you whether you need expert help and how quickly you should get that help. A good lactation consultant or La Leche League Leader can usually tell by asking questions over the phone how serious your problem is and whether you need to be seen.

Medela, the breast pump company, also has an 800 number you can call (1-800-TELL-YOU) for lists of local lactation consultants.

### How Much Do Lactation Consultants Charge?

A lactation consultant's fee depends on where you live (urban, suburban, or rural) and who you choose, but it's usually based on an hourly rate. If your doctor prescribes a visit to a consultant, your insurance company may pay for it.

If any of your friends or relatives don't know what to give you for a baby gift and have between $30 and $100 bucks to spend, tell them to give you a one-time lesson from a lactation consultant. Jill, mother of two, got this for a gift. "It was much better than the four hundred pink outfits I got—for my son!"

## Other Support People

Before the birth of your baby, you may think you won't need support. But since we're social beings and most of us don't like feeling ostracized (this does not apply to you if you have purple, green, or tri-colored hair), it is easier if people close to you support you. Your best support is other breastfeeding mothers. Breastfeeding is much easier if you're not the only one doing it, so you may find that an organized group such as La Leche League can offer camaraderie and a way to trade stories if you don't have a single close friend or relative (whom you like) who's breastfeeding or has breastfed.

### The Famous La Leche League

The La Leche League (1-800-LA-LECHE), contrary to popular mythology usually repeated by women who don't breastfeed, is not a militant organization that forces you to sign on for five years of nursing duty or risk court martial. It's an organization of mothers set up to support other mothers who are trying to breastfeed. The women who go to the meetings are not zealots, not usually, anyway. They are women just like you trying to do their best for their babies.

The leaders are not just women who breastfed. They are highly trained people who've had to pass an exam. That doesn't make them hands-on experts at solving difficult problems the way lactation consultants do. But every leader I've ever interviewed knows her stuff.

Mary Beth didn't like the leader at the first group she attended. She wasn't going to go again until one of her friends coaxed her into trying another group in her area. Five years and two children later, "Some of my best friends and my kid's best friends are women and their kids that we met at La Leche League." If you have a bad experience with one leader, by phone or in a meeting, try another one. You don't have to go to meetings, and telephone advice is free, and keep in mind, that La Leche League leaders are volunteers, so be nice.

Leaders are not available at all hours. This makes sense, because they have families, too. Unfortunately, all of my major medical problems seem to happen just at the close of business hours. The La Leche hotline has regular business hours Monday to Friday, 8 a.m. to 5 p.m. Central Time. You can also be referred to leaders who can help after hours and on weekends. The leaders rotate being on call, and if one isn't available, she'll leave a number (usually on a machine) where you can reach another leader.

## Get to the Telephone Numbers, Already!

### Electric Pump Manufacturers

Medela, Inc.
4610 Prime Parkway
McHenry, IL 60050
1-800-TELL-YOU

Ameda/Egnell, Inc.
765 Industrial Drive
Cary, IL 60013
1-800-323-8750

### Organizations

La Leche League International
1400 North Meacham Road
P.O. Box 4079
Schaumburg, IL 60168-4079
(708) 519-7730 or 1-800-LA-LECHE

Hours for help: weekdays 9:00 a.m. to 5:00 p.m. (Central Time) for help or a referral to an La Leche League leader in your area. Check your white pages, too, under La Leche League, for a local leader's number.

Nursing Mothers Counsel, Inc.
P.O. Box 50063
Palo Alto, CA 94303
415-591-6688

There are also chapters in parts of California; in Denver, Colorado; and in Wayne, Indiana. Call Palo Alto for a number in your area.

Childbirth Education Association of Greater Philadelphia
Nursing Mothers' Support Groups
5 East Second Avenue
Conshohocken, PA 19428
215-828-0131

Boston Association for Childbirth Education (BACE)
Nursing Mothers' Council
184 Savin Hill Avenue
Dorchester, MA 02125
617-244-5102

The Lactation Institute and Breastfeeding Clinic
16430 Ventura Blvd., Suite 303
Encino, CA 91436
818-995-1913

## The Information Superhighway

Check the World Wide Web for information, other parents, chat rooms, and so on. One good resource can be found at: http://www.parentsplace.com. Use your Web Browser and an online search tool such as Infoseek. Begin by looking under key words such as *breastfeeding* or *breast feeding*. Then, if you want more general information, go through the parenting resources. There are parenting sites on America Online and Compuserve.

Keep in mind that some of the people you will be communicating with will be offering their own advice. That is very different from seeking help from a professional. Enjoy the group discussions, but also look for specific articles and experts whose brains you can pick via the Internet.

## Drug Information Hotlines

Brigham and Women's Hospital
Boston, MA
617-732-7166

Rocky Mountain Drug Consultation Center
1-900-285-DRUG
(The charge is about $3.00 for the first minute, $2.00 per minute for each additional minute.)
Stanford University Hospital
Palo Alto, CA
415-723-6422

University of California, San Diego
1-900-288-8273
(The charge is about $3.00 for the first minute, $2.00 per minute for each additional minute.)

University of Chicago
Chicago, IL
312-702-1388

University of Georgia, Augusta
Medical College of Georgia
Augusta, GA
706-721-2887

University of Maryland Medical System
Baltimore, MD
410-706-7568

University of Rochester
Strong Memorial Hospital
Rochester, NY
716-275-3718

University of Texas Medical Center
Galveston, TX
409-772-2734

Washington State University
College of Pharmacy
Spokane, WA
509-456-4409

### Milk Banks

Mother's Milk Unit
Valley Medical Center
751 South Bascome Avenue
San Jose, CA 95128
408-998-4550

For referrals:
Human Milk Banking Association of North America, Inc. (HMBANA)
P.O. Box 370464
West Hartford, CT 06137-0464
203-232-8809

### Clothing

Association for Breastfeeding Fashions (AFBF)
P.O. Box 4378
Sunland, CA 91040
818-352-0697

### Breast Implant Information

There is an organization begun in 1992 called Children Afflicted by Toxic Substances. To contact them, write:

Children Afflicted by Toxic Substances
60 Oser Avenue
Hauppauge, NY 11788
516-273-2287

Jeremiah Levine, M.D., is a pediatric gastroenterologist at Schneider Children's Hospital on Long Island, New York. He has been studying digestive disorders in children born to mothers with implants. If your doctor cannot explain unusual gastrointestinal symptoms, Dr. Levine can be contacted directly by your doctor by calling 718-470-3430.

# References

Ahn CH, MacLean WC. "Growth of the Exclusively Breast-fed Infant." *Am J Clin Nutr.* 1980;33: 183-192.

*Alcohol Topics in Brief: Physiologic Effects of Alcohol.* Rockville, MD: National Institute on Alcohol Abuse and Alcoholism. National Clearinghouse for Alcohol Information, No. RPO 382, 1982; pp. 1-12.

American Academy of Pediatrics and the American College of Obstetricians and Gynecologists. *Guidelines for Perinatal Care.* 3rd ed. Washington, DC: ACOG, AAP; 1992:183

American Academy of Pediatrics, Committee on Drugs. "The Transfer of Drugs and Other Chemicals into Human Milk." *Pediatrics.* 1994;93:137-150.

American Academy of Pediatrics, Committee on Fetus and Newborn, and American College of Obstetricians and Gynecologists. "Maternal and Newborn Nutrition." *Guidelines for Perinatal Care.* 4th ed. Washington, DC: ACOG, AAP; 1997.

American Academy of Pediatrics, Committee on Nutrition. "Fluoride Supplementation for Children: Interim Policy Recommendations." *Pediatrics.* 1995;95:777.

American Academy of Pediatrics, Committee on Nutrition. "Nutritional Needs of Low-birth-weight Infants." *Pediatrics.* 1985;75:976-986.

American Academy of Pediatrics, Committee on Nutrition. *Pediatric Nutrition Handbook.* 3rd ed. Elk Grove Village, IL: AAP; 1993:7.

American Academy of Pediatrics, Committee on Nutrition. "The Use of Whole Cow's Milk in Infancy." *Pediatrics.* 1992;89:1105-1109.

American Academy of Pediatrics, Committee on Nutrition. "Vitamin and Mineral Supplement Needs in Normal Children in the United States." *Pediatrics.* 1980;66:1015-1021.

American Academy of Pediatrics, Committee on Pediatric Aids. "Human Milk, Breastfeeding, and Transmission of Human Immunodeficiency Virus in the United States." *Pediatrics.* 1995;96:977-979.

American Academy of Pediatrics, Committee on Practice and Ambulatory Medicine. "Recommendations for Preventive Pediatric Health Care." *Pediatrics.* 1995;96:373.

American Dietetic Association. "Position of the American Dietetic Association: Promotion of Breast Feeding." *Am Diet Assoc Rep.* 1986;86:1580-1585.

Anderson GC. "Risk in Mother-Infant Separation Postbirth." *IMAGE: J Nurs Sch.* 1989:21:196-199.

Anderson W. Little RE. "Maternal Alcohol Use During Breastfeeding and Infant Development at One Year." *New England Journal of Medicine,* 1989. 321, 425-430.

Angier, Natalie. "Mother's Milk Found to Be Potent Cocktail of Hormones." *The New York Times,* March 24, 1994.

Aniansson G, Alm B, Andersson B, et al. "A Prospective Cohort Study on Breast-feeding and Otitis Media in Swedish Infants." *Pediatr Infect Dis J* 1994;13:183-188.

Arnon SS. "Breast-feeding and Toxigenic Intestinal Infections: Missing Links in Crib Death?" *Rev Infect Dis* 1984;6:S193-S201.

Arthur PG, Hartmann PE, Smith M. "Measurement of the Milk Intake of Breast-fed Infants." *J Pediatric Gastroenterol Nutrition* 1987; 6:758-763.

Arthur PG, Jones TR, Spruce J, Hartmann PE. "Measuring Short-term Rates of Milk Synthesis in Breast-feeding Mothers." *Quarterly Journal Exp Physiology* 1989; 74:419-428.

Ashraf RN, Jalil F, Aperia A, et al. "Additional Water Is Not Needed for Healthy Breast-fed Babies in a Hot Climate." *Acta Paediatr Scand.* 1993;82:1007-1011.

Barger, Jan, and Pat Bull. "A Comparison of the Bacterial Composition of Breastmilk Stored at Room Temperature and Stored in the Refrigerator." *IJCE,* August, 1987.

Beaudry M, Dufour R, Marcoux S. "Relation Between Infant Feeding and Infections During the First Six Months of Life." *J Pediatr.* 1995;126:191-197.

Braveman P, Egerter S, Pearl M, et al. "Problems Associated with Early Discharge of Newborn Infants." *Pediatrics.* 1995;96:716-726.

Brown KH, Black RE, Robertson AD, Akhtar KA, Ahmed G, Becker S. "Clinical and Field Studies of Human Lactation: Methodological Considerations." *American Journal Clinical Nutrition* 1982; 35:745-756.

Butte NF, Garza C, O'Brien Smith JE, et al. "Effect of Maternal Diet and Body Composition on Lactational Performance." *Am J Clin Nutr.* 1984;39:296-306.

Butte NF, Garza C, O'Brian Smith E, Nichols B. "Human Milk Intake and Growth in Exclusively Breast-fed Infants." *Journal Pediatric.* 1984; 104:187-195.

Butte NF, Garza C, Smith EO, Nichols BL. "Evaluation of the Deuterium Dilution Technique Against the Test-weighing Procedure for the Determination of Breast Milk Intake." *American Journal Clinical Nutrition.* 1983; 37:996-1003.

Butte NF, Wills C, Jean CA, O'Brian Smith E, Garza C. "Feeding Patterns of Exclusively Breast-fed Infants During the First Four Months of Life." *Early Human Development.* 1985; 12:291-300.

Centers for Disease Control and Prevention. "Recommendations for Assisting in the Prevention of Perinatal Transmission of Human T-lymphotropic Virus Type III/lymphadenopathy-associated Virus and Acquired Immunodeficiency Syndrome." *MMWR.* 1985;34:721-732.

Chen Y. "Synergistic Effect of Passive Smoking and Artificial Feeding on Hospitalization for Respiratory Illness in Early Childhood." *Chest.* 1989;95:1004-1007.

Chua S, Arulkumaran S, Lim I, et al. "Influence of Breastfeeding and Nipple Stimulation on Postpartum Uterine Activity." *Br J Obstet Gynaecol.* 1994;101:804-805.

Coates MM. "Tides in Breastfeeding Practice." Riordan J, Auerbach KG, eds. *Breastfeeding and Human Lactation.* Boston: Jones and Bartlett Publishers, 1993; pp. 3-48.

Cobo E. "Effect of Different Doses of Ethanol on the Milk Ejecting Reflex in Lactating Women." *Am J Obstet Gynecol.* 1973; 115:817-821.

Cochi SL, Fleming DW, Hightower AW, et al. "Primary Invasive *Haemophilus influenzae* Type b Disease: A Population-based Assessment of Risk Factors." *J Pediatr.* 1986;108:887-896.

Comfort A. *What About Alcohol?* Burlington, NC: Carolina Biological Supply Company, 1983; pp. 8-12.

Covert RF, Barman N, Domanico RS, et al. "Prior Enteral Nutrition with Human Milk Protects Against Intestinal Perforation in Infants Who Develop Necrotizing Enterocolitis." *Pediatr Res.* 1995;37:305A; abstract.

Coward WA, Sawyer MB, Whitehead RG, Prentice AM. "New Method for Measuring Milk Intakes in Breast-fed Babies." *Lancet* 1979; 2 (8132):13-14.

Cumming RG, Klineberg RJ. "Breastfeeding and Other Reproductive Factors and the Risk of Hip Fractures in Elderly Woman." *Int J Epidemiol* 1993;22:684-691.

Cunningham, Allan S., Derrick B. Jelliffe, and E.F. Patrice Jeliffe. "Breastfeeding and Health in the 1980s: A Global Epidemiologic Review." *The Journal of Pediatrics*, May, 1991.

Dallman PR. "Progress in the Prevention of Iron Deficiency in Infants." *Acta Paediatr Scand Suppl.* 1990;365:28-37.

Daly, Steven E.J. Ph.d. "Infant Demand and Milk Supply," Parts 1 & 2, and Hartmann Peter E., PhD. *Journal of Human Lactation.* 11 (1) 1995 21-27.

Daly SEJ, Kent JC, Huynh DQ, Owens RA, Alexander BF, Ng KC, et al. "The Determination of Short-term Breast Volume Changes and the Rate of Synthesis of Human Milk Using Computerized Breast Measurement." *Exp Physiol.* 1992; 77:79-87.

Daly SEJ, Owens RA, Hartmann PE. The Short-term Synthesis and Infant-regulated Removal of Milk in Lactating Women. *Exp Physiology.* 1993; 78:209-220.

Davis MK, Savitz DA, Graubard BI. "Infant Feeding and Childhood Cancer." *Lancet.* 1988;2:365-368.

De Carvalho M, Anderson DM, Giangreco A, Pittard W. "Frequency of Milk Expression and Milk Production by Mothers of Nonnursing Premature Neonates." *American Journal Dis Children.* 1985; 139:483-485.

De Carvalho M, Klaus MH, Merkatz RB. "Frequency of Breast-feeding and Serum Bilirubin Concentration." *Am J Dis Child.* 1982;136:737-738.

De Carvalho M, Robertson S, Friedman A, et al. "Effect of Frequent Breast-feeding on Early Milk Production and Infant Weight Gain." *Pediatrics.* 1983;72:307-311.

Dewey KG, Finley DA, Strode MA, Lönnerdal B. "Relationship of Maternal Age to Breast Milk Volume and Composition." Hamosh M, Goldman AS, eds.

*Human Lactation 2: Maternal and Environmental Factors.* New York: Plenum Press. 1986; pp. 263-73.

Dewey, Kathryn, M. Jane Heinig and Laurie A. Nommsen. "Maternal Weight-loss Patterns During Prolonged Lactation." *Am J Clin Nutr,* 58:162-6. 1993.

—— "Differences in Morbidity Between Breastfed and Formula-fed Infants." *The Journal of Pediatrics,* May, 1995.

Dewey KG, Heinig MJ, Nommsen LA, Lönnerdal B. "Maternal Versus Infant Factors Related to Breast Milk Intake and Residual Milk Volume: The DARLING study." *Pediatrics.* 1991. 87:829-37.

Dewey K, Lönnerdal B. "Infant Self-regulation of Breast Milk Intake." *Acta Paediatr Scand.* 1986; 75:893-98.

Duncan B, Ey J, Holberg CJ, et al. "Exclusive Breast-feeding for at Least 4 Months Protects Against Otitis Media." *Pediatrics.* 1993;91:867-872.

Estes N. *Alcoholism, Consequences and Interventions.* CV Mosby Company. 1982; pp. 95-100.

"Fact Sheet, Drinking Danger Points." Rockville, MD: National Clearinghouse for Alcohol Information, 1979; p. 1.

Fildes V. *Breasts, Bottles and Babies: A History of Infant Feeding.* Edinburgh: Edinburgh University Press, 1986; pp. 118-22.

Finley DA, Lönnerdal B, Dewey KG, Grivetti LE. "Breast Milk Composition: Fat Content and Fatty Acid Composition in Vegetarians and Non-vegetarians." *American Journal Clinical Nutrition* 1985; 41:787-800.

Ford RPK, Taylor BJ, Mitchell EA, et al. "Breast-feeding and the Risk of Sudden Infant Death Syndrome." *Int J Epidemiol.* 1993;22:885-890.

Frank AL, Taber LH, Glezen WP, et al. "Breastfeeding and Respiratory Virus Infection." *Pediatrics.* 1982;70:239-245.

Frederick IB, Auerback KG. "Maternal-infant Separation and Breast-feeding: The Return to Work or School." *J Reprod Med.* 1985;30:523-526.

Freed, Gary L., Sarah J. Clark, James Sorenson, Jacob A. Lohr, Robert Cefalo, and Peter Curtis. "National Assessment of Physicians' Breastfeeding Knowledge, Attitudes, Training, and Experience." *Journal of the American Medical Association,* February 8, 273: 6. 1995.

Freed, J. Gary L., Kennard Fraley, and Richard J. Schanler. "Accuracy of Expectant Mothers' Predictions of Fathers' Attitudes Regarding Breastfeeding." *The Journal of Family Practice.* 3:2. 1993.

Freed GL, McIntosh Jones T, Fraley JK. "Attitudes and Education of Pediatric House Staff Concerning Breast-feeding." *South Med J.* 1992;85:484-485.

Freed GL, Clark SJ, Sorenson J, et al. "National Assessment of Physicians' Breastfeeding Knowledge, Attitudes, Training, and Experience." *JAMA.* 1995; 273;472-476.

Freed GL, Clark SJ, Lohr JA, et al. "Pediatrician Involvement in Breast-feeding Promotion: A National Study of Residents and Practitioners." *Pediatrics.* 1995; 96:490-494.

Gartner LM. Introduction. Gartner LM, ed. "Breastfeeding in the Hospital." *Semin Perinatol.* 1994;18:475.

Gearhart J. "Alcoholism in Women." *American Family Physician*. 44:907-13. 1991.

Gerlin, Andres. 1994. "Hospital's Wean from Formula Makers' Freebies." *The Wall Street Journal*, December 29.

Gerstein HC. "Cow's Milk Exposure and Type 1 Diabetes Mellitus." *Diabetes Care*. 1994;17:13-19.

Gielen AC, Faden RR, O'Campo P, et al. "Maternal Employment During the Early Postpartum Period: Effects on Initiation and Continuation of Breastfeeding." *Pediatrics*. 87:298-305. 1991.

Glover, Jacalynne, and Mark Sandilands. "Supplementation of Breastfeeding Infants and Weight Loss in Hospitals."*Journal of Human Lactation*, vol. 6. 1990.

Goldberg NM, Adams E. "Supplementary Water for Breast-fed Babies in a Hot and Dry Climate—Not Really a Necessity." *Arch Dis Child*. 1983;58:73-74.

Gray RH, Campbell OM, Apelo R, et al. "Risk of Ovulation During Lactation." *Lancet*. 1990;335:25-29.

Greco L, Auricchio S, Mayer M, et al. "Case Control Study on Nutritional Risk Factors in Celiac Disease." *J Pediatr Gastroenterol Nutr*. 1988;7:395-399.

Gross L. *How Much is Too Much? The Effects of Social Drinking*. New York: Random House. 1983; p. 141.

Gunther M. "Instinct and the Nursing Couple." *Lancet*. 575-578. 1955.

Halken S, Host A, Hansen LG, et al. "Effect of an Allergy Prevention Programme on Incidence of Atopic Symptoms in Infancy." *Ann Allergy*. 1992;47:545-553.

Hahn-Zoric M, Fulconis F, Minoli I, Moro G, Carlsson B, Böttiger M, et al. "Antibody Responses to Parenteral and Oral Vaccines Are Impaired by Conventional and Low Protein Formula as Compared to Breast Feeding." *Acta Pediatric Scandinavia*. 1990; 79:1137-42.

Hartman PE, Arthur PG. "Assessment of Lactation Performance in Women." Hamosh M, Goldman AS, eds. *Human Lactation 2: Maternal and Environmental Factors*. New York: Plenum Press. 1986; pp. 215-30.

Hartmann PE, Saint L. "Measurement of Milk Yield in Women." *Journal Pediatric Gastroenterol Nutrition* 1984; 3:270-74.

Hartmann PE, Rattigan S, Prosser CG, Saint L, Arthur PG. "Human Lactation: Back to Nature." Peaker M, Vernon RG, Knight CH, Eds. *Physiological Strategies in Lactation*. London: Academic Press. 1984; pp. 337-68.

*Healthy People 2000: National Health Promotion and Disease Prevention Objectives*. Washington, DC: Government Printing Office. 1990:379-380. US Dept of Health and Human Services publication PHS 91-50212.

Heck H, de Castro JM. "The Caloric Demand of Lactation Does Not Alter Spontaneous Meal Patterns, Nutrient Intakes, or Moods of Women." *Physiol Behav*. 1993;54:641-648.

Heesom KJ, Souza PFA, Ilic V, Williamson DH. "Chain-length Dependency of Interactions of Medium-chain Fatty Acids with Glucose Metabolism in Acini Isolated from Lactating Rat Mammary Glands." *Biochem J*. 1992; 281:273-78.

Heinig, M. Jane, Laurie A. Nommsen, Janet M. Peerson, Bo Lonnderdal, and Kathryn G. Dewey. "Intake and Growth of Breastfed and Formula-Fed Infants in Relation to the Timing of and Introduction of Complementary Foods." Davis Area Research on Lactation, Infant Nutrition and Growth (The DARLING study), *Acta Paediatr.* 82. 1993.

—— "Growth of Breastfed and Formula-fed Infants from 0 to 18 Months: The DARLING Study." *Pediatrics.* June, 89:6. 1992.

—— "Breastfed Infants Are Leaner than Formula-Fed Infants at One Year of Age: The DARLING Study." *American Journal of Clinical Nutrition*, 57:140-5. 1993.

"Here's to Your Health: Alcohol Facts for Women." Washington, DC: US Department of Health and Human Services. 1986; entire pamphlet.

Hopkinson JM, Schanler RJ, Garza C. "Milk Production by Mothers of Premature Infants." *Pediatrics.* 1988; 81:815-20.

Howard CR, Howard FM, Weitzman ML. "Infant Formula Distribution and Advertising in Pregnancy: A Hospital Survey." *Birth.* 1994;21:14-19.

Howard FM, Howard CR, Weitzman ML. "The Physician as Advertiser: The Unintentional Discouragement of Breast-feeding." *Obstet Gynecol.* 1993;81:1048-1051.

Howie PW, Forsyth JS, Ogston SA, et al. "Protective Effect of Breast Feeding Against Infection." *Br Med J.* 1990;300:11-16.

Hytten FE. "Clinical and Chemical Studies in Human Lactation." *British Medical Journal* 1954; 1(4855): 175-82 passim.

Idanpaan-Heikkila J, Jouppila P. "Elimination and Metabolic Effects of Ethanol in Mother, Fetus and Newborn Infant." *Am J Obstet Gynecol* 1972; 112:387-93.

Infant Feeding Position Paper. Intl. Lactation Consultant Assc., February, 1991.

Ing, Roy, J.H.C. Ho, and Nicholas Petrakis. 1977. "Unilateral Breastfeeding and Breast Cancer." *Lancet,* July 16.

Istre GR, Conner JS, Broome CV, et al. "Risk Factors for Primary Invasive *Haemophilus influenzae* Disease: Increased Risk from Day care Attendance and School-aged Household Members." *J Pediatr.* 1985;106:190-195.

Jones B, Jones M. "Male and Female Intoxication Levels or Do Women Really Get Higher than Men?" *Alcohol Tech Rep* 1976; 5:11-14.

Karjalainen, Jukka, Julio Martin, Mikael Knip, Jorma Ilonen, Brian Robinson, Erkki Savilahti, Hans Akerblom, and Hans-Michael Dosch. "A Bovine Albumin Peptide as a Possible Trigger of Insulin-Dependent Diabetes Mellitus." *The New England Journal of Medicine,* July, 1992.

Kennedy KI, Visness CM. "Contraceptive Efficacy of Lactational Amenorrhoea." *Lancet.* 1992;339:227-230.

Kennel, Dietmar A.J. DDS, http://www.flash.net/~dkennel/bottle.htm.

Kinney J. *Loosening the Grip: A Handbook of Alcohol Information.* St. Louis: CV Mosby Company. 1978; pp. 34-35.

Klaus MH. "The Frequency of Suckling—Neglected but Essential Ingredient of Breast-feeding." *Obstet Gynecol Clin North Am.* 1987;14:623-633.

Knott D. *Alcohol Problems: Diagnosis and Treatment.* New York: Pergamon Press, 1986; p. 125.

Koletzko S, Sherman P, Corey M, et al. "Role of Infant Feeding Practices in Development of Crohn's Disease in Childhood." *Br Med J.* 1989;298:1617-1618.

Kovar MG, Serdula MK, Marks JS, et al. "Review of the Epidemiologic Evidence for an Association Between Infant Feeding and Infant Health." *Pediatrics.* 1984;74:S615-S638.

L'Esperance, Carol, and Kittie Frantz. 1985. "Time Limitation for Early Breastfeeding." *JOGNN*, March/April.

Labbock MH, Colie C. "Puerperium and Breast-feeding." *Curr Opin Obstet Gynecol.* 1992;4:818-825.

Labbok M, Krasovec K. "Toward Consistency in Breastfeeding Definitions." *Stud Family Planning.* 1990; 21:226-230.

Lau C, Henning SJ. "A Noninvasive Method for Determining Patterns of Milk Intake in the Breast-fed Infant." *Journal Pediatric Gastroenterol Nutrition.* 1989; 9:481-487.

Lemons P, Stuart M, Lemons JA. "Breast-feeding the Premature Infant." *Clin Perinatol.* 1986;13:111-122.

Linzell JL. "Measurement of Udder Volume in Live Goats as an Index of Mammary Growth and Function." *Journal Dairy Science* 1966; 49:307-311.

Little RE, Anderson W. "Maternal Alcohol Use During Breast-feeding and Infant Mental and Motor Development at One Year." *N Engl J Med* 1989; 321:425-430.

Lucas, A., R. Morley, T.J. Cole, G. Lister, and C. Leeson-Payne. "Breastmilk and Subsequent Intelligence Quotient in Children Born Preterm." *Lancet.* February 1, vol. 339. 1992.

Lucas A, Brooke OG, Morley R, et al. "Early Diet of Preterm Infants and Development of Allergic or Atopic Disease: Randomised Prospective Study." *Br Med J.* 1990;300:837-840.

Lucas A, Cole TJ. "Breast Milk and Neonatal Necrotising Enterocolitis." *Lancet.* 1990;336:1519-1523.

Lucas A, Ewing G, Roberts SB, Coward WA. "How Much Energy Does the Breast-Fed Infant Consume and Expend?" *British Medical J.* 1987; 295 (6590): 75-77.

Lucas A, Morley R, Cole TJ, Lister G, Leeson-Payne C. "Breast Milk and Subsequent Intelligence Quotient in Children Born Preterm." *Lancet.* 1992; 339(8788):261-264.

Marmet, Chele, and Ellen Shell. "Breastfeeding Is Important." Lactation Institute, Encino, Calif. 1991.

—— "Collection and storage of breastmilk." Lactation Institute.

—— "Manual Expression of Breastmilk —The Marmet Technique." Lactation Institute. 1988.

Mayer EJ, Hamman RF, Gay EC, et al. "Reduced risk of IDDM Among Breast-fed Children." *Diabetes.* 1988;37:1625-1632

McTiernan, A. and D.B. Thomas, "Evidence for a Protective Effect of Lactation on Risk of Breast Cancer in Young Women." *American Journal of Epidemiology.* 124: 3.

Melton LJ, Bryant SC, Wahner HW, et al. "Influence of Breastfeeding and other Reproductive Factors on Bone Mass Later in Life." *Osteoporos Int.* 1993;3:76-83.

Mitchell EA, Taylor BJ, Ford RPK, et al. "Four Modifiable and other Major Risk Factors for Cot Death, the New Zealand study." *J Paediatr Child Health.* 1992;28:S3-S8.

Mobbs EJ. "Suckling and Milk Production" (letter). *Med J Aust* 1990; 152:616.

Mohrbacher N, Stock J. *The Breastfeeding Answer Book.* Schaumburg, IL: La Leche League International; 1997:60.

Montgomery D, Splett P. "Economic Benefit of Breast-feeding Infants Enrolled in WIC." *J Am Diet Assoc.* 1997;97:379-385.

Morrow-Tlucak M, Haude RH, Ernhart CB. "Breastfeeding and Cognitive Development in the First 2 Years of Life." *Soc Sci Med.* 1988;26:635-639.

Morrow-Tlucak M, Houde RH, Eruhart CB. "Breastfeeding and Cognitive Development in the First Two Years of Life." *Social Science Medicine.* 1988; 26:635-39.

Neifert M, Lawrence R, Seacat J. "Nipple Confusion: Toward a Formal Definition." *J Pediatr.* 1995;126:S125-129.

Neville MC, Oliva-Rasbach J. "Is Maternal Milk Production Limiting for Infant Growth During the First Year of Life in Breast-fed Infants?" Goldman AS, Atkinson SA, Hanson LA, eds. *Human Lactation 3: The Effects of Human Milk on the Recipient Infant.* New York: Plenum Press, 1987; pp. 123-133.

Newcomb PA, Storer BE, Longnecker MP, et al. "Lactation and a Reduced Risk of Premenopausal Breast Cancer." *N Engl J Med.* 1994;330:81-87.

Newton M. "Human lactation." Kon SK, Cowies AT, eds. *Milk: The Mammary Gland and Its Secretion.* New York: Academic Press. 1961; pp. 281-320.

Newton M, Newton NR. "The Normal Course and Management of Lactation." *Clinical Obstetrics Gynecology* 1962; 5:44-63.

Owen MJ, Baldwin CD, Swank PR, et al. "Relation of Infant Feeding Practices, Cigarette Smoke Exposure, and Group Child Care to the Onset and Duration of Otitis Media with Effusion in the First Two Years of Life." *J Pediatr.* 1993;123:702-711.

Paradise JL, Elster BA, Tan L. "Evidence in Infants with Cleft Palate that Breast Milk Protects against Otitis Media." *Pediatrics.* 1994;94:853-860.

Phillips V. *Successful Breastfeeding,* 6th ed. Nunawading: Nursing Mother's Association of Australia. 1991; pp. 38-39, 99.

Pinilla, Teresa, and Leann L. Birch. 1993. "Help Me Make it Through the Night: Behavioral Entrainment of Breastfed Infants' Sleep Patterns." *Pediatrics.* 91:436-444.

Pisacane, Alfredo, and colleagues. "Breastfeeding and Appendicitis."*British Medical Journal.* March, 1995.

Pisacane A, Graziano L, Mazzarella G, et al. "Breast-feeding and Urinary Tract Infection." *J Pediatr.* 1992;120:87-89.

Pisacane A, De Visia B, Valiante A, et al. "Iron Status in Breast-fed Infants." *J Pediatr.* 1995;127:429-431.

Popkin BM, Adair L, Akin JS, et al. "Breast-feeding and Diarrheal Morbidity." *Pediatrics.* 1990;86:874-882.

Powers NG, Naylor AJ, Wester RA. "Hospital Policies: Crucial to Breastfeeding Success." *Semin Perinatol.* 1994;18:517-524.

Procianoy RS, Fernandes-Filho PH, Lazaro L, et al. "The Influence of Rooming-in on Breastfeeding." *J Trop Pediatr.* 1983;29:112-114.

Rheingold, Joseph C. *The Fear of Being a Woman: A Theory of Maternal Destructiveness.* New York: Grune & Stratton. 1964.

Rigas A, Rigas B, Glassman M, et al. "Breast-feeding and Maternal Smoking in the Etiology of Crohn's Disease and Ulcerative Colitis in Childhood." *Ann Epidemiol.* 1993;3:387-392.

Righard, D., and Margaret Alade. "Delivery Self-Attachment." *Lancet*, 336:1105-07. 1990.

Righard L, Alade MO. "Sucking Technique and Its Effect on Success of Breastfeeding." *Birth.* 1992;19:185-189.

Riordan, Jan, and Kathleen G. Auerbach. 1993. *Breastfeeding and Human Lactation.* London: Jones and Bartlett.

Roe D. *Alcohol and the Diet.* Westport, CT: AVI Publishing Company, 1979; pp. 42-47.

Rohr FJ, Levy HL, Shih VE. "Inborn Errors of Metabolism." Walker WA, Watkins JB, eds. *Nutrition in Pediatrics.* Boston, MA: Little, Brown; 1985:412.

Rosenblatt KA, Thomas DB. "WHO Collaborative Study of Neoplasia and Steroid Contraceptives." *Int J Epidemiol.* 1993;22:192-197.

Russo J, Russo IH. "Development of the Human Mammary Gland." *The Mammary Gland: Development, Regulation, and Function.* New York: Plenum Press, 1987; pp. 67-93.

Ryan AS. "The Resurgence of Breastfeeding in the United States." *Pediatrics.* 1997;99(4). URL: http://www.pediatrics.org/cgi/content/full/99/4/e12.

Ryan AS, Martinez GA. "Breast-feeding and the Working Mother: A Profile." *Pediatrics.* 1989;83:524-531.

Saarinen UM. "Need for Iron Supplementation in Infants on Prolonged Breast Feeding." *J Pediatr.* 1978;93:177-180.

Saarinen UM. "Prolonged Breast Feeding as Prophylaxis for Recurrent Otitis Media." *Acta Paediatr Scand.* 1982;71:567-571.

Saarinen UM, Kajosaari M. "Breastfeeding as Prophylaxis Against Atopic Disease: Prospective Follow-up Study until 17 Years Old." *Lancet.* 1995;346:1065-1069.

Saint L, Maggiore P, Hartmann PE. "Yield and Nutrient Content of Milk in Eight Women Breast-feeding Twins and One Woman Breast-feeding Triplets." *British Journal Nutrition* 1986; 56:49-58.

Schanler RJ, Hurst NM. "Human Milk for the Hospitalized Preterm Infant." *Semin Perinatol.* 1994;18:476-486.

Schulte, Pat RN, "Minimizing Alcohol Exposure of the Breastfeeding Infant." *IBCLC, Journal of Human Lactation* November 4, 1995, 317-318.

Scragg LK, Mitchell EA, Tonkin SL, et al. "Evaluation of the Cot Death Prevention Programme in South Auckland." *N Z Med J.* 1993;106:8-10.

Shrago, Linda, and Debi Bocar. 1990. "The Infant's Contribution to Breastfeeding." *JOGNN*, May/June, 19:3.

Shrago L. "Glucose Water Supplementation of the Breastfed Infant During the First Three Days of Life." *J Human Lactation.* 1987;3:82-86.

Shu X-O, Clemens J, Zheng W, et al. "Infant Breastfeeding and the Risk of Childhood Lymphoma and Leukaemia." *Int J Epidemiol.* 1995;24:27-32.

Song J, Zhu YM. "Mental Development Screening Test in Children Under 6 Years of Age." *Mental Development Tests in Children,* 2nd ed. Shanghai: Shanghai Scientific Technology Press, 1987; pp. 275-359.

Sosa R, Kennell JH, Klaus M, et al. "The Effect of Early Mother-infant Contact on Breast Feeding, Infection and Growth." Lloyd JK, ed. *Breast-feeding and the Mother.* Amsterdam: Elsevier; 1976:179-193.

Sosa R, Klaus M, Urrutia JJ. "Feed the Nursing Mother, Thereby the Infant." *Journal Pediatric.* 1976; 88:688-70.

Spisak S, Gross SS. Second Follow-up Report: *The Surgeon General's Workshop on Breastfeeding and Human Lactation.* Washington, DC: National Center for Education in Maternal and Child Health. 1991.

Sugarman M, Kendall-Tackett KA. "Weaning Ages in a Sample of American Women Who Practice Extended Breastfeeding." *Clin Pediatr.* 1995;34:642-647.

Sveger T. "Breast-feeding, $A_1$-antitrypsin Deficiency, and Liver Disease?" *JAMA.* 1985;254:3036. Letter.

Takala AK, Eskola J, Palmgren J, et al. "Risk Factors of Invasive *Haemophilus influenzae* Type b Disease Among Children in Finland." *J Pediatr.* 1989; 115:694-701.

Tucker HA. "Factors Affecting Mammary Gland Cell Numbers." *Journal Dairy Science.* 1969; 52:720-29.

Tuttle CR, Dewey KG. "Potential Cost Savings for Medi-Cal, AFDC, Food Stamps, and WIC Programs Associated with Increasing Breast-feeding among Low-income Hmong Women in California." *J Am Diet Assoc.* 1996;96:885-890.

Udall JN, Dixon M, Newman AP, et al. "Liver Disease in $A_1$-antitrypsin Deficiency: Retrospective Analysis of the Influence of Early Breast- vs Bottle-feeding." *JAMA.* 1985;253:2679-2682.

Van Den Bosch CA, Bullough CHW. "Effect of Early Suckling on Term Neonates' Core Body Temperature." *Ann Trop Paediatr.* 1990;10:347-353.

Victora, Cesar, Elaine Tomasi, Maria Olinto, and Fernando Barros. 1993. "Use of Pacifiers and Breastfeeding Duration." *Lancet.* 341: 404-06.

Virtanen SM, Rasanen L, Aro A, et al. "Infant Feeding in Finnish Children <7 yr of Age with Newly Diagnosed IDDM." *Diabetes Care.* 1991;14:415-417.

Wang YS, Wu SY. "The Effect of Exclusive Breastfeeding on Development and Incidence of Infection in Infants." *J Hum Lactation.* 1996;12:27-30.

Wang YS, Wu SY. "An Analysis of the Factors Leading to Failure in Persistent Exclusive Breastfeeding During Four Months after Delivery." *Maternal Child Health Care, China.* 1994; 1:15-17.

Whitehead RG, Paul AA, Rowland MGM. "Lactation in Cambridge and in The Gambia." Wharton B, ed. *Topics in Paediatrics 2: Nutrition in Childhood.* Pitman Medical. 1980; pp. 22-33.

Wiberg B, Humble K, de Chateau P. "Long-term Effect on Mother-infant Behavior of Extra Contact During the First Hour Post Partum v Follow-up at Three Years." *Scand J Soc Med.* 1989;17:181-191.

Widstrom AM, Wahlberg V, Matthiesen AS, et al. "Short-term Effects of Early Suckling and Touch of the Nipple on Maternal Behavior." *Early Hum Dev.* 1990;21:153-163.

Wilde CJ, Peaker M. "Autocrine Control of Milk Secretion." *Journal Agricultural Science, Cambridge.* 1990; 114:235-38.

Williams EL, Hammer LD. "Breastfeeding Attitudes and Knowledge of Pediatricians-in-training." *Am J Prev Med.* 1995;11:26-33.

Williams LR, Cooper MK. "Nurse-managed Postpartum Home Care." *JOGNN.* 1993;22:25-31.

Wilson MH. "Feeding the Healthy Child." Oski FA, DeAngelis CD, Feigin RD, et al., eds. *Principles and Practice of Pediatrics.* Philadelphia, PA: JB Lippincott. 1990:533-545.

Wong GHW, Goeddel DV. "Tumour Necrosis factors a and b Inhibit Virus Replication and Synergize with Interferons." *Nature.* 1986; 323 (6091):819-822.

Woolridge MW, Butte N, Dewey KG, Ferris AM, Garza C, Keller R. "Methods for the Measurement of Milk Volume Intake of the Breast-fed Infant." Jenson RG, Neville MC, eds. *Human Lactation: Milk Components and Methodologies.* New York: Plenum Press. 1985; pp. 5-21.

Woolridge MW, How TV, Drewett RF, Rolfe P, Baum JD. "The Continuous Measurement of Milk Intake at a Feed in Breast-fed Babies." *Early Human Development.* 1982; 6:365-73.

Woolridge MW, Phil D, Baum JD. "Recent Advances in Breast Feeding." *Acta Paediatr Japonica.* 1993; 35:1-12.

World Health Assembly. *International Code of Marketing of Breast-milk Substitutes. Resolution of the 34th World Health Assembly.* No. 34.22, Geneva, Switzerland: WHO, 1981.

World Health Organization. "Consensus Statement from the Consultation on HIV Transmission and Breastfeeding." *J Hum Lactation.* 1992;8:173-174.

World Health Organization. *Protecting, Promoting and Supporting Breast-Feeding: The Special Role of Maternity Services.* Geneva, Switzerland: WHO, 1989:13-18.

Wright AL, Holberg CJ, Martinez FD, et al. "Breast-feeding and Lower Respiratory Tract Illness in the First Year of Life." *Br Med J.* 1989;299:945-949.

Wright AL, Holberg CJ, Taussig LM, et al. "Relationship of Infant Feeding to Recurrent Wheezing at Age 6 Years." *Arch Pediatr Adolesc Med.* 1995;149:758-763.

Wright AL, Holberg CJ, Martinez FD, Morgan WJ, Taussig LM, Bean J, et al. "Breastfeeding and Lower Respiratory Tract Illness in the First Year of Life." *British Medical Journal* 1989; 299(6705):946-49.

Zucali JR, Broxmeyer HE, Gross MA, Dinarello CA. "Recombinant Human Tumor Necrosis Factors a and b Stimulate Fibroblasts to Produce Hemopoietic Growth Factors in Vitro." *Journal Immunology* 1988; 140:840-844.

Zuckerman B, Hingson R. "Alcohol Consumption During Pregnancy, a Critical Review." *Dev Med Child Neurol* 1986; 28:649-661.

# Index